Fingerprint Development Techniques

Fingerprint Development Techniques

Theory and Application

Stephen M. Bleay

Home Office Centre for Applied Science and Technology, Sandridge, UK

Ruth S. Croxton

School of Chemistry, University of Lincoln, UK

and

Marcel de Puit

Ministerie van Veiligheid en Justitie, Nederlands Forensisch Instituut, Digitale Technologie en Biometrie, The Hague, The Netherlands

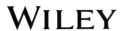

Registered Offices
John Wiley & Sons, Inc., 111 River Street, Hoboken, NJ 07030, USA
John Wiley & Sons Ltd, The Atrium, Southern Gate, Chichester, West Sussex, PO19 8SQ, UK

Editorial Office
The Atrium, Southern Gate, Chichester, West Sussex, PO19 8SQ, UK

For details of our global editorial offices, customer services, and more information about Wiley products visit us at www.wiley.com.

Wiley also publishes its books in a variety of electronic formats and by print-on-demand. Some content that appears in standard print versions of this book may not be available in other formats.

Library of Congress Cataloging-in-Publication data applied for

Hardback ISBN - 9781119992615

Cover design by Wiley
Cover images: (Background) © chokkicx/Gettyimages; (Fingerprint images) Courtesy of Stephen M. Bleay

Set in 10.5/12.5pt Times by SPi Global, Pondicherry, India

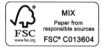

Contents

Series Preface

Developments in forensic science

Practising forensic scientists are constantly striving to deliver their very best in the service of national and international justice. As many types of forensic evidence come under increased scrutiny, the onus is on the forensic science community in partnership with academic researchers, law enforcement and the judiciary to work together to address these challenges. We must have confidence in the scientific validation of the methods used to develop forensic evidence and in how that evidence is correctly and scientifically interpreted within a case context so that it can be admitted within our criminal justice systems with confidence.

As we develop new knowledge and address the research and practical application of science within the forensic science fields, the consolidation, scientific validation and dissemination of new technological innovations and methods relevant to forensic science practice also become essential.

The texts developed in this book series aim to highlight and report the areas where scientific validation is in place as well as areas where challenges remain. It is the objective of this book series to provide a valuable resource for forensic science and law enforcement practitioners and our legal colleagues and in so doing provide a realistic scientific position of the evidence types presented in our courts.

The books developed and published within this series come from some of the leading researchers and practitioners, and I am indebted to them as they make their forensic science disciplines, warts and all, accessible to the wider world.

Professor Niamh Nic Daeid
Leverhulme Research Centre for Forensic Science
University of Dundee
UK, 2017

Acknowledgements

This book would not have been possible without the contributions of several groups of people, and I'd like to acknowledge them here:

Firstly, to my predecessors and past and present colleagues in the Home Office Centre for Applied Science and Technology Fingerprint Research Group, without whose dedication and innovation the forensic science field would be a much poorer place and several of the processes reported in this book would not be available. In particular I'd like to thank Dr Helen Bandey, the late Dr Val Bowman, Rory Downham, Lesley Fitzgerald, Andrew Gibson, Sheila Hardwick, Terry Kent and Vaughn Sears for their inspiration, challenge and support to me and to each other in the provision of a fingermark visualisation and imaging capability the United Kingdom can be proud of.

I'd also like to acknowledge all the placement year, Masters and PhD students that have provided the underpinning and groundbreaking research on which the Home Office work is founded, much of which is described here. Our academic colleagues have been generous in providing their time and expertise to this area, often for little funding, and particular thanks are due to Dr Melanie Bailey, Dr Simona Francese, Prof Sergei Kazarian, Dr Paul Kelly, Mrs Sophie Park and Prof Geraint Williams for the provision of illustrations for this book.

Fingerprint research would be of little value unless it meets the needs of practitioners, and we have been fortunate to have input from laboratory managers and specialists with a genuine interest in new techniques and improving the way things are done. David Charlton, Martin Cox, Paul Deacon, Kenny Laing, Nick Marsh, John O'Hara and Tim Watkinson are just some of those that have made a difference during my time working with fingerprints and have shown me how laboratory research gets put into practice – thanks to you all.

The international fingerprint research community has always been a welcoming one, and I value greatly the discussions and interchange of ideas that I have had with IFRG colleagues. I now understand the trials and tribulations that several have already faced in writing textbooks and hope that this text complements rather than rivals what has gone before.

Finally, to my wife Deborah, family and friends, thank you for your understanding while I have been immersed in preparing this book and for providing a range of welcome diversions!

1

Introduction

Stephen M. Bleay[1] and Marcel de Puit[2]

[1] Home Office Centre for Applied Science and Technology, Sandridge, UK
[2] Ministerie van Veiligheid en Justitie, Nederlands Forensisch Instituut, Digitale Technologie en Biometrie, The Hague, The Netherlands

---

Key points

- The traces left by contact between the hands and other surfaces are an essential tool in forensic investigations.

- Such traces can be used in several ways: to provide contextual information about the contact event and to identify individuals.

- All potential forensic applications of such contact traces rely on them being visualised by some means.

There are several books that deal with how latent fingermarks, and to some level the visualisation thereof, are used for identification purposes. To a great extent, the comparison and identification of latent fingermarks in criminal investigations remains their principal application.

In this book we will describe the chemistry (and other properties) of fingermarks in more depth and describe how fingermarks can be used for more than just identification purposes. We will describe how fingermarks may be deposited, the chemical and biological composition of the fingermark and its physical properties, the chemical and physical techniques used to visualise latent fingermarks and the importance of combining fingermark visualisation with recovery of other forensic evidence. Consideration is also given to the importance of communication between individuals visualising fingermarks and those responsible for their comparison and identification.

Fingerprint Development Techniques: Theory and Application, First Edition.
Stephen M. Bleay, Ruth S. Croxton and Marcel de Puit.
© 2018 John Wiley & Sons Ltd. Published 2018 by John Wiley & Sons Ltd.

The traces that may be left by the contact between the palmar regions of hands and a surface are potentially the most informative forms of evidence available to the forensic scientist. The skin on the inside of the hands can flex and adapt to perform a wide range of manipulative tasks, and there are few actions (legal or illegal) that can be carried out without holding objects and/or touching surfaces. The nature of each of these contacts will be different, but in all cases Locard's exchange principle (Locard, 1934) applies, and there is the potential for the transfer of material between the hand and the surface.

In the context of crime investigation, there are many levels of information that can potentially be extracted from these areas of contact if it is possible for a forensic scientist to first locate and then enhance and analyse them.

At the coarsest level, the configuration of the palm and fingers during the contact with the surface and their position on it can provide useful contextual information about how the surface was touched or gripped. This can be particularly useful in corroborating or disproving particular accounts of events. Figure 1.1 illustrates a situation where the one individual claimed that an assailant had grasped his shirt, whilst the other individual claimed that he had merely pushed the wearer of the shirt away.

The mark that has been revealed suggests that the fabric of the shirt has been gathered together by the hand, and therefore the account of the shirt being grasped by an assailant is more likely than a push with an open hand. Figure 1.2 shows two different orientations of fingermarks on a glass bottle.

In the first case, the bottle has been held whilst drinking from the neck of the bottle. In the second case, the bottle has been gripped as if the bottle has been picked

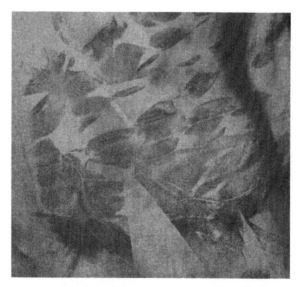

Figure 1.1   A contact (grab) mark on a black cotton shirt developed using vacuum metal deposition. Reproduced courtesy of the Home Office.

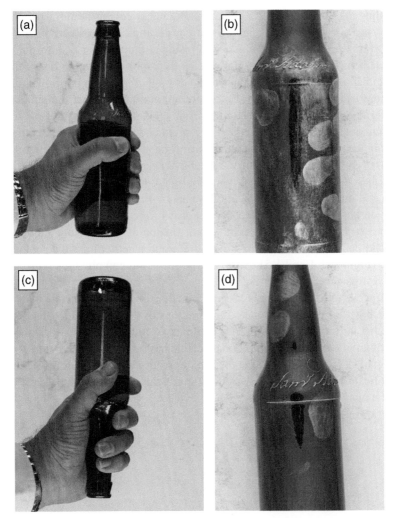

Figure 1.2 The orientation of fingermarks on a glass bottle originating from different actions. (a) Bottle being held to drink from. (b) Fingermarks developed using aluminium powder after drinking. (c) Bottle being held as if to strike. (d) Fingermarks developed using aluminium powder after use as a weapon.

up for use as a weapon. Again, by examination of the configuration of the marks, it may be possible to infer how an item was handled, and this may become evidentially important.

Obviously, there are many more possible scenarios than the two examples presented here, and it should be noted that these are merely illustrative examples. In real casework the propositions (hypotheses) and subsequent examinations are likely to be more complex.

Revealing the distribution of a contaminant (an exogenous material) on the hand may also provide useful information that can be indicative of certain actions. In another example, the firing of a gun will result in the transfer of gunshot residue onto the hands (Figure 1.3). Although the hands can be swabbed to reveal the presence of gunshot residue, if its distribution across the hand can be shown, this may be far more useful in showing that it was much more likely that the gun was held and fired rather than the residue coming from accidental contact. This distribution of contaminant may also be subsequently reproduced in any marks left by the hand.

At a slightly finer level, a closer analysis of the areas of palm and finger contact can also reveal information about the events during the time of contact. Although many of these events may consist of single, light contacts, others may be of longer duration and may include movement of the hand or multiple contacts, for example, as a grip on an object is readjusted. By analysis of the traces left by the contacts, it is possible to obtain information about factors including the pressure applied during contact, slippage of the hand across the surface and whether multiple contacts have occurred (Figures 1.4 and 1.5). All of this information can add context to the case being investigated.

At a finer level of analysis is the examination of the ridge detail that may be reproduced within the fingers and palmar regions of the contact area. These are the features that have traditionally been the primary source of information for identification of individuals. The information available has been described in terms of 'levels' of detail (SWGFAST, 2013), although in practice all of these levels are utilised by identification specialists whilst drawing conclusions about the identity of the donor of a mark.

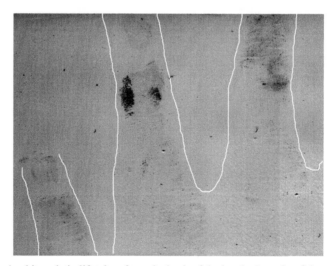

Figure 1.3 A white gelatin lift taken from the back of the hand taken after firing a gun and enhanced using a chemical selectively targeting traces of lead. Reproduced courtesy of the Home Office.

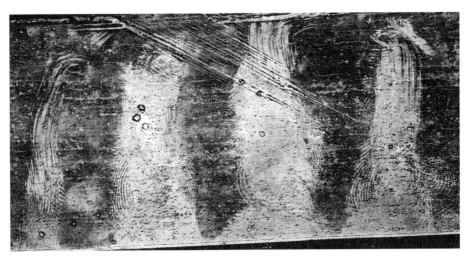

Figure 1.4 A sequence of fingermarks developed using aluminium powder showing evidence of slippage on the surface. Reproduced courtesy of the Home Office.

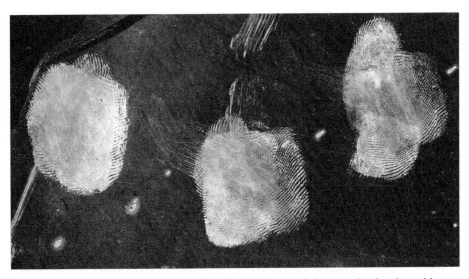

Figure 1.5 A sequence of fingermarks developed using aluminium powder showing evidence of multiple contacts on the surface. Reproduced courtesy of the Home Office.

'Level 1 detail' describes the pattern formed by the flow of the ridges, and three general patterns are generally used to define marks, these being the whorl, loop and arch (Figure 1.6). Further detailed definitions of the general patterns and variations of them have been previously described in specialist texts on fingerprint comparison and identification; this information is however beyond the scope of this book.

'Level 2 detail' describes the features that arise due to disruptions in the flow of the ridges, which include ridge endings and bifurcations where a single ridge forks

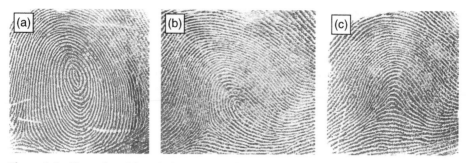

Figure 1.6   Examples of the principal types of fingerprint pattern. (a) The whorl. (b) The loop. (c) The arch.

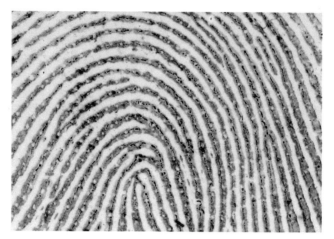

Figure 1.7   An area of a fingerprint showing a number of second-level details.

into two. Other features can be described in terms of combinations of ridge endings and bifurcations (Figure 1.7). These features are sometimes also described as 'minutiae' or 'Galton details'. Level 2 details are those that are most used by identification specialists during comparison and that are automatically marked up by fingerprint database algorithms for automated searching of fingerprints.

'Level 3 detail' includes features associated with friction ridges that may also exist within a fingermark and can be used in conjunction with first- and second-level details to infer identity. These features may include pores, the shape of ridge edges and discontinuities within the ridge (Figure 1.8). Permanent scars and creases within the mark may also sometimes be included in this category. The use of fingermarks in identification has been extensively covered in other publications, and it is not the intention of this book to deal further with the comparison and identification process. However, the second-level and third-level details in fingerprints do play a crucial role in the chemistry and other properties of the fingermarks they produce. They are, respectively, responsible for the distribution and the excretion of sweat over and from the skin.

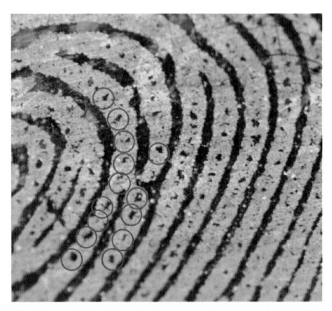

Figure 1.8 A fingermark enhanced using white powder suspension showing level 3 details (in this case pores, illustrated using circles) in the ridges.

Even in cases where the hands and palms are protected with gloves, it may still be possible to obtain useful evidence from the contact area. Not all gloves are totally impervious, and migration of sweat through certain types of glove has been recorded (Willinski, 1980). Similarly, natural deposits may build up on the outside of gloves, and where gloves are thin, the pattern of the fingerprint may still be left on the surface. For thicker gloves, the pattern of the surface of the glove may be left on the surface (Figure 1.9). The resultant glove marks may still contain sufficient features for the glove to be matched to the mark left on the surface (Lambourne, 1984; Sawyer, 2008).

More recently, it has become possible to obtain additional contextual information to that provided by the ridge detail, including information about the donor of the mark, regardless of whether they can be identified from the ridge detail.

Fingermarks often contain shed skin cells (Figure 1.10). It has been recognised for several years that DNA can be extracted from shed skin cells in fingermarks and cell-free nucleic acids have also shown to be present in sweat (Quinones and Daniel, 2012). This gives the scientist another opportunity to establish identity from a contact area, even in situations where there is insufficient ridge detail present for identification. Indeed, the knowledge that a particular area has been touched enables DNA recovery to be targeted, thus giving an increased likelihood of obtaining a profile compared with speculative swabbing over a wider area.

Advanced analytical techniques can be employed to establish both the chemical species present in a fingermark and to map their distribution, both of which can be

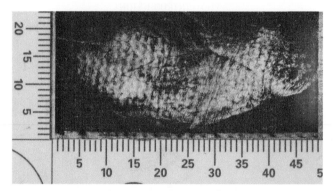

Figure 1.9 An example of a glove mark left by a knitted woollen glove and enhanced with aluminium powder. Reproduced courtesy of the Home Office.

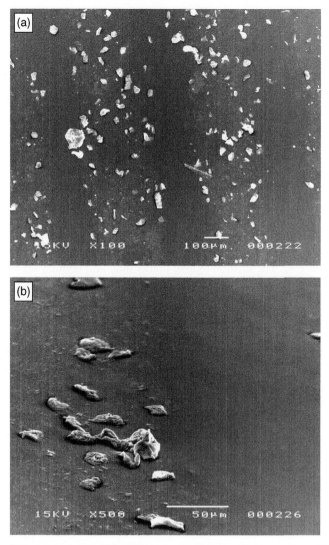

Figure 1.10 Skin cells present within ridges of a mark on an adhesive surface. (a) Low magnification and (b) high magnification. Reproduced courtesy of the Home Office.

extremely valuable pieces of information. From a chemical analysis it may be possible to establish the following:

- The sex of an unknown donor (e.g. Ferguson et al., 2012)

- Whether they are taking illicit or medication drugs (and the nature of those drugs) (e.g. Hazarika et al., 2008; Rowell et al., 2009)

- The nature of the contaminants (e.g. drugs, explosives) (e.g. Tripathi et al., 2011; Rowell et al., 2012) that may have been handled by the donor

The full range of publications in this area is far more extensive than the examples provided. Mapping the distribution of these contaminants may also be able to establish whether the contaminant is present as individual particles that may have been picked up by an accidental contact or are intimately and uniformly associated with the ridges, implying a more direct handling of the substance (Figure 1.11).

It is apparent that although there is a wealth of information in these contact traces that could be utilised by the forensic scientist, none of them will be available if they cannot be made visible to the human eye or a detection system. The aim of this book is to describe the wide variety of processes by which marks can be visualised and how they are selected, how the effectiveness of these processes can be established and how they can be used in sequence with each other and other forensic recovery processes.

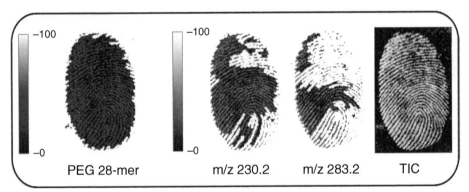

Figure 1.11 MALDI MS images of a condom lubricant-contaminated fingermark. The mark was subjected to gelatin primary lift for analysis via ATR-FTIR. Subsequently a secondary lift of the mark residue was analysed by MALDI MSI enabling imaging of PEG (one of the polymers in the condom lubricant, represented here by the 28-mer) and of endogenous compounds. Here images of 13-aminotridecanoic acid (m/z 230.2) and oleic acid (m/z 283.2) are reported. The mass image of the three total ion currents yielded the complete ridge pattern of the mark (TIC). Reproduced and adapted from Bradshaw et al. (2013) with permission from the Royal Society of Chemistry.

References

Bradshaw, R, Wolstenholme, R, Ferguson, L S, Sammon, C, Mader, K, Claude, E, Black-ledge, R D, Clench, M R, Francese, S, 'Spectroscopic imaging based approach for condom identification in condom contaminated fingermarks', Analyst, vol 138, (2013), p 2546–2557.

Ferguson, L S, Wulfert, F, Wolstenholme, R, Fonville, J M, Clench, M R, Carolan, V A, Francese, S, 'Direct detection of peptides and small proteins in fingermarks and determination of sex by MALDI mass spectrometry profiling', Analyst, vol 137, (2012), p 4686–4692.

Hazarika, P, Jickells, S M, Wolff, K, Russell, D A, 'Imaging of latent fingerprints through the detection of drugs and metabolites', Angew. Chem. Int. Ed., vol 47, (2008), p 10167–10170.

Lambourne, G, 'The Fingerprint Story', Harrap, London, 1984.

Locard, E. 'La police et les méthodes scientifiques', Presses Universitaires de France, Paris, 1934.

Quinones, I, Daniel, B, 'Cell free DNA as a component of forensic evidence recovered from touched surfaces', Forensic Sci. Int. Genet., vol 6, (2012), p 26–30.

Rowell, F, Hudson, K, Seviour, J, 'Detection of drugs and their metabolites in dusted latent finger-marks by mass spectrometry', Analyst, vol 134, (2009), p 701–707.

Rowell, F, Seviour, J, Lim, A Y, Elumbaring-Salazar, C G, Loke, J, Ma, J, 'Detection of nitro-organic and peroxide explosives in latent fingermarks by DART- and SALDI-TOF-mass spec-trometry', Forensic Sci. Int., vol 221(1–3), (2012), p 84–91.

Sawyer, P, 'Police use glove prints to catch criminals', Daily Telegraph, 13 December 2008. http://www.telegraph.co.uk/news/uknews/law-and-order/3740688/Police-use-glove-prints-to-catch-criminals.html (accessed 22 April 2017).

Scientific Working Group on Friction Ridge Analysis, Study and Technology (SWGFAST), Document 19 'Standard Terminology of Friction Ridge Examination (Latent/Tenprint)', Issued 14 March 2013. https://www.nist.gov/sites/default/files/documents/2016/10/26/swgfast_standard-terminology_4.0_121124.pdf (accessed 16 October 2017).

Tripathi, A, Emmons, E D, Wilcox, P G, Guicheteau, J A, Emge, D K, Christesen, S D, Fountain, A W, 3rd, 'Semi-automated detection of trace explosives in fingerprints on strongly interfer-ing surfaces with Raman chemical imaging', Appl. Spectrosc., vol 65(6), (2011), p 611–619.

Willinski, G, 'Permeation of fingerprints through laboratory gloves', J. Forensic Sci., vol 25(3), (1980), p 682–685.

2

Formation of fingermarks

Stephen M. Bleay[1] and Marcel de Puit[2]

[1] Home Office Centre for Applied Science and Technology, Sandridge, UK
[2] Ministerie van Veiligheid en Justitie, Nederlands Forensisch Instituut, Digitale Technologie en Biometrie, The Hague, The Netherlands

---

Key points

- Fingermarks are formed as the result of an interaction between a finger and a surface.

- Several outcomes are possible from this interaction, including deposition of positive marks, removal of material to leave negative marks and formation of impressions on the surface.

- The type of mark resulting from the interaction is determined by the properties of the finger and the surface and the nature of the contact (e.g. pressure, angle).

2.1 Introduction

The generation and recovery of fingermarks (and equivalent areas of ridge detail such as palm marks) from surfaces can be described in terms of several stages that involve different types of interactions. The nature of these interactions is fundamental in determining whether it will ultimately be possible to recover fingermarks, and, if recovery is possible, which visualisation processes are most likely to be effective. This book will consider both the events that occur prior to the initial examination of the surface bearing the fingermark and the interactions that occur during the application of the enhancement process.

Fingerprint Development Techniques: Theory and Application, First Edition.
Stephen M. Bleay, Ruth S. Croxton and Marcel de Puit.
© 2018 John Wiley & Sons Ltd. Published 2018 by John Wiley & Sons Ltd.

The 'timeline' from fingermark deposition to recovery involves four distinct stages, with the ultimate aim of providing an image of the mark that is fit for the purposes of comparison. These stages are as follows:

Formation – the generation of a fingermark on a surface, where the mark is a reproduction of a portion of the palmar ridge pattern that has made contact with the surface.

Ageing – the time period from the moment the fingermark is generated to when it is initially examined. During this time period, the fingermark and the surface it is deposited on will potentially be exposed to a range of varying environmental conditions.

Initial examination – the initial examination of the substrate the fingermark was deposited on with the naked eye, with or without the assistance of additional light sources. The fingermark may already be sufficiently visible for an image of it to be captured at this stage.

Enhancement – the use of a process to enhance the contrast of the fingermark relative to that of the surface so that any ridge detail present can be more readily seen. The processes used for this purpose may be chemical, physiochemical or physical in nature.

This chapter focuses on the formation stage, in particular the interactions that occur between the finger and the surface during initial contact.

2.2 Initial contact

Initial contact involves an interaction between the finger and a surface. The nature of this initial contact will determine whether or not a potentially identifiable mark is formed.

The contact event can be broken down into three stages:

1. Application of the finger to the surface

2. Transfer of material between the finger and the surface

3. Removal of the finger from the surface

During the application of the finger to the surface, positive pressure is applied by the finger until both the finger and the surface have deformed to their full extent.

Transfer of material can occur during the contact. Whether material is transferred from the finger to the surface or vice versa will depend on what substances are present and their relative affinities for the finger and the surface.

During removal of the finger from the surface, the pressure is released and any elastic recovery that the finger and surface can undergo will occur. The transfer of material between finger and surface will also be completed.

2.3 Interaction outcomes

The three principal outcomes that can arise from the interaction between the finger and the surface during initial contact are summarised in Sections 2.3.1–2.3.3.

2.3.1 Positive marks

In the process of the formation of positive fingermarks, residue is transferred from the finger to the surface (Figure 2.1). The mark is either visible or invisible to the naked eye depending upon a number of factors including the composition of the residue, the colour and reflectivity of the surface and the lighting conditions used to examine the surface. The vast majority of fingermarks encountered in crime investigation are positive marks.

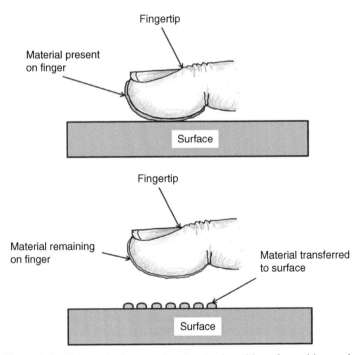

Figure 2.1 Schematic diagram showing the deposition of a positive mark.

Positive fingermarks may be described as 'patent' or 'latent' marks, depending on whether the mark is readily visible or not.

'Patent' marks are defined as those that are obvious to the eye because they have been deposited with a contaminant that contrasts in colour with the background, such as blood or dirt (Figure 2.2).

'Latent' marks are defined as those that are not immediately obvious to a cursory visual examination and require enhancement by some other means to be detected.

Latent marks are encountered much more regularly than patent marks.

2.3.2 Negative marks

Negative marks may be encountered if the surface is covered in loose particulate material (e.g. dust) or a thin continuous layer of contaminant. During contact the finger may pick up some of these particles or contaminant, thus leaving a negative impression of the ridge detail in the material remaining on the surface (Figures 2.3 and 2.4).

Negative marks are considerably less common than positive marks on operational material and are often extremely fragile.

2.3.3 Impressions

Impressions may be formed in cases where the surface can melt or deform during contact. Surfaces made of soft substances (e.g. putty, wet paint) may permanently deform, leaving an impression of the ridge detail in the surface (Figures 2.5 and 2.6). Fingermarks deposited in this way are sometimes referred to as 'plastic'

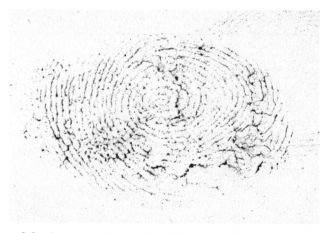

Figure 2.2 A patent mark deposited with mud on white-painted chipboard.

fingermarks, because the deformation caused by the interaction of the finger with the surface is plastic, that is, irreversible.

Impressions are also encountered much less often than positive marks on operational material.

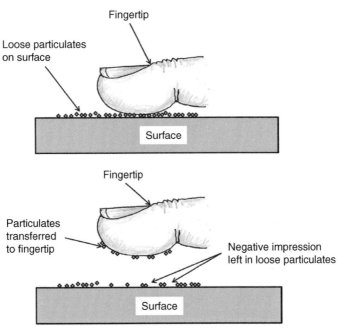

Figure 2.3 Schematic diagram showing the formation of a negative mark.

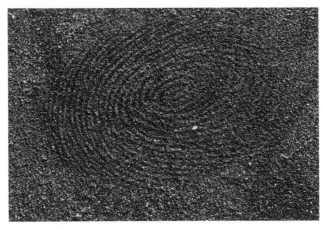

Figure 2.4 Example of a negative mark left by contact with a dusty surface and enhanced with oblique lighting.

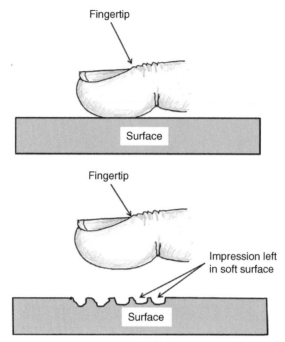

Figure 2.5 Schematic diagram showing the formation of an impression in a soft surface.

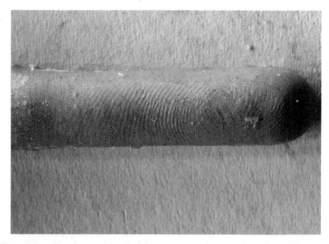

Figure 2.6 Example of an impression left by contact with a soft surface (chocolate) and enhanced with oblique lighting.

The factors that affect which of these outcomes are most likely to occur as a result of the initial contact can be grouped into those that are associated with the finger (e.g. finger deformation, cleanliness) and the surface (e.g. shape, texture, rigidity, elasticity). These factors will be considered in turn in the succeeding text.

2.4   The finger

There are several attributes of the finger that have an influence during the formation of fingermarks. These include the following:

- Mechanical properties
- Cleanliness
- Temperature

2.4.1   Mechanical properties

The mechanical properties of the finger determine its ability to deform on contact with a surface. This in turn will have an effect on the final contact area and therefore on the area over which material transfer can occur and the size and shape of the resultant fingermark. The most comprehensive reported studies on the deformation the finger during fingermark generation have been conducted by Maceo (2009), who relates the structure of the skin in the region of the finger to the way in which this structure influences finger deformation.

The structure of skin has been extensively studied and reported, and authoritative texts on the subject are available (Montagna and Parrakal, 1974). In the particular context of the friction ridge skin, how it is formed and how it grows into the familiar whorl, loop and arch patterns in the womb has been comprehensively described (Wertheim and Maceo, 2002). An outline of those skin features associated with friction ridge skin that are most relevant to the interactions that occur during initial contact is given in the succeeding text.

The skin consists of three distinct layers, the hypodermis, dermis and epidermis, which are illustrated schematically in Figure 2.7.

The epidermis is the outermost protective layer of the skin and performs a barrier function. It is a thin but relatively rigid elastic layer that consists of closely packed keratinocytes, which migrate over time from the base of the epidermis to the surface, where they are ultimately shed as dead skin cells (a process known as desquamation).

The dermis consists of connective tissues including collagen fibres and other elastic fibres held together by an extrafibrillar matrix. It also incorporates sweat glands, blood vessels and touch and heat receptors. Its purpose is to provide flexibility and elasticity to the skin.

The hypodermis primarily contains fat, the varying thickness of which provides contours to the fingers and palm. The fatty tissue is distributed as lobules (small divided compartments) separated by connective tissue fibres. The fatty tissue in the hypodermis provides a cushioning function for the body and behaves as a viscous medium.

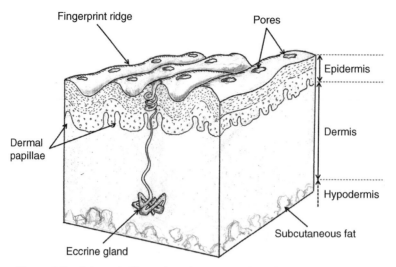

Figure 2.7   Schematic illustration of a cross section of skin on the fingertip.

The distribution of the fatty tissues in the hypodermis is most important in determining the deformation of the finger, and the distribution of these tissues can be
more easily seen by reference to schematic representations of the cross section of
the finger (Figure 2.8).

Maceo (2009) describes two regions of the finger pad on the distal phalanx (i.e.
the final joint of the finger where the fingerprint ridges are present), the rigid distal
finger pulp and the flexible proximal pulp. The distal pulp is found towards the tip
of the finger, in the region beyond the 'tuft' in the distal phalanx bone. The proximal pulp occurs between the joint crease and the tuft in the distal phalanx bone
(Figure 2.8b).

When the finger is applied to a surface with a compressive force, the compartments (lobules) of fatty tissue deform to more evenly distribute the stress across the
finger, bringing more of the pad on the distal phalanx in contact with the surface.
Most deformation can occur within the flexible proximal pulp where the lobules are
larger, but the maximum level of deformation that can occur is constrained by the
elasticity of the dermis and more rigid epidermis, which places an upper limit on the
boundary of the area over which contact occurs. Skin elasticity, subsurface fat and
finger geometry will vary from person to person, with some corresponding variation
in the maximum deformation that the fingertip can undergo.

Research conducted by Serina and co-workers (1997, 1998) to examine
repeated tapping of the finger on a surface (as in typing) showed that the maximum contact area between a finger and a flat surface is obtained at a force of
~5.3 N. During compression, the pulp exhibited viscoelastic behaviour. For
applied forces below 1 N, the pulp was compliant and could undergo large dis-
placements, with between 62 and 74% of the maximum contact area being

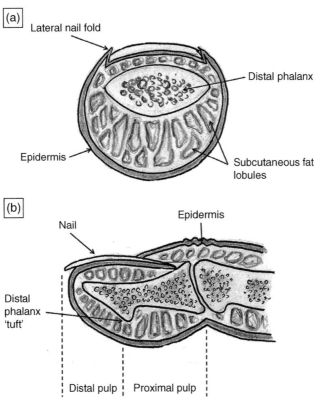

Figure 2.8   Schematic illustrations of the cross section through a finger, showing some of the features of significance for fingermark formation. (a) Refers to a cross section perpendicular to the finger and (b) refers to a cross section parallel to the direction of the finger.

achieved by the time the force applied had reached 1 N. The contact angle between the fingertip and the surface was observed to have a noticeable effect on the results observed. As the applied force was increased from 1 N, the pulp stiffened rapidly with a minimal addition in contact area being observed when force increases further. A series of images showing the effect of applied force on the contact area is shown in Figure 2.9.

Although the force with which the finger is applied to the surface determines the perimeter of the contact area, it also has a major influence on the contact that occurs on a fine scale. Even when the upper limits on the area of deformation of the finger have been reached, further increases in the force applied during contact (compressive stress) can have an impact on the appearance of the ridges. The series of images and schematic diagrams in Figure 2.10 illustrate the effect of increasing force on the ridges and furrows.

For low applied forces only the very highest points of the ridges will make contact with the surface, and therefore the contact may be intermittent.

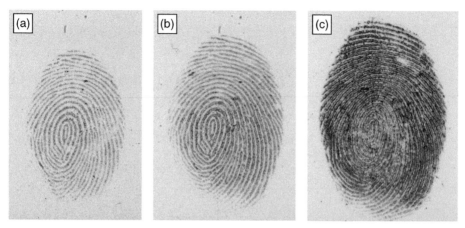

Figure 2.9 The effect of increasing applied force on the contact area of a fingertip with a surface. Inked fingers applied to a ceramic tile. (a) Low force (<1 N). (b) Medium force (1–5 N). (c) High force (>5 N). Reproduced courtesy of the Home Office.

At medium levels of applied force, all of the ridges may make contact giving continuous ridges. The appearance of some features may change as more of the ridge makes contact with the surface, for example, what initially appear to be ridge endings may be revealed as bifurcations. This effect can be observed for some of the features in Figure 2.10.

For high applied forces the ridges themselves may begin to deform laterally on the surface (according to the deformability of the finger outlined earlier), and the spacing between ridges may therefore decrease.

If incipient ridges (partially formed ridges that lay within the furrow region) are present, the likelihood of them making contact with the surface and thus appearing in the resultant mark increases as the applied force increases.

The contact between a fingerprint ridge and a surface at a microstructural level has been studied (Scruton et al., 1975). In these studies it was shown that the actual contact between the ridge and the surface only occurs over a small fraction of the apparent ridge area due to the irregular shape of the ridge surface at a microstructural scale. When the finger was cleaned with acetone and dried, <40% of the ridge came into contact with the surface. When sweat deposits were present, the sweat film filled some of the air gaps between the ridge and the surface. With sweat deposits present, when a finger was applied to the surface with a force of 0.5 N, the typical ridge width was 125 μm with an apparent contact area of ~55%, and when the force was increased to 10 N, the ridge width increased to 250 μm with a corresponding increase in apparent contact area to ~80%.

Maceo (2009) noted that, on a coarser scale, as the applied force increased, the thickening of the ridges was associated with a change in the shape of the ridge edges in the deposited mark. This was attributed to the compression of the ridge against the surface, bringing the edge profile of a deeper section of the

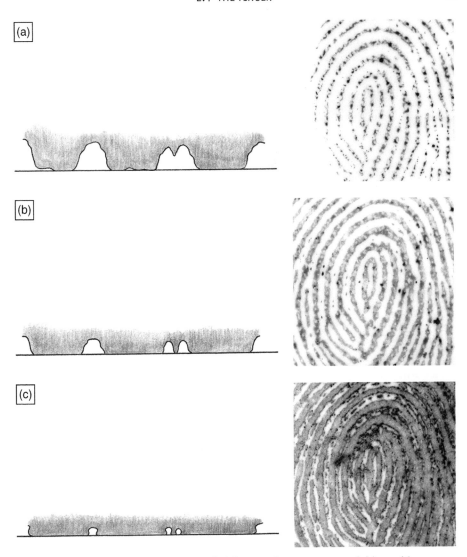

Figure 2.10 The effect of increasing applied force on the contact area of ridges with a surface. Schematic illustrations of ridges and corresponding images of inked fingers applied to a ceramic tile. (a) Low force (<1 N). (b) Medium force (1–5 N). (c) High force (>5 N).

ridge into contact with the surface. This potential change in ridge shape could be an important consideration in cases where 'edgeoscopy' (Chatterjee, 1962), using the shape of ridge edges as level 3 detail, may be used in identification.

It can therefore be seen that the mechanical properties of the finger determine its deformation in response to an applied force and are therefore important in defining the contact area. The description given here is a simple one and only considers the most basic case of a finger applied to the surface with a pure downward (compressive) force. In the more detailed studies conducted by Maceo (2009), other types of force such as torque and shear are considered and are also shown to have a major influence on contact area, deformation and slippage of the finger across the surface. Contact angle during contact is also another important factor that needs to be considered, as demonstrated by the results of Serina et al. (1997).

2.4.2 Cleanliness

The cleanliness of the finger will influence what material is transferred between the finger and surface during contact. In this respect, the nature and quantity of any material present on the finger will be important during initial contact.

The fingers may be relatively 'clean' in that the material present contains primarily natural secretions or may be dominated by contaminants picked up on the hands by prior contact with other surfaces. These contaminants may be liquid or solid in nature and may either strongly adhere to the finger or be loosely bound to it.

When the finger comes into contact with the surface, transfer of material will occur if the material can form bonds with the surface. Liquid substances that wet the surface will generally leave residue, and so will loosely bound solid material on the finger. The cleanliness of the surface relative to the finger will also be an important factor in this transfer process. Examples of some of the materials that may be found on a fingertip are shown in Figure 2.11.

The force applied during contact can influence the way in which any material transferred from the finger becomes distributed on the surface. As the applied force increases, any beads of liquid residue (e.g. eccrine sweat) will initially be compressed and may spread along the ridges away from their original position. Where large quantities of liquid contaminant are present on the finger at high applied forces, the liquid may be driven from the ridges into the furrows. Liquid will also be pushed away from the flexible core region of the finger pad towards the periphery of the finger (Figure 2.12). The viscosity of the liquid present will influence the extent to which this occurs.

The composition of the natural secretions and the contaminants that are commonly encountered on the fingertip are described in greater detail in Chapter 3.

2.4.3 Temperature

The temperature of the finger may also play a limited role during contact. The elasticity of the skin on the finger is affected by temperature, the skin becoming less flexible as temperature decreases (Middleton and Allen, 1973). As a consequence,

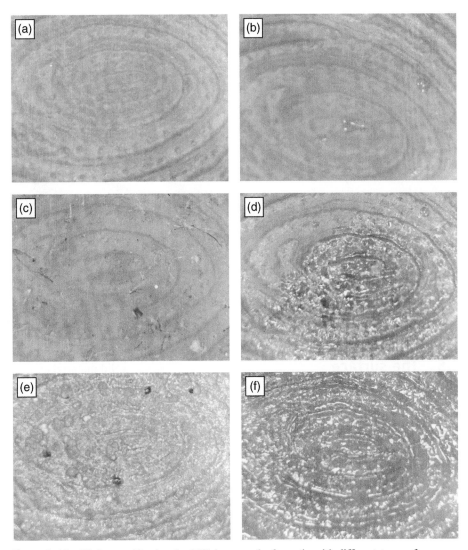

Figure 2.11 High magnification (~×250) images of a fingertip with different types of contaminant present. (a) A clean finger. (b) Beads of eccrine sweat. (c) Solid dust particles. (d) Blood. (e) Food residues (flavoured potato crisps). (f) Butter.

the deformation a finger can undergo during contact may be reduced if the surface temperature of the finger is low (e.g. after prolonged exposure to cold environments).

In most situations, however, the surface of the skin is relatively warm, and the temperature of the finger may even be sufficient to cause localised melting on certain surfaces where the combination of heat and pressure raise the surface temperature to above its melting point (e.g. chocolate; Figure 2.6).

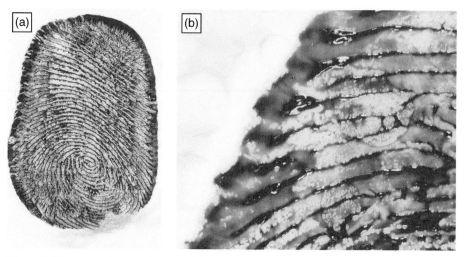

Figure 2.12 A thumb contaminated with butter applied to a ceramic tile with high force and enhanced using Solvent Black 3. (a) Showing the concentration of butter around the periphery of the mark. (b) Higher magnification image showing higher concentration of butter forced into the furrows.

2.5 The surface

The other contributing element to the initial contact is the surface. How the surface is able to respond to the force applied to it by the finger has a significant influence on the outcome of this interaction. The attributes of the surface that are considered most important during initial contact are as follows:

- Mechanical properties

- Shape and texture

- Cleanliness

- Temperature

2.5.1 Mechanical properties (stiffness, yield strength, elasticity)

The resistance provided by the surface to the force applied to it by the finger can be defined in terms of its bulk mechanical properties. Where the surface is a solid (which will be the case in the vast majority of contact interactions), the resistance to an applied force can be described in terms of a stress–strain graph (Figure 2.13).

In this form of plot, stress (σ) is defined as the applied force divided by the area over which the force is applied and has the units of Nm^{-2} (Pa). In terms

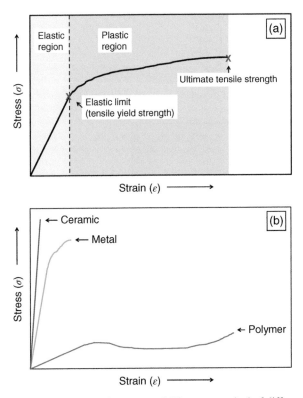

Figure 2.13 (a) A generic stress–strain curve and (b) curves typical of different generic types of material (not to scale).

of fingermark deposition, it is the force applied by the finger divided by its contact area (Figure 2.14):

$$\sigma = \frac{F}{A}$$

Strain (ε) is the dimensional change caused by the applied force, divided by the original dimension in the direction of the applied force (Figure 2.15). Strain is a dimensionless parameter.

$$\varepsilon = \frac{\delta l}{l_o}$$

The modulus of the material (E) is defined as the stress divided by the strain and gives a measure of the stiffness of the material (i.e. how much deformation it is likely to undergo when a given force is applied to it).

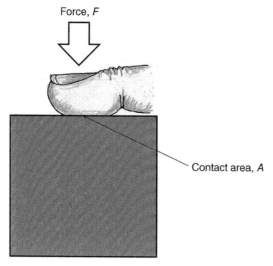

Figure 2.14   Schematic diagram illustrating stress in the context of fingermark deposition.

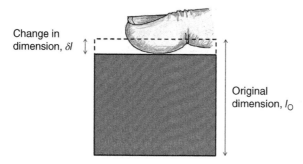

Figure 2.15   Schematic diagram illustrating strain in the context of fingermark deposition.

$$E = \frac{\sigma}{\varepsilon}$$

Materials with high values of modulus (e.g. ceramics, metals) are stiff and undergo minimal deformation under applied stress, whilst materials with low values of modulus (e.g. rubber, expanded polystyrene) may deform by a significant amount under low levels of applied stress (Wyatt and Dew-Hughes, 1974).

Another feature of note in the stress–strain curve is the elastic limit, the point beyond which any further increase in applied stress ceases to produce a linear increase in strain. For applied stress levels below the elastic limit, the deformation is reversible, and the material returns to its original dimensions on the removal of the applied stress. When applied stress exceeds the elastic limit, some irreversible 'plastic' deformation can occur. In the context of initial contact between a finger and a surface, it is at this point that a permanent impression can be left in the surface. As noted earlier, the finger itself can also deform, and it is essentially the modulus of the surface in relation to the finger (i.e. which material is stiffer) that determines what the outcome of such a contact will be. The relationship between the mechanical properties of the surface and their expected responses to the finger during initial contact are summarised in the succeeding text.

Hard, high modulus surfaces such as glass and metals will deform very little, if at all during initial contact and all of the deformation will occur in the finger. The surface is highly unlikely to experience stress levels that exceed the elastic limit, and therefore any deformation that does occur will be elastic and reversible.

Soft, low modulus surfaces may deform appreciably during initial contact. In many cases the applied stress may still be below the elastic limit, in which case the surface will regain its original shape and dimensions once the finger is removed. If extensive deformation takes place during formation of the fingermark, the developed mark may appear heavily distorted in comparison to the original contact area, and this may need to be taken into account during any subsequent comparison for identification purposes. Thin rubber sheet (such as that used to make balloons) is an example of a soft, elastic surface that may undergo extensive deformation during initial contact (Figure 2.16).

Soft, low modulus surfaces may also undergo plastic deformation during fingermark deposition, leaving a permanent impression of the finger in the surface. Examples of soft, plastic surfaces are putty, plasticine and 'Blu Tack'. Plastic deformation may also occur where the surface consists of a viscous liquid above its melting point (e.g. heated chocolate, hot wax) or liquid solutions with a solvent that subsequently evaporates to leave a solid surface (e.g. wet paint).

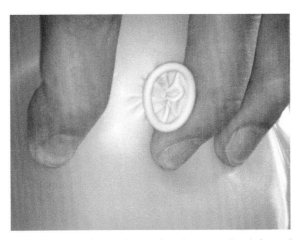

Figure 2.16   A rubber surface undergoing extensive deformation.

2.5.2 Shape and texture

Surface shape and texture is of primary importance during the moment of contact with the finger and influences (in combination with skin and surface elasticity) how much contact actually occurs between the finger and the surface.

On a flat, 'smooth' surface, if the finger is applied with sufficient pressure, contact can occur over the entire surface area, and a full record of the ridge detail on the fingertip can be deposited, as shown in Figure 2.1.

A surface may be smooth on a microscopic level, but it may also be formed into a shape that involves tight curvatures in relation to the dimensions of the finger, for example, writing pens and cartridge cases. When such surfaces are held by the fingers, only a limited portion of the finger actually makes contact with the surface and a partial mark results (Figure 2.17).

For 'rough' surfaces with larger surface features, the ridges on the finger may only make contact with the uppermost features of the surface topography, even if the finger is applied to the surface with significant pressure (Figure 2.18).

The result of such a contact is an intermittent distribution of fingermark residue, even when high applied forces are used during deposition (Figure 2.19). This means that on highly textured surfaces, it may only be possible to develop discontinuous ridge detail, and this may not be sufficient for identification.

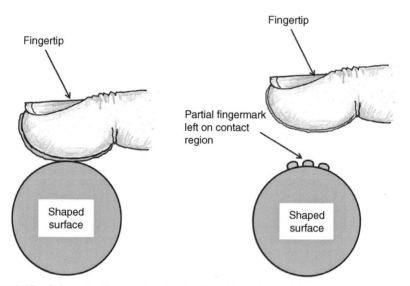

Figure 2.17 Schematic diagram showing the deposition of a partial fingermark on a smooth, curved surface where only a small portion of the finger makes contact with the surface.

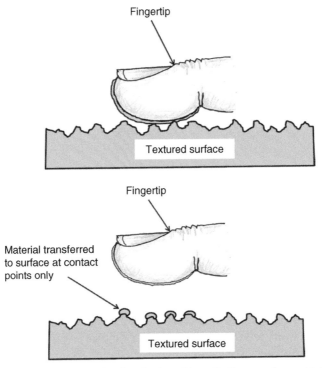

Figure 2.18   Schematic diagram showing the deposition of a fingermark on a highly textured surface where the finger only makes contact with the uppermost surface features.

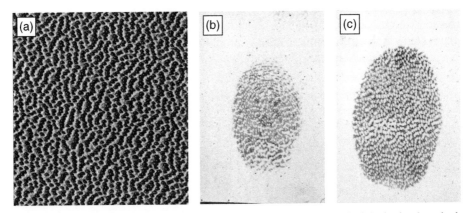

Figure 2.19   (a) A highly textured surface under oblique lighting. (b) An inked print deposited on the textured surface with a low (<1 N) applied force and lifted using a white gelatin lifter. (c) An inked print deposited using a high (>5 N) force and lifted in the same way.

2.5.3 Cleanliness

The cleanliness of the surface relative to the finger influences the transfer of material. For surfaces that are covered in particulates such as dust (Figure 2.20a) or a layer of solid or liquid contaminant (Figure 2.20b), it becomes more likely that the dominant transfer mechanism will be the transfer of the material from the surface to the finger, as opposed to from the finger to the surface. When the surface is clean, it is more likely that material is transferred from the finger to the surface. In most cases an intermediate situation exists where material can be transferred in both directions.

2.5.4 Temperature

In some cases the temperature of the surface material may determine its properties and response to the finger, whereas in other cases it may also have an influence on the finger itself. For materials close to their melting point, such as chocolate, small increases in temperature may make the surface soft and more likely to undergo plastic deformation when a finger comes into contact with it, leaving an impression.

Surfaces at the extremes of temperature may also affect the outcome of the contact process, with very cold and very hot surfaces increasing the likelihood that skin cells may adhere to the surface and therefore be left behind when the finger is removed.

2.6 Removal of the finger from the surface

The most commonly encountered scenario is the formation of a positive mark, where some of the film of the material initially present on the finger is transferred to a relatively clean surface.

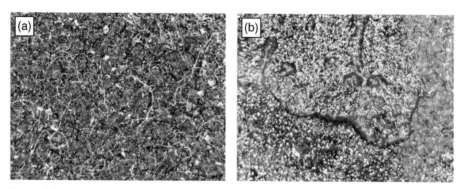

Figure 2.20 High magnification (~×250) images of contaminated surfaces. (a) Dust. (b) Grease.

The mechanism of deposition as the finger is lifted from the surface has been studied by Scruton et al. (1975). They observed that as the finger is removed, a meniscus is formed at the periphery of the film of sweat trapped between the fingerprint ridge and the surface. This meniscus recedes as the finger is lifted until it necks and contact is finally broken, leaving a deposit on the surface along the ridge contact area that may be a continuous pool or a series of droplets. Scruton et al. (1975) established that whether the resultant ridge was a continuous pool or a series of droplets was strongly influenced by the composition of the sweat film, the type of substrate present, and the speed at which the finger was lifted.

It was found that for rapid lifting of the finger, marks deposited in purely eccrine sweat formed a series of droplets with diameter 1–30 µm (Figure 2.21). Similar behaviour was observed for sebaceous sweat on certain surfaces (glass, metals, PTFE), whereas on many other materials including a range of polymers, a continuous pool was formed along the ridges.

For slow lifting of the finger, similar behaviour was observed for eccrine and sebaceous sweat on all surfaces, and a series of large, isolated droplets were observed to form (Figure 2.22).

Scruton et al. (1975) proposed a model for retraction of the film on removal of the finger and considered that the observed behaviour could be explained by a balance between viscous and surface tension forces. Thin adsorbed layers of materials such as fatty acids could also locally modify the behaviour of the surface from that expected from the bulk substrate. When the finger was lifted slowly, viscous resistance was negligible and the geometry of the meniscus determined according to local surface tension and wetting conditions. For faster

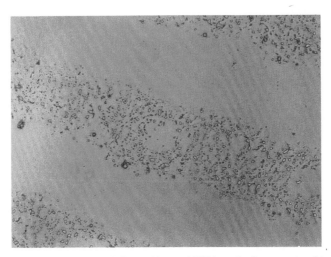

Figure 2.21   The type of fingermark formed by rapid lifting of a finger covered in eccrine sweat. Reproduced courtesy of the Home Office.

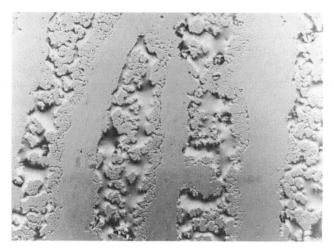

Figure 2.22 The type of fingermark formed by slow lifting of a finger covered in sebaceous sweat. Reproduced courtesy of the Home Office.

lifting of the finger, viscous forces were thought to dominate how the film between the finger and the substrate flowed and ultimately retracted onto the surface once contact was broken.

2.7   Summary of the initial contact

As has been described earlier, the combination of the finger and the surface determines the following:

- The type of mark deposited (positive mark, negative mark, impression)
- The contact area
- Degree of slippage, movement, etc.
- Whether sufficient continuous ridge detail has been deposited in the mark to enable identification
- The composition of the mark

The initial contact may leave a potentially identifiable fingermark or contact traces that are too smudged or fragmentary to enable identification. Such contact traces may still yield useful forensic information, as outlined in the Introduction. In some cases, both finger and surface may be clean and dry, and little or no transfer of material occurs. Viable fingermarks are not produced by every contact, and the absence of fingermarks should not be used to infer that contact has not taken place.

Even in cases where the ridge detail in the mark is sufficient for identification immediately after deposition, it may become degraded by subsequent exposure to the environment and therefore may no longer be available for enhancement at the time of initial examination. The degradation processes that may occur during this ageing period are described in detail in Chapter 4. However, to appreciate fully what degradation processes may occur, it is first necessary to understand the chemical composition and other properties that may be associated with fingermark residue. These are further discussed in Chapter 3.

References

Chatterjee, S K, 'Edgeoscopy', Finger Print Identif. Mag., vol 44(3), (1962), p 3–13.

Maceo, A V, 'Qualitative assessment of skin deformation: A pilot study', J. Forensic Identif., vol 59(4), (2009), p 390–440.

Middleton, J D, Allen, B M, 'The influence of temperature and humidity on stratum corneum and its relation to skin chapping', J. Soc. Cosmet. Chem., vol 24, (1973), p 239–243.

Montagna, W, Parrakal, P F, 'The Structure and Function of Skin', 3rd edn, Academic Press, New York, 1974, p 172–258.

Scruton, B, Robins, B, Blott, B H, 'The deposition of fingerprint films', J. Phys. D Appl. Phys., vol 8, (1975), p 714–723.

Serina, E R, Mote, C D, Jr, Rempel, D, 'Force response of the fingertip pulp to repeated compression – effects of loading rate, loading angle and anthropometry', J. Biomech., vol 30(10), (1997), p 1035–1040.

Serina, E R, Mockensturn, E, Mote, C D, Jr, Rempel, D A, 'Structural model of the forced compression of the fingertip pulp', J. Biomech., vol 31(7), (1998), p 639–646.

Wertheim, K, Maceo, A, 'The critical stage of friction ridge and pattern formation', J. Forensic Identif., vol 52(1), (2002), p 35–85.

Wyatt, O H, Dew-Hughes, D, 'Metals, Ceramics and Polymers', Cambridge University Press, Cambridge, 1974.

3

Composition and properties of fingermarks

Ruth S. Croxton[1], Stephen M. Bleay[2] and Marcel de Puit[3]

[1] School of Chemistry, University of Lincoln, Lincoln, UK

[2] Home Office Centre for Applied Science and Technology, Sandridge, UK

[3] Ministerie van Veiligheid en Justitie, Nederlands Forensisch Instituut, Digitale Technologie en Biometrie, The Hague, The Netherlands

Key points

- Fingermarks have a complex chemical composition that may contain both natural secretions and contaminants.

- The chemicals present are not necessarily homogeneously distributed, both at a microscopic and macroscopic level.

- The chemical composition will change after deposition of the mark.

- In addition to the chemical properties, fingermarks also have both physical and biological properties that can be exploited during fingermark enhancement.

3.1 Chemical composition of fingermarks

3.1.1 Introduction

Latent fingermarks have a complex chemical composition. They are composed of natural secretions (predominantly sweat) from glands in the skin, and environmental contaminants, for example, bacterial spores, cosmetics, dust, hair products and tobacco compounds, may also contribute (Cuthbertson, 1965). The amount of

Fingerprint Development Techniques: Theory and Application, First Edition.
Stephen M. Bleay, Ruth S. Croxton and Marcel de Puit.
© 2018 John Wiley & Sons Ltd. Published 2018 by John Wiley & Sons Ltd.

residue deposited in a latent fingermark is very small, typically <2–20 μg (Croxton, 2008) of which 0.3–2.5 mg L⁻¹ is a complex mixture of organic and inorganic components (Ramotowski, 2001). Compositional information from extensive studies of sweat and skin surface residues may be extrapolated and applied to latent fingermark residue with caution. It is only since the 1960s that studies have been conducted to specifically examine the chemical composition of fingermark residue. The number of studies is ever growing, and developments in technology mean that the type of information we can obtain from a latent fingermark is ever increasing also.

Latent fingermarks can consist of components from a range of sources as outlined in Table 3.1. The relative contribution of each of these sources varies for each fingermark. As a consequence, no two fingermarks have the exact same chemical composition, although there can be similarities in the relative composition. It should be noted that this poses challenges when conducting research into the enhancement or chemical analysis of latent fingermarks and the methods used to generate the fingermark samples. 'Natural' fingermarks are used to describe those for which no prior treatment has been carried out, that is, fingermarks are deposited by donors who have conducted their normal daily routine. 'Groomed' or 'loaded' fingermarks

Table 3.1 Summary of latent fingermark residue sources.

Source	Location	Constituents
Eccrine sweat	Eccrine sweat glands found all over the body and particularly abundant on the palms of hands and fingertips	Water, urea, uric acid, creatinine, amino acids, ammonia, choline, glucose and other reducing sugars, lactic acid and lactate, sodium, chloride, potassium, calcium, trace metal ions, phosphate, sulphate, enzymes, peptides, proteins, vitamins
Sebum	Sebaceous glands on the face, head and other locations associated with hair follicles	Free fatty acids (C_7–C_{22}, saturated and unsaturated), cholesterol esters, mono-, di- and triacylglycerols, wax esters, cholesterol, squalene and other hydrocarbons
Apocrine sweat	Apocrine sweat glands found in the axillary regions of the body, namely, the armpits and genital area	Ammonia, androgenic steroids, cholesterol, glycogen (carbohydrates), iron, proteins and water
Epidermal (skin surface) lipids	From touching other areas of the body (the epidermis) and migration of material from the non-palm side of hand	Free fatty acids, glycerides, proteins, sterols, sterol esters
External contaminants (exogenous substances)	Picked up as a consequence of touching other objects and surface	Illicit drugs, nicotine, cosmetics, explosives, foodstuffs, dust, grease

are generated whereby donors have carried out a specific pre-treatment, for example, washing their hands and then wearing gloves or plastic bags over the hands to allow eccrine sweat to accumulate and therefore generate eccrine-rich fingermarks. More commonly, sebaceous-loaded fingermarks are used whereby donors wipe their fingers across their face and/or forehead where sebaceous glands are abundant. As might be expected, the lipid content of these fingermarks can be significantly higher than 'natural' fingermarks encountered at crime scenes. Research has shown increases of as much as 2000% for some compounds (Croxton et al., 2010). Whilst eccrine- and sebaceous-loaded fingermarks have their place, they are not representative of real fingermarks found at crime scenes, and it is necessary to consider carefully how fingermarks are collected in an experiment.

3.1.2 Natural sweat overview

Three types of gland can contribute to latent fingermark residue: eccrine, sebaceous and apocrine sweat glands. Eccrine sweat glands are found all over the body, varying in size and density between individuals and anatomical site. They are found in highest density on the palms of the hands and soles of the feet and are the only glands found in this location (Saga, 2002). Eccrine sweat can, therefore, be a predominant component of latent fingermark residue.

Sebaceous glands are found predominantly associated with hair follicles. They also vary in abundance with anatomical site, being most abundant on the scalp and face. Sebaceous sweat (sebum), together with the epidermal lipids, form the skin surface lipids. Although the palmar regions are devoid of sebaceous glands, sebum and other epidermal lipids are found in latent fingermark residue as a consequence of touching other parts of the body such as the face (Downing and Strauss, 1974; Strauss et al., 1991). There is also some migration of material from the dorsal surfaces of the hand. The lipid component of fingermarks has been most extensively studied due to its greater abundance and ease of analysis. It is important with respect to some visualisation techniques since it provides the fingermark's 'stickiness' for powders and remains present in fingermarks that have been exposed to water. Apocrine sweat glands are found in the axillary regions of the body, namely, the armpit and genital areas. They are not active until puberty and are controlled by adrenergic nerves (Robertshaw, 1991; Saga, 2002). Apocrine sweat has been reported to contain proteins, ammonia, carbohydrates, ferric ions, cholesterol and androgen steroids (Saga, 2002). It may contribute to latent fingermark residue again as a result of the fingertips touching those parts of the body where these glands are found.

Latent fingermark residue is an emulsion and a heterogeneous mixture of a wide range of chemical components. Ultimately the composition of each deposited latent fingermark is unique. The extent to which the eccrine, sebaceous and apocrine glands contribute to latent fingermark residue depends on a number of factors such as physiological and psychological state, the level of sweating and time since hands were last washed. It takes time for the residues on the skin surface to be replenished following

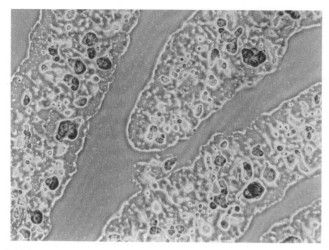

Figure 3.1 A high magnification interference micrograph of a fingermark ridge showing heterogeneous distribution of constituents. Reproduced courtesy of the Home Office.

washing as a result of eccrine sweat gland secretion and/or touching other parts of the body. Whilst there will be similarities between fingermarks in terms of relative quantities of a large number of chemical constituents, quantitatively there will be differences, and the overall profile of all constituents present will be a unique representation of the immediate history of the fingertip and what it has come into contact with.

When a latent fingermark is deposited, the chemical components are not necessarily homogeneously distributed. When viewed under a microscope, discrete regions of eccrine and sebaceous sweat can be seen (Figure 3.1). Eccrine fingermarks typically consist of discrete droplets of material, and sodium chloride crystals are often evident (see Figure 4.10). Conversely, sebum-rich fingermarks consist of continuous pools of material forming the ridges. In mixed fingermarks, the sebaceous material forms irregularly shaped intermittent pools of material (Scruton et al., 1975; Thomas and Reynoldson, 1975a; Thomas, 1978). In addition, particles of skin may be visible in latent fingermarks. Chemical imaging techniques such as Fourier transform infrared (FTIR) spectroscopy and matrix-assisted laser desorption/ionisation mass spectrometry (MALDI-MS) have shown that the two-dimensional (2D) distribution of individual chemical components within a fingermark also varies, largely due to differences in their source of origin. Fingermarks also have a third dimension, which is particularly prominent on porous surfaces such as paper. Differences in affinity of different chemical components of the fingermark can result in differential diffusion of compounds into the paper itself (Almog et al., 2004).

3.1.3 Eccrine sweat

Eccrine sweat is the only type of sweat excreted from the glands on the palms of the hands and the fingers (Figure 3.2).

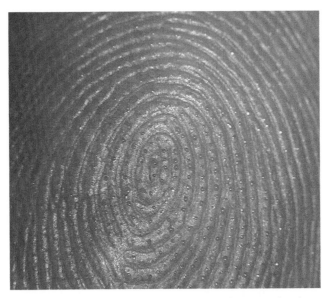

Figure 3.2   The surface of a fingertip, showing beads of eccrine sweat forming at the pores along fingerprint ridges.

Typically a very high proportion of eccrine sweat is water, with organic compounds and inorganic salts forming the remainder (Table 3.2). The composition of eccrine sweat can vary greatly over time (Rothman, 1954; Olsen, 1972).

Amino acids and proteins are prominent organic components of eccrine sweat. The concentration of amino acids in eccrine sweat is reported to be between 0.3 and 2.59 mg L^{-1} (Hansen and Joullié, 2005). Amino acids present on the surfaces of the hands were studied previously in the 1960s (Hamilton, 1965; Oro and Skewes, 1965; Hadorn et al., 1967). Serine, glycine and alanine are the most abundant amino acids. Threonine, leucine, tyrosine, isoleucine, lysine, phenylalanine, methionine and cystine are present in lower amounts (listed in approximate decreasing order). More recent studies using gas chromatography–mass spectrometry (GC-MS) have identified and quantified amino acids in latent fingermarks deposited on non-porous substrates and found composition profiles comparable with those of sweat studies (Croxton et al., 2010).

In addition to amino acids, a variety of other ninhydrin-positive substances have been found in sweat, including cysteic acid, methionine sulphoxide, α-aminoisobutyric acid, glucosamine, cystathionine, ethanolamine and carnosine (Liappis and Hungerland, 1973). A variety of proteins have also been identified including albumin, cathepsin D, immunoglobulins (IgG, IgA, IgD, IgE), keratin 1, keratin 10, glycoproteins and carcinoembryonic antigen (O'Neal Page and Remington, 1967; Nakayashiki, 1990). Antimicrobial proteins and peptides, such as DCD-1 and cathelicidin LL-37, have been detected and have a key role in the innate immune response of the skin and the regulation of skin flora (Flad et al., 2002; Murakami et al., 2002). Drapel et al. (2009) detected keratins 1 and 10, cathepsin D and

Table 3.2 Summary of eccrine sweat composition.

Inorganic (major)		Inorganic (trace)	
Sodium	34–266 mEq L^{-1}	Magnesium	
Potassium	4.9–8.8 mEq L^{-1}	Zinc	
Calcium	3.4 mEq L^{-1}	Copper	
Iron	1–70 mg L^{-1}	Cobalt	
Chloride	0.52–7 mg mL^{-1}	Lead	
Fluoride	0.2–1.18 mg L^{-1}	Manganese	
Bromide	0.2–0.5 mg L^{-1}	Molybdenum	
Iodide	5–12 µg L^{-1}	Tin	
Bicarbonate	15–20 mM	Mercury	
Phosphate	10–17 mg L^{-1}		
Sulphate	7–190 mg L^{-1}		
Ammonia	0.5–8 mM		
Organic (general)		**Organic (lipids)**	
Amino acids	0.3–2.59 mg L^{-1}	Fatty acids	0.01–0.1 µg mL^{-1}
Proteins	15–25 mg dL^{-1}	Sterols	0.01–0.12 µg mL^{-1}
Glucose	0.2–0.5 mg dL^{-1}		
Lactate	30–40 mM		
Urea	10–15 mM	**Miscellaneous**	
Pyruvate	0.2–1.6 mM	Enzymes	
Creatine		Immunoglobulins	
Creatinine			
Glycogen			
Uric acid			
Vitamins			

Ramotowski (2001). Reproduced with permission of Taylor and Francis.

dermcidin in deposited latent fingermarks using immunodetection methods. Peptides and small proteins have also been detected and identified in latent fingermarks by MALDI-MS profiling (Ferguson et al., 2012). Additional organic compounds that can be found in eccrine sweat include glucose (typically at very low concentrations), pyruvic and lactic acid (the levels of the latter increase during exercise and thermogenic sweating), urea, uric acid, creatinine, creatine and ammonia. Water-soluble vitamins have also been shown to be present in small amounts in eccrine sweat.

Chloride (Cl$^-$) is the most abundant inorganic salt, predominantly in the form of sodium chloride but also as potassium chloride. Bromide, iodide and fluorides are also found. Eccrine sweat chloride concentration varies depending on a number of variables, including the rate and duration of sweating, skin surface and environmental temperatures, dietary and water intake and anatomical site (Rothman, 1954; Olsen, 1972). Cuthbertson (1969) found that the chloride concentration in latent fingermarks varied between donors and on different substrates, with larger amounts being deposited on filter paper compared with aluminium foil. Age, occupation (probably related to the amount of hand washing) and digit used significantly affected chloride concentration also.

Small amounts of copper and manganese and moderate amounts of magnesium and phosphorus have been found in eccrine sweat. Large amounts of iron and calcium are present, whilst other minerals may also be found depending on dietary intake. Negligible amounts of sulphates and phosphates have been reported (Rothman, 1954; Olsen, 1972). Aluminium, arsenic, nickel and titanium may be found in trace amounts and generally arise from external sources, for example, coins, jewellery and watches (Liden and Carter, 2001).

3.1.4 Sebaceous sweat (sebum)

Sebaceous glands are holocrine structures. Sebocytes (specialised epithelial cells) produce lipid droplets and then rupture to release sebum, the secretory product of the sebaceous gland (Zouboulis, 2004) (Figure 3.3). Sebum and epidermal lipids (predominantly from stratum corneum cells) form the skin surface lipids (Nicolaides, 1974; Nikkari, 1974). Resident skin bacteria and apocrine and eccrine sweat contribute relatively small amounts to the skin surface lipids (Nicolaides, 1974).

Sebum composition is highly complex (Table 3.3). The vast array of synthesis pathways, affected by genetics and to some extent diet, result in the highly unlikely probability that two individuals have identical sebum compositions. Skin surface lipids are highly abundant, can be easily sampled and have consequently been studied extensively using a variety of methods. The general compounds that make up skin surface lipids are fatty acids, wax esters, triacylglycerols, cholesterol and squalene (Table 3.4). Squalene, wax esters and triglycerides are major components of sebum. Epidermal lipids consist of large amounts of sterols, sterol esters, glycerides and phospholipids (Downing and Strauss, 1974; Downing et al., 1977).

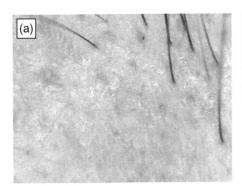 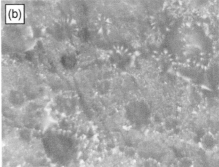

Figure 3.3 High magnification (~×250) images of the surface of the skin, showing sebum being formed on the surface. (a) Hair follicles at the hairline on the forehead and (b) the side of the nose.

Table 3.3   A summary of the composition of sebaceous secretions.

Organic (major)		Organic (trace)
Triglycerides	30–40%	Aldehydes
		Ketones
Free fatty acids	15–25%	Amines
Saturated	50%	Amides
Monounsaturated	48%	Alkanes
Polyunsaturated	2%	Alkenes
		Alcohols
Wax esters	20–25%	Phospholipids
		Pyrroles
Squalene	10–12%	Pyridines
		Piperidines
Cholesterol	1–3%	Pyrazines
		Furans
Cholesterol esters	2–3%	Haloalkanes
		Mercaptans
		Sulphides

Ramotowski (2001). Reproduced with permission of Taylor and Francis.

Table 3.4   Approximate composition of sebum and surface epidermal lipids (Downing and Strauss, 1974).

Constituent	Sebum (% weight)	Surface epidermal lipid (% weight)
Glycerides and free fatty acids[a]	57.5	65.0
Wax esters	26.0	–
Squalene	12.0	–
Cholesterol esters	3.0	15.0
Cholesterol	1.5	20.0

Downing and Strauss (1974). Reproduced with permission of Elsevier.
[a] Total glycerides (mono-, di- and tri-) and free fatty acids given to eliminate variable affect of triglyceride hydrolysis.

It has been established that skin surface lipid composition varies with age, in correspondence with the activity of the sebaceous glands, which are stimulated by androgens. Pathological conditions such as acne, diet and environmental conditions (such as local temperature and ultraviolet (UV) irradiation) affect skin surface lipid composition and production. Microorganisms that colonise the skin surface also play an important role in determining skin surface lipid composition (Bojar and Holland, 2002). For example, free fatty acids found on the skin surface arise from the hydrolysis of triglycerides by bacterial lipase, which occurs as the sebum travels from the follicle onto the surface.

The reported relative abundance of fatty acids in skin surface lipids ranges between 16 and 33%. Over a third of the fatty acids are 'biologically valuable' acids, namely, myristic (tetradecanoic, $C_{14:0}$), palmitic (hexadecanoic, $C_{16:0}$), stearic (octadecanoic, $C_{18:0}$), oleic (*cis*-9-octadecenoic, $C_{18:1}$) and linoleic (*cis*-9,12-octadecadienoic, $C_{18:2}$) acids (Nicolaides, 1974). The remaining consists of over 200 hundred species. Palmitic acid is the most abundant fatty acid in skin surface lipids, followed by palmitoleic (*cis*-9-hexadecenoic acid, $C_{16:1}$) and oleic acid (Boniforti et al., 1973; Nazzaro-Porro et al., 1979). Variation has been found in the relative abundance of fatty acids with age, and some fatty acids have only been determined in individuals with pathological conditions, for example, octadeca-5,8-dienoic acid, which has been found to be present in high amounts in the triglycerides of patients with acne vulgaris (Krakow et al., 1973).

Wax esters are produced exclusively by the sebaceous glands and form approximately 20–27% of skin surface lipids. Wax ester secretion rates vary between individuals and have been found to exhibit an age-related decline (Jacobsen et al., 1985). Squalene (2,6,10,15,19,23-hexamethyl-2,6,10,14,18,22-tetracosahexaene) is an intermediate in the synthesis of cholesterol. It forms 10–15% of skin surface lipids. Cholesterol (cholest-5-en-3β-ol) is the most abundant sterol and constitutes 0.7–2.4% of skin surface lipids, and sterol esters, predominantly cholesterol ester, constitute 2–3.3%. A variety of other organic compounds, many of which are volatile and readily lost, including carboxylic acids, short-chain alcohols, aldehydes, alkane, alkenes, ketones, aromatic amides, amines and heterocyclics, have also been identified in skin surface residue.

The most abundant fatty acids found in latent fingermarks are palmitic ($C_{16:0}$), stearic ($C_{18:0}$), oleic ($C_{18:1}$) and palmitoleic ($C_{16:1}$) acids. Cholesterol, squalene, wax esters and a number of triacylglycerides and diacylglycerides have also been identified in deposited latent fingermarks using a range of analytical techniques (Mong et al., 1999; Archer et al., 2005; Wolstenholme et al., 2009; Croxton et al., 2010; Emerson et al., 2011). The lipid component of latent fingermarks is dependent on a large number of variables including the frequency of touching the face, the amount present on the face, those factors affecting skin surface lipid composition as described previously and the presence of cosmetics, amongst others. Consequently the lipid composition of latent fingermarks has been shown to vary between individuals in terms of amount and relative abundance of components present and to vary between different fingermarks collected from the same individual over a period of time (Archer et al., 2005; Croxton et al., 2010; Weyermann et al., 2011). The amount and composition of sebaceous material found has also been shown to vary with the age of the donor, with children found to produce higher levels of the more volatile components such as free fatty acids compared with adult fingermarks that contain higher levels of less volatile long-chain fatty acid esters (Buchanan et al., 1996; Mong et al., 1999). As seen previously for eccrine-based components, the amount of lipid material deposited in a latent fingermark also varies with type of substrate, with greater amounts deposited on porous substrates compared with nonporous ones (Weyermann et al., 2011).

3.1.5 External contaminants

A wide variety of contaminants, which come into contact with the fingertip, can be deposited in a latent fingermark (Table 3.5 and Figure 3.4).

   These contaminants can be detected and their source identified, which may be of forensic value and demonstrate that an individual has handled a particular substance

Table 3.5 Examples of exogenous contaminants that can contribute to latent fingermark residue and affect its properties or provide intelligence information.

Exogenous compounds secreted in sweat	External skin contaminants	Environmental contaminants
Ethanol	Biological fluids	Bacterial spores
Illicit drugs or their metabolites	Cosmetics, for example, facial creams and hair gel	Cigarette smoke
Nicotine or its metabolite cotinine	Explosives	Dust
Pharmaceutical drugs or their metabolites	Foodstuffs	Exhaust fumes
	Illicit drugs and cutting agents	Grease (food or mechanical)
	Pharmaceutical drugs	Trace material, for example, fibres, pollen and soil particles
	Tobacco products	Water

Source: Bandey (2014). Licensed under open government 3.0, https://www.nationalarchives.gov.uk/doc/open-government-licence/version/3/ (accessed 21 October 2017).

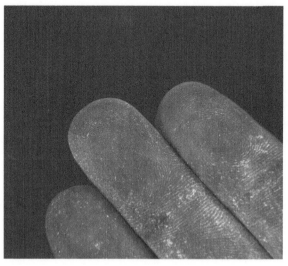

Figure 3.4 Fingertips viewed under long-wave ultraviolet radiation, showing distribution of a fluorescent contaminant arising from peeling an orange.

such as explosives or illicit drugs or in the case of the presence their metabolites indicate that the individual has taken/consumed a particular substance, for example, illicit drugs, nicotine and caffeine. Some contaminants may affect how the fingermark ages, for example, cosmetic creams and lotions containing oily compounds could prolong the age of the fingermark by slowing mechanisms such as water loss. There may also be environmental contaminants either on the substrate prior to fingermark deposition or in the air that then deposit on the deposited fingermark, for example, dust and bacterial spores. A range of external contaminants have been detected and identified in deposited latent fingermarks.

Infrared (IR) spectroscopy- and Raman spectroscopy-based techniques have been used to identify and map powder contaminants in fingermarks such as pharmaceutical and illicit drugs (Day et al., 2004a; Grant et al., 2005; Ricci et al., 2006; West and Went, 2008, 2009). The presence of powder particles could indicate recent handling. It has also been shown that this analysis can be carried out on latent fingermarks that have been recovered from a crime scene using a gelatin lifter (Ricci et al., 2007b) or that have been enhanced with powders and lifted (West and Went, 2008, 2009) or with superglue (Day et al., 2004b). It is well established that a variety of drugs, and in some cases their metabolites, can be detected in sweat, indicating consumption of that drug. This has been shown to also be possible with latent fingermarks. Surface-assisted laser desorption/ionisation mass spectrometry (SALDI-MS) has been used also for the detection drugs and their metabolites, for example, cocaine, methadone, nicotine and cotinine, in latent fingermarks that have been lifted or after cyanoacrylate fuming (Rowell et al., 2009; Benton et al., 2010a, 2010b; Sundar and Rowell, 2014). MALDI-MSI has also been used to detect the presence of caffeine, cocaine, procaine and pseudoephedrine (Bradshaw et al., 2012; Francese et al., 2013; Kaplan-Sandquist et al., 2014). Time-of-flight secondary ion mass spectrometry (ToF-SIMS) has been employed to detect amphetamine-type drugs in deposited latent fingermarks (Szynkowska et al., 2009, 2010). Liquid chromatography–tandem mass spectrometry (LC-MS/MS) has been used to detect, identify and quantify methadone and its metabolite EDDP (2-ethylidene-1,5-dimethyl-3,3-diphenylpyrrolidine) in deposited latent fingermarks (Jacob et al., 2008). Lorazepam and its metabolite have similarly been studied (Goucher et al., 2009). Antibody–gold nanoparticle conjugates and antibody–magnetic particle conjugates have been developed to detect and enhance the fingermarks of drugs users, targeting parent drugs, for example, nicotine, methadone and cocaine, as well as their metabolites, that is, cotinine, EDDP and benzoylecgonine, respectively (Leggett et al., 2007; Hazarika et al., 2009; Boddis and Russell, 2012).

Ricci and Kazarian (2009) have shown that it is possible to detect and identify by attenuated total reflection Fourier transform infrared (ATR-FTIR) spectroscopic imaging different cosmetic products (viz. face creams and body lotion) in fingermarks either deposited directly onto the ATR crystal, deposited on fabric or lifted from a non-porous surface using a gelatin tape lift. Species such as the dimethyldioctadecylammonium ion, arising from cosmetic products such as lotions, hair products and body washes, have also been mapped in fingermarks by MALDI-MSI

(Wolstenholme et al., 2009). Previously Mong et al. (1999) detected hydrocarbons, small glycerides and wax esters typical of cosmetics by GC-MS in the fingermarks of those donors that had used cosmetics prior to sampling. Condom lubricants have also been identified and mapped in latent fingermarks by MALDI-MSI, which may be of value in sexual assault cases (Bradshaw et al., 2011, 2013a).

The detection and identification of explosive residues in latent fingermarks can similarly provide useful forensic intelligence and also evidence of handling these materials. As for other contaminants discussed, a number of techniques have been used to detect explosives such as RDX (1,3,5-trinitro-1,3,5-triazine), HMX (octahy-dro-1,3,5,7-tetranitro-1,3,5,7-tetrazocine), PETN (pentaerythritol tetranitrate), TNT (2,4,6-trinitrotoluene) and ammonium nitrate in deposited latent fingermarks including Raman spectroscopy (Cheng et al., 1995; Tripathi et al., 2011), FTIR spectroscopy (Chen et al., 2009; Banas et al., 2012), SALDI-MS (Rowell et al., 2012) and MALDI-MS (Kaplan-Sandquist et al., 2014). Ion chromatography has been used to detect gunshot residue in latent and enhanced fingermarks (Gilchrist et al., 2012; Love et al., 2013), as well as ToF-SIMS (Szynkowska et al., 2010).

As the stratum corneum is sloughed off, corneocytes (biologically dead, nuclei-free horny cells) are predominantly lost. Nucleated epithelial cells may also be lost in vastly smaller numbers (Balogh et al., 2003a). These cells may be deposited in a fingermark and it may consequently be possible to obtain a DNA profile (Schulz and Reichert, 2002; Balogh et al., 2003b; Schulz et al., 2004). Variation exists between individuals in their 'DNA-shedding' ability, that is, the ability to leave DNA in fingermarks (touch DNA) (Van Oorschot and Jones, 1997; Ladd et al., 1999; Lowe et al., 2002), and variations have also been found in the shedding ability from different parts of the palmar region (Oleiwi et al., 2015). This has important implications on latent fingermark enhancement. For example, DNA has been found on fingermark brushes and shown to be deposited on subsequently brushed surfaces (Van Oorschot et al., 2005). There is also potential for contamination of reagent solutions used for fingermark enhancement particularly in the case of biological samples such as blood (Bowman, 2004).

3.1.6 The individuality of latent fingermark residue

The complex nature of latent fingermark residue and the large number of variables that can affect its composition mean that no two fingermarks will have the exactly the same composition, even from the same digit (Table 3.6). Those factors that affect the composition of skin surface lipids and eccrine sweat will in turn affect latent fingermark residue composition.

Many of the donor-dependent variables are known to affect sweat composition and consequently will affect latent fingermark residue composition. The initial composition of latent fingermark residue is affected by the donor's genetic make-up and in turn their physiology, for example, race, sex and age. The personal lifestyle of the donor may also affect the composition or be apparent in the composition, for

Table 3.6 Factors that may affect latent fingermark composition.

Variables that affect initial composition		Variables that affect how a latent fingermark ages
Donor dependent	Deposition dependent	
Age	Pressure applied	Initial composition
Sex	Substrate properties, for example, temperature, porosity, surface topography, etc.	Humidity
Diet	Time of year, that is, season and associated weather conditions	Temperature (of substrate and environment)
Health	Pre-treatment, for example, washing of hands or deliberate touching of other parts of the body	Lighting
Smoking	Activity prior to deposition, for example, exercising and sedentary lifestyle	Aeration
Cosmetics		Substrate properties, for example, temperature, porosity, surface topography, etc.
Psychological state		
Medication		
Racial origin		

example, their occupation, their dietary intake and whether they smoke or take drugs. The health of the donor will also have an effect, and abnormal levels of some components in sweat are associated with particular disease states.

It has been shown in a number of studies that latent fingermarks differ in chemical composition depending on the age of the donor. The main difference between the latent fingermarks of children and young adults and those of older people is that the former have a high abundance of free fatty acids, whilst the latter have a high abundance of longer-chain fatty acid esters, which are less volatile. A number of studies using ATR-FTIR and IR microspectroscopy combined with mathematical modelling have shown that it is possible to distinguish between latent fingermarks from children and those from adults and to potentially predict the age of the fingermark donor (Hemmila et al., 2008; Antoine et al., 2010; Williams et al., 2011).

Work has been carried out to try to identify markers in latent fingermark residue that can be used to determine the sex of the donor. For example, Ferguson et al. (2012) demonstrated that it is possible to determine the sex of an individual based on the peptide profile of their latent fingermark using MALDI-MSP. Emerson et al. (2011) found significant sex differences in four triacylglycerols identified in deposited sebaceous-loaded fingermarks. However, significant variation was also observed in replicate samples collected from the same donor over several months, which could limit the use of triacylglycerols for sex determination. Fritz et al. (2013) also studied sex differences in lipid composition using synchrotron IR microscopy and found no significant differences associated with the sex of the fingermark donor. They also found no significant differences associated with the age of the fingermark or the age of the donor.

It has long been known that sweat composition can vary depending on the health of the individual. One example of how fingermarks could in the future be used to determine the current health of someone is a study by Khedr (2010), who looked at the free amino acid profiles of water washings from the fingertips of healthy volunteers and beta-thalassaemic volunteers. Clear differences were observed in the amino acid profiles of the beta-thalassaemic volunteers compared with those of the healthy donors with significantly lower amounts of selected amino acids (aspartic acid, glycine, isoleucine, phenylalanine, ornithine and lysine) and significantly higher amounts of others (glutamic acid, asparagines, citrulline, serine, arginine, proline, tryptophan and ammonia). This identified potential markers for the detection of beta-thalassaemia.

Deposition-dependent variables will also impact on the latent fingermark composition including the time since the fingertips were washed, what they were washed with, time of day, ambient temperature and humidity and substrate. The amount of pressure applied when depositing a fingermark has been shown to affect the area of the fingermark and would therefore affect the amount of material deposited (Cuthbertson, 1971; Thomas, 1978). The effect of the substrate on the amount of material deposited was demonstrated in the work of Cuthbertson (1969). Following deposition environmental conditions to which the fingermarks are exposed will also affect the composition and how it changes (Chapter 4).

3.1.7 Analytical techniques used to study latent fingermark composition

There has been a marked increase in the number of studies conducted looking at the chemistry of latent fingermarks, with a view to (i) understanding field observations, for example, why children's fingermarks appear to vanish soon after deposition; (ii) developing novel enhancement techniques, for example, to enhance marks on surfaces exposed to very high temperatures or to determine the age of a fingermark; and (iii) trying to derive intelligence about an unknown suspect, for example, whether they smoke or take illicit substances. A wide variety of techniques have been applied to study the chemical composition of latent fingermark residue, and each has their advantages and disadvantages.

Chromatographic techniques such as gas chromatography (GC) and liquid chromatography (LC) allow bulk fingermark residue to be separated into its individual components. In GC the sample is first vaporised and then separated on a column into its component constituents. Whilst GC is suitable for volatile compounds that are thermally stable, not all compounds can be successfully analysed by this technique. LC separates sample mixtures in the liquid phase on a column. It permits the analysis of larger or thermally labile molecules not suitable for GC. When GC and LC are combined with mass spectrometry, the separated components of the sample mixture can be identified. The sample components are first ionised, forming ionised parent molecules and/or ion fragments. The abundance and mass-to-charge (m/z) ratio of these ions is determined, and a mass spectrum produced, which can then be used, together with retention time, to identify the individual components of the sample. It is also possible to quantify individual components, an advantage over many of the other techniques used to analyse latent fingermarks. The disadvantage of GC-MS and LC-MS for the analysis of latent fingermarks is that they are destructive and require the fingermarks to be removed from the substrate. Sample preparation can require derivatisation, particularly in the case of GC-MS to form volatile compounds more amenable to analysis, and consequently be lengthy. Also in some studies, multiple fingermarks are required for one sample due to the detection limits of the instrument. Whilst qualitative and quantitative information is determined for the bulk fingermark residue, no imaging information is provided. GC-MS and LC-MS have been used for the identification and quantification of endogenous components of latent fingermarks including amino acids, fatty acids, squalene, squalene degradation products, cholesterol and wax esters (Mong et al., 1999; Archer et al., 2005; Mountfort et al., 2007; Croxton et al., 2010; Weyermann et al., 2011) and exogenous components including methadone and lorazepam and their metabolites and nicotine (Jacob et al., 2008; Goucher et al., 2009).

ATR-FTIR spectroscopy and Raman spectroscopy are vibrational spectroscopy techniques that permit *in situ* analysis and imaging, whereby the fingermark can be analysed either on the substrate on which it has been deposited or after being lifted from the surface. FTIR spectroscopy is based on the absorption of IR radiation, which is characteristic of the molecular structure and consequently the chemical composition of the sample being analysed. The spectrum can provide a 'fingerprint' pattern of the sample and can be used for identification in some circumstances.

In the ATR-FTIR process, the surface being analysed is placed on top of an ATR crystal (typically germanium or diamond) and in intimate contact with it. In the ATR mode a beam of IR radiation is passed into the crystal so that it is totally internally reflected from the surface of the crystal that is in contact with the surface being analysed. This internal reflection event results in the formation of an evanescent wave that extends 0.5–2 μm into the sample (depending on the angle of incidence and refractive index of the crystal used). This wave interacts with the molecular species present, and the modified beam that exits the crystal is collected by a detector and analysed (Figure 3.5). By using an array of sensors, IR absorption spectra can be simultaneously collected for each pixel over a relatively large area.

Once the chemical information has been collected, the absorption spectra can be analysed, and absorption peaks associated with naturally occurring constituents or contaminants present in the fingermark residue (e.g. triglycerides, illicit drugs) can be identified. These can then be displayed as a map showing the distribution of the constituent and its relative abundance.

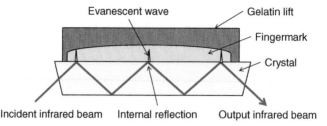

Figure 3.5   Schematic diagram of a fingermark on a gelatin lift being analysed by ATR-FTIR.

When combined with microscopy, this spectroscopic technique can be used to study individual components of the fingermark, for example, droplets of eccrine sweat or sebaceous material, skin cells or particles of contaminants, on the basis of characteristic features of their IR spectrum (Ricci et al., 2006, 2007a; Williams et al., 2011). FTIR microspectrometry can also be used for imaging a fingermark with typical spatial resolution of a few microns. An IR spectrum can be collected at regular points in the latent fingermark, creating a 3D digital image whereby each pixel is represented by a full IR spectrum of the mixture of chemical compounds in that location. Consequently the technique provides both chemical and visual information, permitting an image of the ridge detail to be produced and consequently identified by traditional means. Whilst it is generally not possible to identify single compounds within fingermark residue using this technique, specific regions of the spectrum correspond to particular functional groups. The intensity of particular spectral bands can be attributed to the abundance of certain chemical compounds, for example, lipids or amino acids and proteins, and the distribution of the particular component can be mapped to give a 2D image of the fingermark ridge detail without the need to use reagents to enhance it (Tahtouh et al., 2005, 2007; Crane et al., 2007; Ricci et al., 2007b). Changes in the intensity of particular spectral bands can be monitored over time to study the chemical changes in the fingermark residue. The technique can also be used to image fingermarks that have been enhanced, for example, with ethyl cyanoacrylate (Tahtouh et al., 2005). Synchrotron-sourced IR microscopy has also been used for the analysis of latent fingermarks, and this technique offers improved signal to noise and therefore greater sensitivity compared with conventional IR sources (Perry et al., 2004; Fritz et al., 2013). FTIR spectroscopy offers the advantages that it is non-destructive (at the macro-scale) and enables 2D mapping of latent fingermarks. It can be used for fingermarks that have been lifted from a crime scene (Ricci et al., 2007b). The disadvantage of this technique is that whilst chemical information can be obtained, for example, for a discrete particle such as illicit drugs within the fingermark ridge that permits identification, identification of the individual components that make up the fingermark ridge is not possible, although inferences can be made. The technique also only provides semi-quantitative data, and absolute quantification is not possible.

Raman spectroscopy can similarly be used to detect and map materials in latent fingermarks. Analogous to FTIR, particulates of exogenous material can be identified on the basis of their Raman spectrum (Day et al., 2004a; West and Went, 2008,

2009), and fingermarks can be mapped using selected vibrational band intensities. Surface-enhanced Raman spectroscopy (SERS) has enhanced sensitivity compared with Raman spectroscopy and has been used to map endogenous components such as skin surface lipids and proteins in doped latent fingermarks (Connatser et al., 2010; Song et al., 2012).

A number of mass spectrometry-based techniques have been used to chemically map latent fingermarks including desorption electrospray ionisation (DESI) mass spectrometry (DESI-MS), MALDI-MS, SALDI-MS and secondary ion mass spectrometry (SIMS). Whilst these techniques have their differences, they all permit the *in situ* analysis of latent fingermarks with no or minimal sample preparation and, like the vibrational spectroscopic imaging techniques, provide the means to chemically map a fingermark. A 3D digital image can be created using these techniques whereby each pixel is represented by a full mass spectrum of the mixture of chemical compounds in that location. A further advantage of these techniques is that the mass spectrometry component provides the ability to identify individual components of the fingermark residue by providing molecular weight information and in some cases structural information, allowing unequivocal identification. A disadvantage of some of these techniques is that traditionally the fingermark must be deposited onto a specific type of substrate. However, researchers are developing methods of lifting fingermarks from a crime scene, which can then be analysed in the laboratory, in order for the methods to be applicable to real-life forensic applications. In other cases techniques such as SIMS are being adapted for use in ambient conditions, removing the restriction on exhibit size.

DESI-MS allows chemical mapping of latent fingermarks *in situ* on a substrate under ambient conditions. Charged solvent droplets are electrosprayed onto the surface, and compounds of interest are then released from the sample as secondary scattered droplets and form ions. The m/z ratios of the ions formed are measured by the mass spectrometer and permit the generation of a mass spectrum and identification. By rastering the electrosprayed stream of charged solvent droplets across the surface of the item being analysed, a chemical map is created. DESI-MS has been used to map endogenous compounds, for example, fatty acids (including palmitic, stearic and oleic) and triacylglycerols, and exogenous compounds, for example, cocaine, Δ^9-tetrahydrocannabinol and the explosive RDX (trinitrohexahydro-1,3,5-triazine), on porous and non-porous substrates (Ifa et al., 2008).

In terms of latent fingermark analysis, MALDI-MS can be used in two modes – profiling (MALDI-MSP) and imaging (MALDI-MSI). In both cases a UV-absorbing matrix is added to the sample by either spotting in discrete locations for MALDI-MSP or spray coating across the whole sample for MALDI-MSI. The matrix solution is selected so that it is capable of dissolving the molecules of interest on the surface, and as the solvent evaporates, the matrix recrystallises and incorporates molecules from the surface.

A suitable matrix material meets several requirements: it needs to be capable of strongly absorbing energy from the laser being used for excitation, it needs to be polar so that it can dissolve in aqueous solutions and it needs to be of relatively low molecular weight to vaporise easily under the laser beam. Most matrices used are acidic, thus providing protons to aid ionisation of the molecules from the surface that have become co-crystallised in the matrix. The matrix material most generally suited to the analysis of the constituents of fingermarks is α-cyano-4-hydroxycin-namic acid (α-CHCA).

Once the matrix has been applied to the surface, it is irradiated with a laser operating in the UV region of the spectrum, such as nitrogen lasers (output at 337 nm) and frequency-tripled and frequency-quadrupled Nd:YAG lasers (outputs at 355 and 266 nm, respectively). The effect of the laser on the surface is magnified by the matrix enhancer, which absorbs the energy of the laser and directs it into the surface where ablation of the surface layers occurs. The ablation process produces a heated plume of matrix molecules and related species close to the surface, and this heated plume then contributes to the ionisation of the molecules from the surface, producing the fragments that pass into the mass spectrometer (Figure 3.6). Typically protonated molecular species or adduct ions are formed, which can be identified on the basis of their m/z ratio.

For imaging the laser is systematically rastered across the sample, creating a 3D dataset. The spatial resolution that can be obtained ranges between 10 and 150 μm depending on the instrumentation used (Francese et al., 2013). MALDI-MS can provide two types of information. Fingermarks can be imaged by generating 2D molecular images and selecting key species, for example, fatty acids, fatty acid degradation products, cholesterol and diacylglycerols known to be abundant in fingermark residue, thereby providing a physical image of the ridge detail that can be identified using traditional comparison methods of level 1 and level 2 ridge detail (Wolstenholme et al., 2009). In addition to this, chemical information can be obtained about what the individual has consumed, for example, caffeine, or handled, for example, drugs,

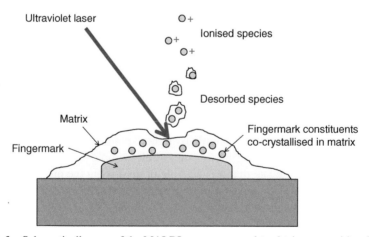

Figure 3.6   Schematic diagram of the MALDI process as used to obtain compositional information about a fingermark.

condom lubricants and toiletries (Wolstenholme et al., 2009; Bradshaw et al., 2011, 2012, 2013a). MALDI-MS has a large m/z range, meaning it can be used to detect a wide range of compounds from small volatile compounds to large peptides and proteins. Work has also shown that it is possible to integrate MALDI-MS into the standard forensic workflow whereby a fingermark can be lifted from a crime scene, photographed and imaged using UV and fluorescence detection before being analysed by MALDI-MS (Bradshaw et al., 2013b). Currently it is not possible to quantify using MALDI-MS, but research is ongoing in this area. MALDI-MS is non-destructive to the extent that not all of the fingermark is desorbed from the surface during analysis. It is possible to remove the matrix by washing and to process the sample using other techniques (Wolstenholme et al., 2009). Laser desorption/ ionisation time-of-flight mass spectrometry (LDI-TOF-MS) is a similar technique to MALDI-MS but does not require the application of a matrix. It has been used to successfully detect endogenous triacylglycerols and diacylglycerols in deposited sebaceous-loaded latent fingermarks (Emerson et al., 2011). Exogenous compounds thought to be derived from cosmetic products, namely, polyethylene glycol (PEG) derivatives and polypropylene glycol (PPG) derivatives, were also identified.

In SALDI-MS deposited latent fingermarks are powdered using hydrophobic silica nanoparticles (which can also be functionalised to bind to specific components of interest), producing a visible fingermark for recovery and identification. The fingermark can then subsequently be analysed by SALDI-MS, providing chemical information similar to that obtained using MALDI-MS, whereby the silica nanoparticles act as a laser desorption/ionisation-enhancing agent. The fingermark can be analysed directly or lifted first, making it possible to analyse fingermarks deposited on a range of surfaces and recovered from crime scenes. The technique has been used to detect both endogenous components such as amino acids, fatty acids and squalene (Lim et al., 2011) and exogenous components such as cocaine, methadone, nicotine and their metabolites in deposited and lifted latent fingermarks (Rowell et al., 2009; Benton et al., 2010a).

ToF-SIMS has also been used to generate chemical images of fingermarks, mapping the presence of both endogenous and exogenous compounds.

In the SIMS process, an energetic (keV–MeV) beam of ions is used to bombard the surface. For the more established keV process, the sample is kept under high vacuum, whilst for the more recent MeV process, it may be possible to employ ambient conditions. As the energetic particles impinge upon the surface, collisions occur with the molecules in the surface layer. These collisions produce a number of charged atoms, neutral species, molecules and molecular fragments that are ejected from the surface and are characteristic of the molecules present in the surface layers (Figure 3.7). The process by which these species are ejected is known as sputtering, and the ejected species are known as secondary ions. The secondary ions may be positively or negatively charged. The secondary ions are identified on the basis of their m/z ratio.

Once ejected from the surface, the secondary ions can be focused into a mass spectrometer where they are separated and identified according to their m/z ratio.

The conditions can be adjusted so that minimal fragmentation of the surface molecules occurs and the molecular ions present can be more readily identified.

The SIMS instrument can be operated in a scanning mode, scanning the ion beam across the surface and recording the molecular species ejected at each point. This mode is useful in building up distribution maps of particular constituents across the surface.

The more well-established SIMS process using incident ions in the keV energy range (e.g. 25 keV Bi_3^+) requires the sample to be placed into the vacuum chamber of the SIMS instrument. This tends to be relatively small and may necessitate the area of interest to be cut from the item. In MeV SIMS, the energy of the incident ions is much higher, and therefore they are capable of passing through air to interact with the surface. This means that in theory larger items could be examined by bringing them in close proximity to the instrument, negating the need to cut areas from the item. MeV SIMS systems are less mature than keV systems, and the process is not readily available.

The technique removes a few monolayers of material from the surface and is reported to be less destructive than other techniques such as MALDI-MS and DESI. It also has the best resolution of submicron (Bailey et al., 2012). ToF-SIMS has been used to map a range of inorganic and organic endogenous components in deposited latent fingermarks including sodium, potassium, fatty acids and squalene (Bailey et al., 2012, 2013). It has been shown to be able to further enhance fingermarks developed with traditional enhancement techniques such as cyanoacrylate fuming and wet powders (Bailey et al., 2013). MeV SIMS is a high energy variant of ToF-SIMS and employs at high energy oxygen primary ion beam (e.g. 3 MeV $^{16}O^{3+}$). The advantage of this technique is that it can be carried out under ambient conditions, like DESI-MS, rather than requiring vacuum conditions. It has been

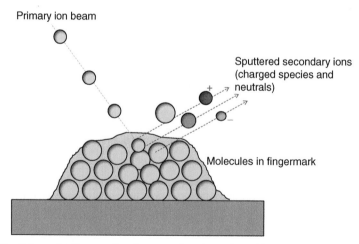

Figure 3.7   Schematic diagram showing secondary ions ejected from surface layers of a fingermark by action of primary beam.

shown that when subjected to vacuum conditions, fingermarks lose approximately 26% of their mass and that there are compositional changes, with the loss of fatty acids and their esters, as well as squalene and water (Bright et al., 2013). The ability to work under ambient conditions also means that the exhibit size is no longer a restriction.

Alternatively, SIMS can be run in a spot analysis mode, focusing the ion beam on a single point and collecting molecular information over time as the ion beam etches deeper into the surface. This mode is more useful in providing depth profiling information that may assist in determining the order of deposition of overlapping fingermarks and inks (Bright et al., 2012; Attard-Montalto et al., 2014).

A small number of studies have been conducted studying the elemental composition of latent fingermarks, with a particular focus on inorganic elements. Worley et al. (2006), for example, imaged latent fingermarks using micro-X-ray fluorescence spectroscopy to map the distribution of inorganic elements such as sodium, potassium and chlorine. The advantage of using inorganic ions is that they are nonvolatile and will not degrade with time and as such will be present in aged fingermarks. X-ray photoelectron spectroscopy has also been used to detect a range of elements in latent fingermark samples including sodium, calcium, potassium, chlorine, carbon, oxygen and nitrogen (Bailey et al., 2012).

Whilst the different analytical techniques described previously differ in their spatial resolution, chemical specificity and analysis conditions, and each has its advantages, no single technique can at present provide a complete chemical profile of a latent fingermark, in terms of qualitative and quantitative data. They all provide complementary information and if applied in combination would provide the ultimate package to help improve our understanding of latent fingerprint chemistry, as demonstrated by Bailey et al. (2012).

3.2 Biological properties of fingermarks

All regions of the skin, including the friction ridges on the palms of the hands and soles of the feet, can play host to a range of microbial flora, which include bacteria, fungi and possibly viruses (Marples, 1969; Noble, 1981) (Figure 3.9). These microbes may be categorised as 'transient', 'temporary residents' or 'residents' (Noble, 1981), depending on whether the microbe originates from the skin or from an external contaminant and whether it can multiply and persist on the skin for a prolonged period of time. Some microbes can utilise water-soluble substances in eccrine sweat such as lactic acid and amino acids as energy sources during growth, making areas such as the palm where eccrine sweat predominates a suitable environment for colonies to form. Other microbes utilise lipid-soluble substances or the breakdown products of keratin and cell debris as nutrients.

In certain circumstances there may be high contents of bacteria or fungi within the fingermark residue, and growth of these microbes may be promoted under favourable conditions (Figures 3.8 and 3.9).

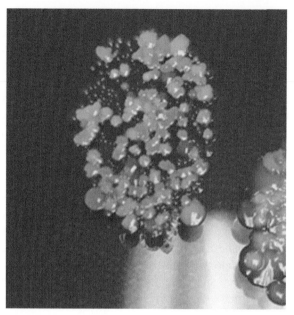

Figure 3.8 Growth of bacterial colonies from a fingermark deposited on agar gel. Reproduced courtesy of Loughborough University.

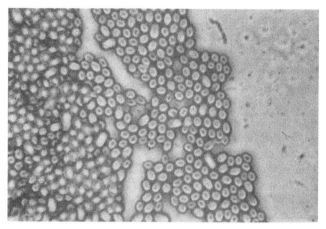

Figure 3.9 Optical micrograph showing the growth of a bacterial colony within the ridges of a deposited fingermark (Thomas, 1974). Reproduced courtesy of the Home Office.

Together with the chemicals present on the hand, these microbes can be transferred from the finger to the surface by contact. Although it was observed (O'Neill, 1941) that bacteria transferred to a nutrient agar from a finger could be cultivated to produce an identifiable fingermark, there was no reported attempt to utilise the microbial content of fingermarks in forensic investigation until the work by Harper et al. published in 1987. Harper et al. (1987) identified a range of microbes present on the skin that were capable of growing and forming colonies on sebaceous material and used several of these in agar gel overlays that were placed over fingermarks deposited on polythene sheet. On removal of the gel overlays after 48 h incubation, the colonies grown on the fingermark ridges were enhanced by staining with Solvent Black 3 (a process used for fingermark enhancement described in Chapter 11). Fingermarks with clearly identifiable ridge detail were successfully enhanced by this route. The microbe that developed the fingermarks with the most distinct ridge detail was subsequently identified as *Acinetobacter calcoaceticus*, a recognised species of human bacteria distributed over the entire body. However, the concept of biological enhancement of fingermarks does not appear to have been pursued further.

With advances in detection and analysis techniques that have made identification of microbial species easier, an alternative approach has been proposed for using the biological composition of fingermarks for personal identification. Fierer et al. (2008) conducted an initial assessment of the bacteria species present by swabbing both hands of 51 adults using a PCR technique to amplify the bacterial DNA recovered by the swabs and then a novel high throughput sequencing process known as pyrosequencing to characterise the species present. This study distinguished 332 000 bacteria types belonging to 4742 different species across the set of volunteers, on average each volunteer having 3200 different bacteria from >150 species on their hands. The diversity found between individuals and between different hands on the same individual was significant. Only five species, including the recognised skin bacteria *Streptococcus*, *Staphylococcus* and *Lactobacillus*, were found on all hands. Almost half of the species identified were rare with hands from the same individual having only 17% of their species in common, with hands of different individuals sharing only 13% of their bacterial species. This high diversity led to the proposal that analysis of the bacterial species left by the contact from a finger could be used for personal identification.

In a follow-on study in 2010, Fierer et al. took swabs from articles including computer keyboards and mice that had been touched by a set of volunteers and also swabs from similar surfaces that had not been handled. They also took swabs from the fingers of the volunteers and from 270 randomly selected individuals not participating in the handling experiments. By using the pyrosequencing approach, they were able to use the sets of bacterial species identified on each swab to differentiate the individual that had handled the surfaces with an accuracy of between 70 and 90%. This analysis was shown to be feasible for swabs taken up to 2 weeks after handling. It has been proposed that further advances in technology could lead to improvements in the ability to differentiate between individuals and make this a viable approach for forensic investigation (Fierer et al., 2010).

3.3 Physical properties of fingermarks

In addition to their complex chemistry, the natural sweat secretions deposited by the finger on the surface also have a range of physical properties that can potentially be utilised by enhancement processes. There are far fewer reported studies of the physical properties of fingermarks, and a summary of what has been evaluated is given in the following sections.

3.3.1 Topography

The residues left on the surface by the finger have physical dimensions, and it is possible to measure the magnitude of these dimensions relative to the baseline of a smooth, non-porous surface. Thomas and Reynoldson (1975a) made use of quantitative interference microscopy to measure droplet topography.

The maximum thickness of fingermark residues estimated by this route varied from 10 nm to approximately 2 μm, although this was increased to 5–10 μm when fingers were deliberately loaded with sebaceous material (e.g. by wiping the fingers across the nose or forehead). The topography of a typical droplet within a fingermark deposit and its change over time is illustrated in Figure 3.10.

On naturally deposited fingermarks on glass, it can be seen that the topography of the droplets was smooth and initially 1 μm maximum. As the droplet aged and dried out, the deposit became more viscous, and topography became increasingly irregular with the mean height decreasing to ~100 nm.

Dorakumbura et al. (2016) have recently used PeakForce quantitative nanomechanical mapping (PF QNM) atomic force microscopy (AFM) to revisit the variations in topography of latent fingermark droplets over time. It proved possible to observe the topographical variation of eccrine droplets using this technique, and the lateral spread of the fingermark over time was also observed, with a thin film of material propagating from the fingermark ridges into the furrows almost as soon as the mark had been deposited.

3.3.2 Adhesion

Fingermark residues have adhesive properties, and it is thought that several constituents may contribute to this and more than one mechanism of adhesion may operate. Thomas (1978) reported work by Blott and Scruton that measured the force of detachment for an aluminium powder particle from a powdered mark. In these studies, a sheet of aluminised mylar was placed over the mark, and a voltage applied until the particles were detached. Using this method, fields of 10^9 Vm^{-1} could be applied to the surface, which equated to forces of 10^7 Nm^{-1} on the areas of ridge where aluminium particles were present.

Particles were removed from the surface in the region of the furrows at forces of 10^3 Nm^{-1}, whereas from the ridges applied forces of 2.2×10^6 Nm^{-1} were required to remove particles, although some still remained attached to the surface.

Dorakumbura et al. (2016) also studied adhesion using AFM and found that adhesive properties could vary significantly within fingermark ridges, even within a single droplet, reinforcing the heterogeneous nature of fingermarks. It was also found that the adhesive properties of fingermark droplets changed significantly as they aged.

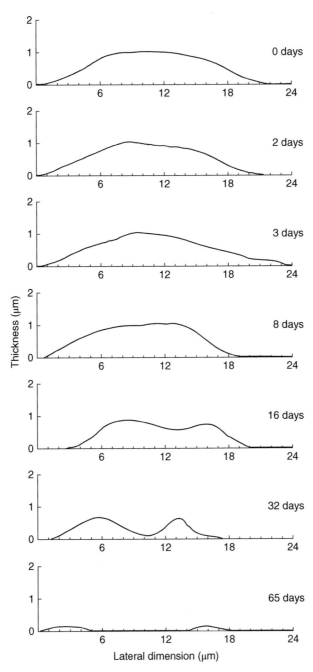

Figure 3.10   A cross section across a typical droplet of finger deposit and its temporal variation (Thomas and Reynoldson, 1975b). Reproduced courtesy of the Home Office.

3.3.3 Electrical resistivity

The resistivity (ρ) of a material is a measure of the resistance of the material to the flow of electric charge through it. Materials with low values of electrical resistivity are those that allow charge to flow through them easily (i.e. are good conductors).

Thomas (1975) utilised a resistivity cell specially designed for very small volumes of material to measure the resistivity of sweat collected from the fingers of a small pool of donors. He found that the resistivity of fresh fingermark residue had a resistivity of 10 Ωm and this increased to between 100 and 400 Ωm after approximately 4 h, after which it remained reasonably constant.

3.3.4 Surface potential

Scruton and Blott (1973) developed a high resolution electrostatic probe that could be combined with a scanning system and used it to measure the difference in surface potential between surfaces and the fingermark residue deposited on them. Differences in surface potential of several 100 mV were observed between the ridges (where fingermark residue was present) and furrows (where no residue was present and the surface properties dominate). This difference was consistent on a range of smooth, insulating surfaces such as glass. However, on paper the measured difference between ridges and furrows was ~20 mV, and on fabric it was ~10 mV, neither value changing significantly over 24 h. In both cases, the variation was small in comparison with local fluctuations in surface potential that could arise from variations in surface texture, and therefore it was considered that the presence of fingermarks would be difficult to detect by means of surface potential measurements alone.

In further measurements conducted by Thomas (1978) using Scruton and Blott's probe, it was shown that on smooth conducting surfaces (in this case gold), the surface potential difference was 300 mV, which decreased to 100 mV after 2 days.

3.3.5 Relative permittivity (dielectric constant)

The relative permittivity (ε_r) of a material is a measure of how much electrical energy can be stored by a material in response to an applied voltage, in comparison with how much energy would be stored by a vacuum. Materials that are polar and are readily polarised by an applied voltage (e.g. water) have high values of relative permittivity, whereas non-polar materials have values closer to 1.

Permittivity can be described in terms of both real and imaginary components, although often only the value of the real component is quoted. The real component may also sometimes be described as the 'dielectric constant'.

The relative permittivity of sweat has not been extensively researched, but the growing need for 'liveness' detection of fingerprints to prevent 'spoofing' of biometric fingerprint readers has initiated studies in this area (Chizmadzhev et al., 1998). Eccrine sweat has high value of relative permittivity ($\varepsilon_r \sim 60$–80), which is related to the high water content of the sweat. Lipids, such as those found in sebaceous sweat, may have values of relative permittivity approximately 30 times lower than this. In both cases the relative permittivity of fingermark residue is likely to be different from that of the surface it has been deposited on (e.g. paper $\varepsilon_r \sim 3.85$, polythene $\varepsilon_r \sim 2.25$). It is likely that relative permittivity of fingermark residue will change as water is lost, but the residual salts and lipids remaining may still cause local modification of the relative permittivity, even on surfaces such as paper where the mark can be absorbed into the surface.

3.3.6 Refractive index

The refractive index (n) is a measure of the change in velocity of electromagnetic radiation (in this case visible light) as it propagates through a medium, compared with the speed of light in a vacuum, where

$$n = \frac{c}{v}$$

where c, speed of light in a vacuum; and v, speed of light in the substance.

Thomas and Reynoldson (1975a) used interference microscopy and the interphako method to measure phase changes associated with the presence of fingermark deposits. The refractive index of the fingermark residue was measured at a wavelength 551 nm by comparing the phase shifts in air with those in an aqueous solution of barium mercuric iodide. The average refractive index measured using this method was 1.47, with a distribution over the range 1.40–1.54 (Figure 3.11).

This value differs significantly from that of water ($n = 1.333$), which indicates that the water deposit of the residue may be less than that found in studies of sweat

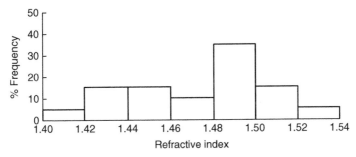

Figure 3.11 Refractive index distribution of fingermark deposits of less than a day old for $\lambda = 551$ nm (Thomas and Reynoldson, 1975b). Reproduced courtesy of the Home Office.

collected from fingers (Kuno, 1956) and the refractive index may be more influenced by the presence of long-chain fatty material. The average value also differs slightly from transparent materials on which fingermarks may be deposited, such as Perspex ($n = 1.49$) and the soda glass used in windows ($n = 1.52$), and therefore it may be possible to exploit these differences to enhance the contrast of the fingermarks.

Many of the studies reported previously have not been revisited since the 1970s, and significant advances in technology have been made since then. The advent of techniques such as AFM, with its wide range of imaging modes (contact, non-contact, tapping), means that it may be possible to obtain more accurate values for some of the parameters measured previously and to map their variation across fingermark residues. The studies reported by Dorakumbura et al. indicate that such studies are beginning to take place.

References

Almog, J., Azoury, M., Elmaliah, Y., Berenstein, L., Zaban, A. 'Fingerprints' third dimension: the depth and shape of fingerprints penetration into paper – cross section examination by fluorescence microscopy', J. Forensic Sci., vol 49, (2004), p 981–985.

Antoine, K.M., Mortazavi, S., Miller, A.D., Miller, L.M. 'Chemical differences are observed in children's versus adults' latent fingerprints as a function of time', J. Forensic Sci., vol 55, (2010), p 513–518.

Archer, N.E., Charles, Y., Elliott, J.A., Jickells, S. 'Changes in the lipid composition of latent fingerprint residue with time after deposition on a surface', Forensic Sci. Int., vol 154, (2005), p 224–239.

Attard-Montalto, N., Ojeda, J.J., Reynolds, A., Ismail, M., Bailey, M., Doodkorte, L., de Puit, M., Jones, B.J. 'Determining the chronology of deposition of natural fingermarks and inks on paper using secondary ion mass spectrometry', Analyst, vol 139, (2014), p 4641–4653.

Bailey, M.J., Bright, N.J., Croxton, R.S., Francese, S., Ferguson, L.S., Hinder, S., Jickells, S., Jones, B., Jones, B.N., Kazarian, S.G., Ojeda, J.J., Webb, R.P., Wolstenholme, R., Bleay, S. 'Chemical characterization of latent fingerprints by matrix-assisted laser desorption ionization, time-of-flight secondary ion mass spectrometry, mega electron volt secondary mass spectrometry, gas chromatography/mass spectrometry, x-ray photoelectron spectroscopy, and attenuated total reflection fourier transform infrared spectroscopic imaging: an intercomparison', Anal. Chem., vol 84, (2012), p 8514–8523.

Bailey, M.J., Ismail, M., Bleay, S., Bright, N., Levin Elad, M., Cohen, Y., Geller, B., Everson, D., Costa, C., Webb, R.P., Watts, J.F., de Puit, M. 'Enhanced imaging of developed fingerprints using mass spectrometry imaging', Analyst, vol 138, (2013), p 6246–6250.

Balogh, M.K., Burger, J., Bender, M., Schneider, P.M., Alt, K.W. 'Fingerprints from fingerprints', Int. Congr. Ser., vol 1239, (2003a), p 953–957.

Balogh, M.K., Burger, J., Bender, M., Schneider, P.M., Alt, K.W. 'STR genotyping and mtDNA sequencing of latent fingerprint on paper', Forensic Sci. Int., vol 137, (2003b), p 188–195.

Banas, A., Banas, K., Breese, M.B.H., Loke, J., Heng Teo, B., Lim, S.K. 'Detection of microscopic particles present as contaminants in latent fingerprints by means of synchrotron radiation-based fourier transform infra-red micro-imaging', Analyst, vol 137, (2012), p 3459–3465.

Bandey, H. (Ed.) 'Fingermark Visualisation Manual', Home Office, London, 2014.

Benton, M., Rowell, F., Sundar, L., Jan, M. 'Direct detection of nicotine and cotinine in dusted latent fingermarks of smokers by using hydrophobic silica particles and MS', Surf. Interface Anal., vol 42, (2010a), p 378–385.

Benton, M., Chua, M.J., Gu, F., Rowell, F., Ma, J. 'Environmental nicotine contamination in latent fingermarks from smoker contacts and passive smoking', Forensic Sci. Int., vol 200, (2010b), p 28–34.

Boddis, A.M., Russell, D.A. 'Development of aged fingermarks using antibody-magnetic particle conjugates', Anal. Methods, vol 4, (2012), p 637–641.

Bojar, R.A., Holland, K.T. 'Review: the human cutaneous microflora and factors controlling colonisation', World J. Microbiol. Biotechnol., vol 18, (2002), p 889–903.

Boniforti, L., Passi, S., Caprilli, F., Nazzaro-Porro, M. 'Skin surface lipids. Identification and determination by thin-layer chromatography and gas-liquid chromatography', Clin. Chim. Acta, vol 47, (1973), p 223–231.

Bowman, V. (Ed.) 'Manual of Fingerprint Development Techniques', revised 2nd edition, Home Office, Sandridge, (2004).

Bradshaw, R., Wolstenholme, R., Blackledge, R.D., Clench, M.R., Ferguson, L.S., Francese, S. 'A novel MALDI MSI based methodology for the identification of sexual assault suspects', Rapid Commun. Mass Spectrom., vol 25, (2011), p 415–422.

Bradshaw, R., Rao, W., Wolstenholme, R., Clench, M.R., Bleay, S., Francese, S. 'Separation of overlapping fingermarks by matrix assisted laser desorption ionisation mass spectrometry imaging', Forensic Sci. Int., vol 222, (2012), p 318–326.

Bradshaw, R., Wolstenholme, R., Ferguson, L.S., Sammon, C., Mader, K., Claude, E., Blackledge, R.D., Clench, M.R., Francese, S. 'Spectroscopic imaging based approach for condom identification in condom contaminated fingermarks', Analyst, vol 138, (2013a), p 2546–2557.

Bradshaw, R., Bleay, S., Wolstenholme, R., Clench, M.R., Francese, S. 'Towards the integration of matrix assisted laser desorption ionisation mass spectrometry imaging into the current fingermark examination workflow', Forensic Sci. Int., vol 232, (2013b), p 111–124.

Bright, N.J., Webb, R.P., Bleay, S., Hinder, S., Ward, N.I., Watts, J.F., Kirkby, K.J., Bailey, M.J. 'Determination of the deposition order of overlapping latent fingerprints and inks using secondary ion mass spectrometry', Anal. Chem., vol 84, (2012), p 4083–4087.

Bright, N.J., Willson, T.R., Driscoll, D.J., Reddy, S.M., Webb, R.P., Bleay, S., Ward, N.I., Kirkby, K.J., Bailey, M.J. 'Chemical changes exhibited by latent fingerprints after exposure to vacuum conditions', Forensic Sci. Int., vol 230, (2013), p 81–86.

Buchanan, M.V., Asano, K., Bohanan, A. 'Chemical characterisation of fingerprints from adults and children', SPIE Proc. Forensic Evid. Anal. Crime Scene Investig., vol 2941, (1996), p 89–95.

Chen, T., Schultz, Z.D., Levin, I.W. 'Infrared spectroscopic imaging of latent fingerprints and associated forensic evidence', Analyst, vol 134, (2009), p 1902–1904.

Cheng, C., Kirkbride, T.E., Batchelder, D.N., Lacey, R.J., Sheldon, T.G. 'In situ detection and identification of trace explosives by Raman microscopy', J. Forensic Sci., vol 40, (1995), p 31–37.

Chizmadzhev, Y.A., Indenborn, A.V., Kuzmin, P.I., Galichenko, S.V., Weaver, J.C., Potts, R.O. 'Electrical properties of skin at moderate voltages: contribution of appendageal macropores', Biophys. J., vol 74, (1998), p 843–856.

Connatser, R.M., Prokes, S.M., Glembocki, O.J., Schuler, R.L., Gardner, C.W., Lewis, S.A., Lewis, L.A. 'Toward surface-enhanced Raman imaging of latent fingerprints', J. Forensic Sci., vol 55, (2010), p 1462–1470.

Crane, N.J., Bartick, E.G., Schwartz Perlman, R., Huffman, S. 'Infrared spectroscopic imaging for noninvasive detection of latent fingerprints', J. Forensic Sci., vol 52, (2007), p 48–53.

Croxton, R.S. 'Analysis of Latent Fingerprint Components by Gas Chromatography-Mass Spectrometry'. PhD Thesis, University of Lincoln, Lincoln, UK, (2008).

Croxton, R.S., Baron, M.G., Butler, D., Kent, T., Sears, V.G. 'Variation in amino acids and lipid composition of latent fingerprints', Forensic Sci. Int., vol 199, (2010), p 93–102.

Cuthbertson, F. *The Composition of Fingerprints*, SSCD Memorandum SAC/2/65, AWRE Report. (1965).

Cuthbertson, F. *The Chemistry of Fingerprints*, AWRE Report No. 013/69. (1969).

Cuthbertson, F. *The Chemistry of Fingerprints*, Report for Period 1 April 1970 to 31 March 1971, SSCD Memorandum 308, AWRE Report. (1971)

Day, J.S., Edwards, H.G.M., Dobrowski, S.A., Voice, A.M. 'The detection of drugs of abuse in fingerprints using Raman spectroscopy I: latent fingerprints', Spectrochim. Acta A Mol. Biomol. Spectrosc., vol 60, (2004a), p 563–568.

Day, J.S., Edwards, H.G.M., Dobrowski, S.A., Voice, A.M. 'The detection of drugs of abuse in fingerprints using Raman spectroscopy II: cyanoacrylate-fumed fingerprints', Spectrochim. Acta A, vol 60, (2004b), p 1725–1730.

Dorakumbura, B., Becker, T., Lewis, S.W., 'Nanomechanical mapping of latent fingermarks: a preliminary investigation into the changes in surface interactions and topography over time', Forensic Sci. Int., vol 267, (2016), p 16–24.

Downing, D.T., Strauss, J.S. 'Synthesis and composition of surface lipids of human skin', J. Investig. Dermatol., vol 62, (1974), p 228–244.

Downing, D.T., Strauss, J.S., Norton, L.A., Pochi, P.E., Stewart, M.E. 'The time course of lipid formation in human sebaceous glands', J. Investig. Dermatol., vol 69, (1977), p 407–412.

Drapel, V., Becue, A., Champod, C., Margot, P. 'Identification of promising antigenic components in latent fingermark residues', Forensic Sci. Int., vol 184, (2009), p 47–53.

Emerson, B., Gidden, J., Lay, Jr., J.O., Durham, B. 'Laser desorption/ionization time-of-flight mass spectrometry of triacylglycerols and other components in fingermark samples', J. Forensic Sci., vol 56, (2011), p 381–389.

Ferguson, L.S., Wulfert, F., Wolstenholme, R., Fonville, J.M., Clench, M.R., Carolan, V.A., Francese, S. 'Direct detection of peptides and small proteins in fingermarks and determination of sex by MALDI mass spectrometry profiling', Analyst, vol 137, (2012), p 4686–4692.

Fierer, N., Hamady, M., Lauber C.L., Knight, R., 'The influence of sex, handedness, and washing on the diversity of hand surface bacteria', Proc. Natl. Acad. Sci. U. S. A., vol 105(46), (2008), p 17994–17999.

Fierer, N., Lauber, C.L., Zhou, N., McDonald, D., Costello, E.K., Knight, R., 'Forensic identification using skin bacterial communities', Proc. Natl. Acad. Sci. U. S. A., vol 107(14), (2010), p 6477–6481.

Flad, T., Bogumil, R., Tolson, J., Schittek, B., Garbe, C., Deeg, M., Mueller, C.A., Kalbacher, H. 'Detection of dermcidin-derived peptides in sweat by ProteinChip technology', J. Immunol. Methods, vol 270, (2002), p 53–62.

Francese, S., Bradshaw, R., Ferguson, L.S., Wolstenholme, R., Clench, M.R., Bleay, S. 'Beyond the ridge pattern: multi-informative analysis of latent fingermarks by MALDI mass spectrometry', Analyst, vol 138, (2013), p 4215–4228.

Fritz, P., van Bronswjik, W., Lepkova, K., Lewis, S.W., Lim, K.F., Martin, D.E., Puskar, L. 'Infrared microscopy studies of the chemical composition of latent fingermark residues', Microchem. J., vol 111, (2013), p 40–46.

Gilchrist, E., Smith, N., Barron, L. (2012) 'Probing gunshot residue, sweat and latent human fingerprints with capillary-scale ion chromatography and suppressed conductivity detection', Analyst, 137, 1576–1583.

Goucher, E., Kicman, A., Smith, N., Jickells, S. 'The detection and quantification of lorazepam and its 3-O-glucuronide in fingerprint deposits by LC-MS/MS', J. Sep. Sci., vol 32, (2009), p 2266–2272.

Grant, A., Wilkinson, T.J., Holman, D.R., Martin, M.C. 'Identification of recently handled materials by analysis of latent human fingerprints using infrared spectromicroscopy', Appl. Spectrosc., 59, (2005), p 1182–1187.

Hadorn, B., Hanimann, F., Anders, P., Curtius, H.C. 'Free amino-acids in human sweat from different parts of the body', Nature, vol 215, (1967), p 416–417.

Hamilton, P.B. 'Amino-acids in hands', Nature, vol 205, (1965), p 284–285.

Hansen, D.B., Joullié, M.M. 'The development of novel ninhydrin analogues', Chem. Soc. Rev., vol 34, (2005), p 408–417.

Harper, D.R., Clare, C.M., Heaps, C.D., Brennan, J., Hussain, J., 'A bacteriological technique for the development of latent fingerprints', Forensic Sci. Int., vol 33, (1987), p 209–214.

Hazarika, P., Jickells, S.M., Russell, D.A. 'Rapid detection of drug metabolites in latent fingermarks', Analyst, vol 134, (2009), p 93–96.

Hemmila, A., McGill, J., Ritter, D. 'Fourier transform infrared reflectance spectra of latent fingerprints – a biometric gauge for the age of an individual', J. Forensic Sci., vol 53, (2008), p 369–376.

Ifa, D.R., Manicke, N.E., Dill, A.L., Cooks, G. 'Latent fingerprint chemical imaging by mass spectrometry', Science, vol 321, (2008), p 805.

Jacob, S., Jickells, S., Wolff, K., Smith, N. 'Drug testing by chemical analysis of fingerprint deposits from methadone-maintained opioid dependent patients using UPLC-MS/MS', Drug Metab. Lett., vol 2, (2008), p 245–247.

Jacobsen, E., Billings, J.K., Frantz, R.A., Kinney, C.K., Stewart, M.E., Downing, D.T. 'Age-related changes in sebaceous wax ester secretion rates in men and women', J. Investig. Dermatol., vol 85, (1985), p 483–485.

Kaplan-Sandquist, K., LeBeau, M.A., Miller, M.L. 'Chemical analysis of pharmaceuticals and explosives in fingermarks using matrix-assisted laser desorption ionization/time-of-flight mass spectrometry', Forensic Sci. Int., vol 235, (2014), p 68–77.

Khedr, A. 'The profile of free amino acids in latent fingerprint of healthy and beta-thalassemic volunteers', J. Chromatogr. B, vol 878, (2010), p 1576–1582.

Krakow, R., Downing, D.T., Strauss, J.S., Pochi, P.E. 'Identification of a fatty acid in human skin surface lipids apparently associated with acne vulgaris', J. Investig. Dermatol., vol 61, (1973), p 286–289.

Kuno, Y. 'Human Perspiration', Charles C. Thomas, Springfield, IL; Blackwell Scientific Publications, Oxford, (1956).

Ladd, C., Adamowicz, M.S., Bourke, M.T., Scherczinger, C.A., Lee, H.C. 'A systematic analysis of secondary DNA transfer', J. Forensic Sci., vol 44, (1999), p 1270–1272.

Leggett, R., Lee-Smith, E.E., Jickells, S.M., Russell, D.A. '"Intelligent" fingerprints: simultaneous identification of drug metabolites and individuals by using antibody-functionalized nanoparticles', Angew. Chem. Int. Ed., vol 46, (2007), p 4100–4103.

Liappis, N., Hungerland, H. 'The trace amino acid pattern in human eccrine sweat', Clin. Chim. Acta, vol 48, (1973), p 233–236.

Liden, C., Carter, S. 'Nickel release from coins', Contact Dermatitis, vol 44, (2001), p 160–165.

Lim, A.Y., Ma, Z., Ma, J., Rowell, F. 'Separation of fingerprint constituents using magnetic silica nanoparticles and direct on-particle SALDI-TOF-mass spectrometry', J. Chromatogr. B, vol 879, (2011), p 2244–2250.

Love, C., Gilchrist, E., Smith, N., Barron, L. 'Detection of anionic energetic material residues in enhanced fingermarks on porous and non-porous surfaces using ion chromatography', Forensic Sci. Int., vol 231, (2013), p 150–156.

Lowe, A., Murray, C., Whitaker, J., Tully, G., Gill, P. 'The propensity of individuals to deposit DNA and secondary transfer of low level DNA from individuals to inert surfaces', Forensic Sci. Int., vol 129, (2002), p 25–34.

Marples, M.J. 'Life on the human skin', Sci. Am., vol 220, (1969), p 108–111.

Mong, G., Petersen, C.E., Clauss, T.R.W. *Advanced Fingerprint Analysis Project. Final Report – Fingerprint Constituents*, Pacific Northwest National Laboratory Report 13019. (1999).

Mountfort, K.M., Bronstein, H., Archer, N., Jickells, S.M. 'Identification of oxidation products of squalene in solution and in latent fingerprints by ESI-MS and LC/ACPI-MS', Anal. Chem., vol 79, (2007), p 2650–2657.

Murakami, M., Ohtake, T., Dorschner, R.A., Schittek, B., Garbe, C., Gallo, R.L. 'Cathelicidin anti-microbial peptide expression in sweat, an innate defense system for the skin', J. Investig. Dermatol., vol 119, (2002), p 1090–1095.

Nakayashiki, N. 'Sweat protein components tested by SDS-polyacrylamide gel electrophoresis followed by immunoblotting', Tohoku J. Exp. Med., vol 161, (1990), p 25–31.

Nazzaro-Porro, M., Passi, S., Boniforti, L., Belsito, F. 'Effects of aging on fatty acids on skin surface lipids', J. Investig. Dermatol., vol 73, (1979), p 112–117.

Nicolaides, N. 'Skin lipids: their biochemical uniqueness', Science, vol 186, (1974), p 19–26.

Nikkari, T. 'Comparative chemistry of sebum', J. Investig. Dermatol., vol 62, (1974), p 257–267.

Noble, W.C., 'Microbiology of Human Skin', Lloyd-Luke Ltd., London, (1981).

O'Neill M.E., 'Bacterial fingerprints', J. Crim. Law Criminol. Police Sci., vol 32, (1941), p 482.

Oleiwi, A., Schmerer, W.M., Morris, M.R., Sutton, R. 'The relative DNA-shedding propensity of palmar and fingerprint surfaces', Sci. Justice, vol 55, (2015), p 329–334.

Olsen, R.D. 'The chemical composition of palmar sweat', Fingerprint Identif. Mag., vol 53, (1972), p 3–16.

O'Neal Page, C., Remington, J.S. 'Immunologic studies in normal human sweat', J. Lab. Clin. Med., vol 69, (1967), p 634–650.

van Oorschot, R.A.H., Treadwell, S., Beaurepaire, J., Holding, N.L., Mitchell, R.J. 'Beware of the possibility of fingerprints techniques transferring DNA', J. Forensic Sci., vol 50, (2005), p 1417–1422.

Oro, J., Skewes, H.B. 'Free amino-acids on human fingers the question of contamination in microanalysis', Nature, vol 207, (1965), p 1042–1045.

Perry, D.L., Wilkinson, T.J., Martin, M.C., McKinney, W.R. *Application of Synchrotron Infrared Microspectroscopy to the Study of Fingerprints*, Ernest Orlando Lawrence Berkeley National Laboratory, Berkeley, (2004).

Ramotowski, R.S. 'Composition of Latent Print Residue', In 'Advances in Fingerprint Technology', 2nd edition, (Eds, Lee, H.C., Gaensslen, R.E.) CRC Press, Boca Raton, FL, chapter 3, (2001).

Ricci, C., Kazarian, S.G. 'Collection and detection of latent fingermarks contaminated with cosmetics on nonporous and porous surfaces', Surf. Interface Anal., vol 42, (2009), p 386–392.

Ricci, C., Chan, K.L.A., Kazarian, S.G. 'Combining the tape-lift method and fourier transform infrared spectroscopic imaging for forensic applications', Appl. Spectrosc., 60, (2006), p 1013–1021.

Ricci, C., Phiriyavityopas, P., Curum, N., Chan, K.L.A., Jickells, S., Kazarian, S.G. 'Chemical imaging of latent fingerprint residues', Appl. Spectrosc., vol 61, (2007a), p 514–522.

Ricci, C., Bleay, S., Kazarian, S.G. 'Spectroscopic imaging of latent fingermarks collected with the aid of a gelatine tape', Anal. Chem., vol 79, (2007b), p 5771–5776.

Robertshaw, D. 'Apocrine Sweat Glands', In 'Physiology, Biochemistry, and Molecular Biology of the Skin', (Ed., Goldsmith, L.A.), Oxford University Press, New York, chapter 27, p 763–775, (1991).

Rothman, S. 'Physiology and Biochemistry of the Skin', University of Chicago Press, Chicago, IL, (1954).

Rowell, F., Hudson, K., Seviour, J., 'Detection of drugs and their metabolites in dusted latent fingermarks by mass spectrometry', Analyst, vol 134, (2009), p 701–707.

Rowell, F., Seviour, J., Lim, A.Y., Elumbaring-Salazar, C.G., Loke, J., Ma, J. 'Detection of nitro-organic and peroxide explosives in latent fingermarks by DART- and SALDI-TOF- mass spectrometry', Forensic Sci. Int., vol 221, (2012), p 84–91.

Saga, K. 'Structure and function of human sweat glands studied with histochemistry and cytochemistry', Prog. Histochem. Cytochem., vol 37, (2002), p 323–386.

Schulz, M.M., Reichert, W. 'Archived or directly swabbed latent fingerprints as a DNA source for STR typing', Forensic Sci. Int., vol 127, (2002), p 128–130.

Schulz, M.M., Wehner, H.-D., Reichert, W., Graw, M. 'Ninhydrin-dyed latent fingerprints as a DNA source in a murder case', J. Clin. Forensic Med., vol 11, (2004), p 202–204.

Scruton, B., Blott, B.H. *Surface Potential of Finger Prints on Paper and Fabrics*, Physics Department, University of Southampton, Report for PSDB, 18 June, (1973).

Scruton, B., Robins, B.W., Blott, B.H. 'The deposition of fingerprint films', J. Phys. D Appl. Phys., vol 8, (1975), p 714–723.

Song, W., Mao, Z., Liu, X., Lu, Y., Li, Z., Zhao, B., Lu, L. 'Detection of protein deposition within latent fingerprints by surface-enhanced Raman spectroscopy imaging', Nanoscale, vol 4, (2012), p 2333–2338.

Strauss, J.S., Downing, D.T., Ebling, F.J., Stewart, M.E. In 'Physiology, Biochemistry, and Molecular Biology of the Skin', (Ed., Goldsmith, L.A.), Oxford University Press, New York, p 712–740, (1991).

Sundar, L., Rowell, F. 'Detection of drugs in lifted cyanoacrylate-developed latent fingermarks using two laser desorption/ionisation mass spectrometric methods', Analyst, vol 139, (2014), p 633–642.

Szynkowska, M.I., Czerski, K., Rogowski, J., Paryjczak, T., Parczewski, A. 'ToF-SIMS application in the visualization and analysis of fingerprints after contact with amphetamine drugs', Forensic Sci. Int., vol 184, (2009), e24–e26.

Szynkowska, M.I., Czerski, K., Rogowski, J., Paryjczak, T., Parczewski, A. 'Detection of exogenous contaminants of fingerprints using ToF-SIMS', Surf. Interface Anal., vol 42, (2010), p 393–397.

Tahtouh, M., Kalman, J.R., Roux, C., Lennard, C., Reedy, B.J. 'The detection and enhancement of latent fingermarks using infrared chemical imaging', J. Forensic Sci., vol 50, (2005), p 64–72.

Tahtouh, M., Despland, P., Shimmon, R., Kalman, J.R., Reedy, B. 'The application of infrared chemical imaging to the detection and enhancement of latent fingerprints: method optimization and further findings', J. Forensic Sci., vol 52, (2007), p 1089–1096.

Thomas, G.L. 'Physical Methods Applied to Fingerprint Problems', In Proceedings of the Conference on the Science of Fingerprints, 24–25 September 1974, PSDB, Home Office, London, UK, p 155–173, (1974).

Thomas, G.L. 'The resistivity of fingerprint material', J. Forensic Sci. Soc., vol 15, (1975), p 133–135.

Thomas, G.L. 'The physics of fingerprints and their detection', J. Phys. E Sci. Instrum., vol 11, (1978), p 722–731.

Thomas, G.L., Reynoldson, T.E. 'Some observations on fingerprint deposits', J. Phys. D Appl. Phys., vol 8, (1975a), p 724–729.

Thomas, G.L., Reynoldson, T.E. *A Quantitative Study of Fingerprint Deposits Using Interference Microscopy*, Home Office PSDB Tech. Memo. 02/75, 1975b.

Tripathi, A., Emmons, E.D., Wilcox, P.G., Guicheteau, J.A., Emge, D.K., Christesen, S.D., Fountain, III, A.W. 'Semi-automated detection of trace explosives in fingerprints on strongly interfering surfaces with Raman chemical imaging', Appl. Spectrosc., vol 65, (2011), p 611–619.

Van Oorschot, R.A.H., Jones, M.K. 'DNA fingerprints from fingerprints', Nature, vol 387, (1997), p 767.

West, M.J., Went, M.J. 'The spectroscopic detection of exogenous material in fingerprints after development with powders and recovery with adhesive lifters', Forensic Sci. Int., vol 174, (2008), p 1–5.

West, M.J., Went, M.J. 'The spectroscopic detection of drugs of abuse in fingerprints after development with powders and recovery with adhesive lifters', Spectrochim. Acta A Mol. Biomol. Spectrosc., vol 71, (2009), p 1984–1988.

Weyermann, C., Roux, C., Champod, C. 'Initial results on the composition of fingerprints and its evolution as a function of time by GC/MS analysis', J. Forensic Sci., vol 56, (2011), p 102–108.

Williams, D.K., Brown, C.J., Bruker, J. 'Characterization of children's latent fingerprint residues by infrared microspectroscopy: forensic implications', Forensic Sci. Int., vol 206, (2011), p 161–165.

Wolstenholme, R., Bradshaw, R., Clench, M.R., Francese, S. 'Study of latent fingermarks by matrix-assisted laser desorption/ionisation mass spectrometry imaging of endogenous lipids', Rapid Commun. Mass Spectrom., vol 23, (2009), p 3031–3039.

Worley, C.G., Wiltshire, S.S., Miller, T.C., Havrilla, G.J., Majidi, V. 'Detection of visible and latent fingerprints using micro-x-ray fluorescence elemental imaging', J. Forensic Sci., vol 51, (2006), p 57–63.

Zouboulis, C.C. 'Acne and sebaceous gland function', Clin. Dermatol., vol 22, (2004), p 360–366.

4

Ageing of fingermarks

Stephen M. Bleay[1] and Marcel de Puit[2]
[1] Home Office Centre for Applied Science and Technology, Sandridge, UK
[2] Ministerie van Veiligheid en Justitie, Nederlands Forensisch Instituut, Digitale Technologie en Biometrie, The Hague, The Netherlands

---

Key points

- What happens to a fingermark after its formation is determined by a 'triangle of interaction' influenced by the composition/properties of the fingermark, the surface it has been deposited on and the environment they are exposed to.

- The nature of these interactions and the time over which they occur determine whether a viable fingermark remains for enhancement.

- Obtaining information about the fingermark, the surface, the environment and the timescales since deposition is an important stage in selecting the most appropriate enhancement process.

- Several methods for dating fingermarks have been researched, although none are yet considered sufficiently reliable for operational use.

4.1 The 'triangle of interaction'

Once a fingermark has been formed on a surface as described in Chapter 2, another set of interactions may begin to occur. Whereas the nature of the initial interaction between the finger and surface determines the area of contact and the type of mark that is formed, the interactions that occur in the subsequent ageing interval determine whether the mark continues to be present and viable for enhancement. They also influence which fingermark enhancement processes are likely to be most effective.

Fingerprint Development Techniques: Theory and Application, First Edition.
Stephen M. Bleay, Ruth S. Croxton and Marcel de Puit.

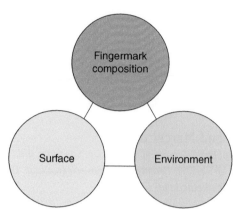

Figure 4.1 A schematic representation of the concept of the 'triangle of interaction'.

The events occurring in this time interval can be described in terms of the concept of the 'triangle of interaction' (Figure 4.1).

The three elements of the 'triangle of interaction' are the composition of the *fingermark*, the nature of the *surface* the mark has been deposited on and the *environment* the surface and the mark are exposed to after deposition. The length of time between deposition and initial examination is also of importance, as it may influence the extent to which a particular interaction occurs. This chapter will describe the factors associated with each of these three elements, both individually and in combination, that are of importance during the ageing process.

4.2 The fingermark

In the case of negative marks and impressions, little or no material is actually transferred to the surface, and therefore it is the interaction between the surface and the environment that will determine whether the impression of the ridges survives until initial examination.

During formation of positive marks, whether 'latent' or 'patent' in nature, material from the finger is transferred to the surface. The composition and properties of this material will influence how it interacts with its surroundings and whether it will still be available for enhancement after the ageing interval. The chemical composition and physical and biological properties of fingermarks have already been described in detail in Chapter 3. The remainder of this chapter will expand upon the ways in which the surface and the environment play a role in determining what happens to the fingermark after deposition and also how this subsequently influences which process(es) is likely to be most effective in enhancing it.

4.3 The surface

During the ageing process, the term 'surface' could be more accurately substituted by 'substrate', because for porous and semi-porous materials, the fingermark will also interact with the bulk material as well as the surface. However, for simplicity the term 'surface' will be used throughout.

The properties of the surface are important both during the initial physical contact with the finger as described in Chapter 2 and also in determining what happens to the fingermark once it has been transferred onto the surface. The surface properties of most importance during the subsequent interactions with the fingermark and environment are

- Surface porosity

- Surface chemistry

Surface porosity (or more accurately a combination of porosity and related properties such as its wettability) determines whether the fingermark will remain upon the surface after deposition or whether it can migrate into it to any extent. For non-porous surfaces, the fingermark deposit cannot penetrate the surface and remains on top of it. The situation for porous surfaces is different. For these materials it is not just the substances present at the surface that interact with the fingermark residues; any additives present in the bulk of the material can also influence what happens to the residues during ageing and subsequent enhancement.

The other important attribute of the surface is the surface chemistry. In this context, 'surface chemistry' is a very general term that covers many properties of the surface. Some examples of chemical properties that could have an influence on what interactions can occur when residues are deposited on the surface include

- Affinity of surface species for water (hydrophobic or hydrophilic)

- How chemically inert the surface is

- Degree of difference between the chemical species at the surface and those in the fingermark

The properties earlier influence how the fingermark spreads (e.g. whether it forms droplets or not), whether any chemical reactions begin to occur at the surface/fingermark interface and whether the chemical differences between the ridge detail in the mark and the surface are sufficient for them to be exploited during a subsequent enhancement process.

There is a huge variety in the type of surface that fingermarks may be deposited on, and it is not possible to provide descriptions of all of them. However, a short summary of some of the representative types of material that may be encountered is given later.

4.3.1 Metals

Metals are non-porous in nature but differ from most other non-porous surfaces in that they may be more chemically active and the presence of fingermarks may initiate corrosion processes on them. There can be significant chemical differences between metal types (Fontana, 1987). Metals such as gold and platinum are chemically inert and usually remain bright and resistant to corrosion. Other metals and alloys including nickel, aluminium, chromium, tin, titanium and stainless steels have thin, coherent oxide layers present on the surface and have reasonable corrosion resistance. Another category of metals including copper, zinc and their alloy brass will progressively lose their brightness under normal atmospheric conditions and are more susceptible to corrosion. Lead oxidises to form thicker but stable layers that can include insoluble lead compounds such as carbonates. In the case of iron, corrosion can readily occur because the oxide formed (rust) is not protective. The metals described earlier may also be treated with processes such as anodising, which may give the surface layer very different characteristics from the metal beneath it.

4.3.2   Glasses and ceramics

Glasses are non-porous surfaces. Most commonly encountered types of glass are silica-based (Wyatt and Dew-Hughes, 1974), but can differ slightly in terms of the elemental additions incorporated to give the desired properties (e.g. sodium to reduce the melt viscosity of the soda glass used for windows, boron and aluminium to increase chemical and heat resistance in borosilicate kitchenware). Continued exposure to water may leach some alkali species from the surface of some types of glass, and some salts in fingermarks may locally modify the glass composition under certain conditions of environmental exposure.

Decorative ceramics such as those found in pottery and wall/floor tiles are generally made from fired clay, which describes a group of minerals with a layered silicate structure that form a plastic substance when mixed with water and can be readily worked into complex shapes (Wyatt and Dew-Hughes, 1974). Such ceramics are typically coated with silica-based glazes to make them non-porous, but these glazes will also contain a variety of other metal ions for pigmentation and other purposes. Glazes may also contain some degree of microscopic porosity and the surface may not be truly non-porous. Some ceramics may be left unglazed (e.g. terracotta) (Figure 4.2), and these will behave more like porous surfaces.

4.3.3   Polymers

Polymers consist of multiple base monomer units that become linked together into long chains by polymerisation reactions (Young, 1981). Cross-links may also be formed between individual polymer chains. There are two fundamental types of polymer: thermoplastics, which become 'plastic' or easily formable when raised above a melting temperature and then return to a solid state on cooling below it, and thermosets, which can be formed to shape in a liquid form but are then cured to produce a rigid solid that can no longer melt but instead chars and burns when exposed to high temperature.

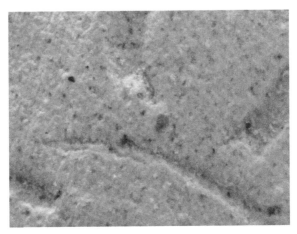

Figure 4.2   Microstructure of an unglazed terracotta surface, ~×250.

Many different types of polymer may be encountered. Polymers may be encountered in a rigid form, for example, the engineering polymers used to form structures such as refuse bins and chairs, as surface layers in laminated structures, or as thin films used for packaging. Rubber can also be considered as a special type of polymeric material. Many of these materials are increasingly being marked with recycling symbols making identification of the basic polymer type easier. Most polymers used in rigid structures (e.g. ABS, polypropylene) are essentially non-porous and inert, although they may retain thin surface layers of mould release agent, for example, where parts are formed to shape. Some of these rigid polymers are less inert; for example, nylon can absorb water and unplasticised PVC may sometimes behave more like a semi-porous surface. The rigid polymers selected for use as the surface layer of laminates (e.g. melamine) can be considered as non-porous and inert.

The most variability in behaviour is experienced with thin polymeric packaging materials, where even different types of the same basic polymer can give very different properties. Polyethylene is a good example of this, with high density polyethylene (HDPE) being found in thin, 'crinkly' plastic bags, low density polyethylene (LDPE) being used for thicker 'waxy' plastic bags and heavily plasticised polyethylene being used as cling film. For all polymers it is necessary to focus on the composition of the surface layer rather than the bulk material, because it is these surface layers that the fingermarks interact with. For example, plastic bags contain additives such as plasticisers and release agents that may migrate to the surface layers (Brydson, 1999), making the surface composition very different from the bulk. In some cases the presence of these additives may inhibit the performance of some fingermark enhancement processes.

Polymers may also be encountered in expanded form, such as the expanded polystyrene foam used for packing. The individual polystyrene beads are effectively non-porous, but the interfaces between the compressed beads may allow the ingress of some liquids into the bulk of the material (Figure 4.3).

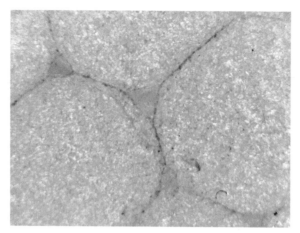

Figure 4.3   The microstructure of expanded polystyrene, showing gaps between the compressed beads that may allow liquid to penetrate, ~×250.

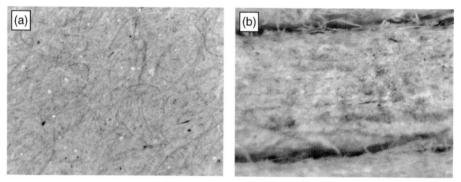

Figure 4.4   The microstructure of cardboard: (a) normal to surface showing random distribution of fibres, (b) cross section showing the porous, layered structure, ~×250.

4.3.4   Paper

The general term 'paper' describes a wide range of materials including the high grade, long-lived material used for currency to low grade recycled newspaper and fine tissue paper. Such materials are produced from fibre pulp mixed with water, which is compressed and dried to form flexible sheets. Cardboard (Figure 4.4) is essentially a thicker, heavy-duty type of paper made using a similar manufacturing process.

Most paper is based on cellulose fibres, although currency paper may contain high contents of other fibres such as cotton, and there are also entirely polymeric 'papers' produced from polymer fibres. Paper also contains additives, for example, calcium carbonate (chalk), which may be added as a bulking filler and also as a whitening agent (Roberts, 1996). The potential presence of such additives should be taken into account when considering enhancement processes. Other additives such as colouring pigments and optical brighteners may also be present. The fundamental paper composition and the additives incorporated into it can vary significantly around the world, it being known that in some countries paper can be acidic and in other countries alkaline. This may affect the way in which enhancement processes work, particularly when pH of the solution is important to the reaction mechanisms that may occur. Various types of coating may be applied to papers to seal them and reduce porosity, or printing may be applied, which can again locally modify the properties.

4.3.5   Wood

Wood and wood-based products such as chipboard and fibreboard also behave as porous surfaces when they are unvarnished. The main materials present are the cellulose and lignin forming the wood structure (Wyatt and Dew-Hughes, 1974), and highly directional porosity is present in the form of structures called vessels, which transport water when part of the living tree (Figure 4.5).

For natural wood, there are variations in the level of porosity according to the type of wood. Soft woods (e.g. pine) are highly porous, whereas harder woods (e.g. mahogany) are significantly less so, and this affects the way in which the fingermark residues are absorbed. Other substances such as wood preservatives and binders (for chipboard) may be present, and these can interact with fingermark enhancement reagents.

4.3.6   Paints

The matt emulsion paints commonly used for interior walls are mostly porous in nature. Modern emulsion paints are predominantly water based and when dry the material consists of polymeric binders and pigments such as titanium dioxide. Gloss

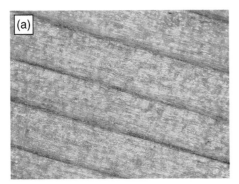 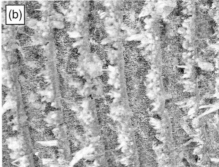

Figure 4.5   The microstructure of wood: (a) normal to surface showing directional fibres, (b) cross section showing the porosity associated with the vessels, ~×250.

paints use a varnish medium as the carrier for the pigments and when dry present an essentially non-porous surface.

4.3.7 Fabrics

Fabrics are a complex surface, and there are few enhancement processes that are capable of reliably developing fingermarks on them. On a macroscopic level, fabrics are porous, with the fibre diameter and weave type affecting the macroscopic porosity level (Figure 4.6).

The fibre type also influences the porosity on a microscopic level, with natural fibres such as cotton and wool being porous and irregular in profile and synthetic fibres such as nylon and polyester being non-porous and having more regular cross sections. Fibres also incorporate dyes and may be treated with substances to make them waterproof or stain resistant. All of these may affect the way in which the surface interacts with the fingermark.

4.3.8 Leather

Leather is produced from a range of different types of animal hide by a process known as tanning, giving a flexible material that is resistant to decomposition (Figure 4.7).

Leather in its natural state is porous and it may be expected that fingermark residues would be absorbed into it. In practice there are many different dyes and surface finishes that can be applied to leather, and the finished product can vary from patent leather (which is hard, smooth and behaves as a non-porous material) to suede (soft, rough and porous in nature). This variability means that each leather article must be treated on the basis of its individual surface characteristics.

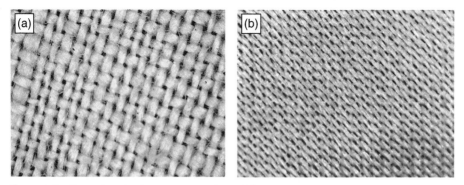

Figure 4.6 Examples of microstructures of two different types of fabric: (a) a section of a linen shirt, (b) a satin weave garment made of polyester fibres, ~×250.

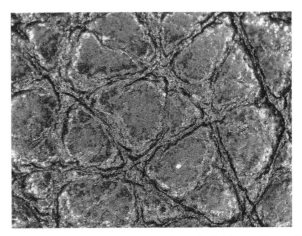

Figure 4.7 Microstructure of the surface of a leather wallet, ~×250.

It may sometimes be difficult to distinguish real leather from simulated leather from an initial examination. Simulated leather is made from plasticised vinyl polymer and is effectively a non-porous surface.

4.3.9 Adhesive surfaces

A range of materials may be encountered that have adhesive surfaces, such as adhesive tapes. Such materials consist of a thin layer of pressure-sensitive adhesive applied to a backing material, which can be paper, polymeric or metal foil. Pressure-sensitive adhesives form a bond between the surface and the backing material upon application of light pressure. The composition of the adhesive can be modified to vary the adhesive properties, from easily removable systems used for materials such as masking tapes and 'post-it' notes to more highly adhesive, permanent systems used for duct tape. The composition of the pressure-sensitive adhesives falls into one of three general categories, rubber based, acrylic based or mixed character. The chemical composition of the adhesive that is present can have a significant influence on the effectiveness of some enhancement processes.

4.3.10 Skin

Reference must also be made to human skin as a surface for fingermark deposition. Through all the history of research into fingerprints, efforts have been made to identify a process that will reliably enhance marks on the skin. Although there are some processes that can enhance marks on the skin, and there are documented cases of the successful application of these processes (Sampson et al., 1997), the nature of the surface itself makes development of fingermarks very unlikely. The fact that living skin continues to secrete sweat means that the survival of fingermark residues from the donor will be short-lived and that it will be difficult to distinguish the deposited mark from the secretions from the skin. Sweat secretion will also continue for several minutes after death. Skin is also highly flexible, and the level of deformation that can occur during contact makes deposition of an identifiable fingermark less likely. The presence of body hair will also disrupt fingermark deposition, and therefore chances of recovery are best on smooth, hairless regions of the body.

4.4 The environment

Once the fingermark has been transferred from the finger onto the surface, the environment that the fingermark and the surface are simultaneously exposed to prior to enhancement becomes important. The 'normal' outdoor environment will include exposure to air at different temperatures, different velocities, different humidity levels (including precipitation as rain), airborne particulates and gaseous products and also exposure to sunlight (Figure 4.8).

The indoor environment is generally more protected and controlled, but there is still the potential for surfaces and fingermarks to be exposed to a range of different environmental conditions.

Each aspect of the 'normal' environment can be considered in more detail.

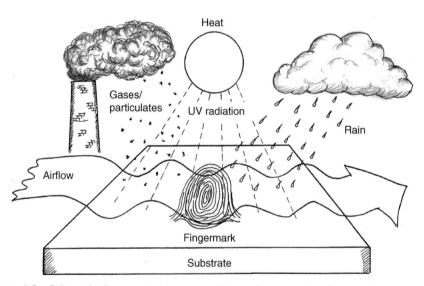

Figure 4.8   Schematic diagram showing some of the environments that fingermarks and substrates may be exposed to.

4.4.1 Temperature

In the United Kingdom, the range of outdoor temperatures experienced is not as extreme as many other parts of the world, with an all-time minimum of −27.2°C and a maximum of 38.5°C. In general temperatures are well within these limits, with average minimum and maximum air temperatures over the year being in the range 1–22°C. However, outside surface temperatures may reach much higher levels, for example, dark surfaces that absorb significant amounts of energy may reach temperatures in excess of 60°C on hot, sunny days. Indoor temperatures are theoretically less variable because of control systems such as central heating and air conditioning but can sometimes reach higher values than outdoor temperatures on the same day, for example, when sunlight passes into buildings with large areas of glass present.

In other parts of the world where more extreme climatic conditions are experienced, both the maximum and minimum temperatures can significantly exceed those experienced in the United Kingdom.

4.4.2 Wind

In outdoor environments wind causes the movement of air across the surface. This motion of air can have a drying effect, but moving air can also act as a carrier for other solid particulates or liquid droplets. Indoor environments are again more controlled, but fans and air conditioning units can result in surfaces being exposed to relatively high velocities of air flow across them.

4.4.3 Humidity

The relative humidity of air can influence interactions subsequent to fingermark deposition. Relative humidity is related to the amount of water vapour present in the air, which is strongly influenced by the air temperature and pressure. Reducing the temperature of air reduces the amount of water that can be accommodated as water vapour, and therefore when warm air of high relative humidity comes into contact with a cold surface, water may condense from the air and water droplets form as a 'dew' on the surface. The relative humidity of the surrounding air may also determine how quickly any water in the fingermark (and/or the surface) evaporates. The relative humidity experienced can again vary significantly around the world and even in different locations within the same country.

Water condensed from the air in the atmosphere can precipitate and fall as rain, which may have a more profound effect on both the fingermark and surface when it impinges upon them. Although rain will only be encountered in outdoor environments, there are also indoor environments where exposure to water droplets can occur, including locations with running water such as bathrooms and kitchens.

4.4.4   Airborne substances

In addition to water vapour, air can contain many other substances in solid, liquid and gaseous form, which can interact with both surfaces and fingermarks. In indoor environments, air can carry dust particles that include shed skin cells, fragments of hair and fibres from textiles and paper products. In outdoor environments, dust composition can differ and the solid particulates present include pollen and fine mineral particles from various sources including eroded sand and soil, volcanic eruptions and industrial pollutants such as soot. All of these particulates may settle from the air onto the surface and the fingermark.

Water is the principal liquid substance that is borne by the air, but other liquids such as oil droplets and the 'honeydew' that drips from lime trees may be carried and redeposited depending on the particular local environment.

Gaseous substances that may be found in various concentrations in the air include a range of gases produced by industrial processes, including carbon dioxide, carbon monoxide, sulphur dioxide, nitrous oxides and other volatile organic compounds. These gases may be preferentially adsorbed into either the fingermark or the surface.

4.4.5   Sunlight

Sunlight consists of electromagnetic radiation that is output over a wide range of wavelengths. In addition to visible radiation, sunlight contains a significant amount of ultraviolet radiation, although in practice short-wavelength UVC radiation is blocked by the atmosphere and it is only the longer wavelength UVB and UVA radiation that reaches ground level. Window glass further filters shorter wavelengths of ultraviolet radiation, and exposure to ultraviolet radiation in indoor environments is significantly less. Sunlight also contains wavelengths of infrared radiation extending beyond 2000 nm, and this can have a considerable heating effect on surfaces that absorb these wavelengths strongly.

Some possible effects of these commonly encountered environmental conditions are outlined in the section on interactions later. The environment experienced by the fingermark and the surface will actually be a combination of the conditions described earlier, for example, high temperature and high relative humidity, in combination with bright sunlight.

In addition to the 'normal' environments previously described, other more extreme environments may be encountered. These may include

- Exposure to potentially more aggressive liquids (e.g. acids, alkalis, fuels, cleaning solvents)

- Exposure to solid contaminants (e.g. mud, drugs, soot)

- Exposure to extremes of temperature (e.g. fires, extreme cold)

- Exposure to chemical and biological agents or decontaminants

- Exposure to ionising radiation

It is not proposed to cover the interactions of such environments in this book, because a detailed summary has been provided elsewhere (Ramotowski, 2013).

4.5 Interactions

It is the interactions that occur post-deposition that determine whether the fingermark (and the surface it has been deposited on) can survive the environments they are exposed to during the ageing interval. It may be the case that although some constituents of both fingermark and surface may survive the environmental exposure, others will not and it is therefore necessary to understand what may still be available for enhancement when selecting a process.

Those that need to be considered during the ageing interval are those defined by the triangle of interaction, namely,

- Interactions that could occur between the fingermark and the surface

- Interactions that could occur between the fingermark and the environment

- Interactions that could occur between the surface and the environment

- Interactions that could occur when the surface, fingermark and environment are present in combination

4.5.1 Interactions between fingermarks and the surface

As has been discussed previously, the interaction between the fingermark and the surface is strongly influenced by surface porosity, surface chemistry and fingermark composition.

For most surfaces that are considered 'non-porous', the fingermark spreads across the surface in a manner determined by factors including the wettability of the surface and the pressure of application, but does not penetrate into it. The physical profile of the mark gradually shrinks as it dries out, and the water content is lost (Champod et al., 2004) (Figure 4.9). Features such as trapped skin cells and salt crystals may become more prominent as the water is lost (Figure 4.10). There may also be compositional changes in the fingermark, as discussed in the section on interactions between the fingermark and the environment.

A different scenario occurs on 'porous' surfaces (e.g. paper). In this case the fingermark wets the surface and most constituents are absorbed into it. A small proportion of the insoluble constituents may remain on the surface, but the water in the residues carries the water-soluble constituents into the interior of the material

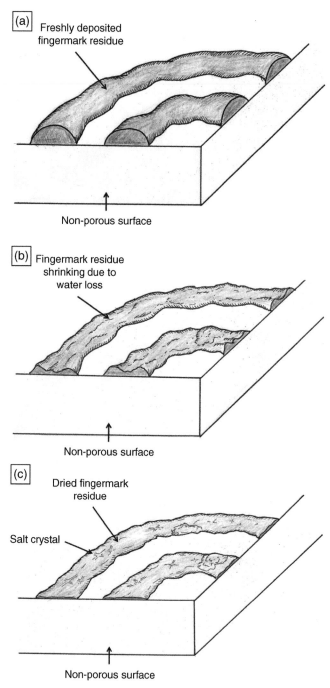

Figure 4.9 Schematic diagrams showing the changes in a fingermark deposited on a non-porous surface at different times after deposition: (a) immediately after deposition, (b) days after deposition and (c) weeks after deposition. Adapted from Champod et al. (2004) and Thomas and Reynoldson (1975).

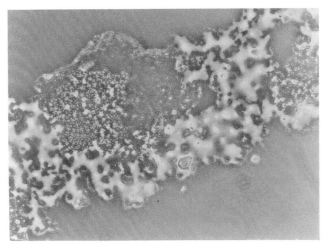

Figure 4.10   A high magnification interference micrograph of salt crystals (small cross-shaped features) formed within a fingermark ridge on drying. Reproduced courtesy of the Home Office.

where they continue to migrate at different rates (Champod et al., 2004) (Figure 4.11). Amino acids can become closely bound to the cellulose present in papers and generally do not migrate far from the original location of the fingertip contact. The depth of penetration of the fingermark into the paper (Figure 4.12) is determined by the smoothness of the paper (Almog et al., 2004); other properties such as porosity are also important. Other constituents such as urea and chlorides may subsequently migrate further (especially under conditions of high humidity), and consequently older fingermarks or fingermarks exposed to high humidity and subsequently developed by processes targeting these constituents may appear diffuse to the extent of being unidentifiable (Figure 4.13).

Intermediate between these two types, there are 'semi-porous' surfaces that exhibit mixed behaviour, where there is only limited wetting of the surface. On such surfaces there is generally some fingermark residue remaining on the surface and a limited amount that diffuses into it. A decision will therefore need to be made regarding whether the surface is likely to be more receptive to treatments specific to porous or non-porous surfaces. There are also surfaces where porous and non-porous regions exist in close proximity, and selection of a single development process is made complicated. An example of this situation can be found on certain printed papers where the printing inks may create non-porous regions on an essentially porous surface. If it is not possible to identify a single treatment for such mixed nature surfaces, selective masking may be carried out to protect areas from the effects of incompatible reagents.

The situations described earlier are cases where the surface is essentially inert, and there is little or no chemical reaction between the fingermark residue and the surface. Certain types of metal surface are capable of chemically reacting with the chemical constituents in the fingermark residues (Bond, 2008). This may result in

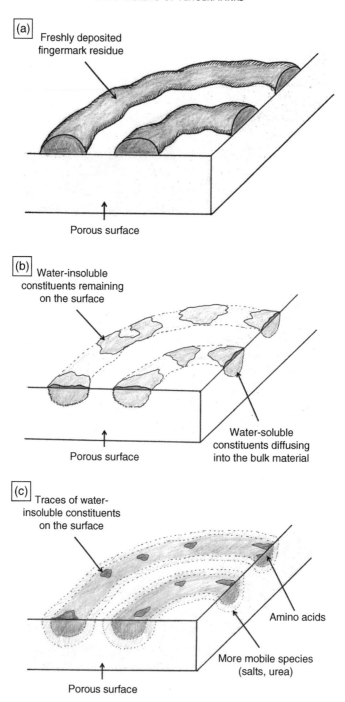

Figure 4.11 Schematic diagrams showing the changes in a fingermark deposited on a porous surface at different times after deposition: (a) immediately after deposition, (b) hours after deposition and (c) weeks after deposition. Adapted from Champod et al. (2004).

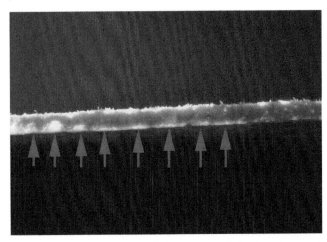

Figure 4.12 A micrograph of a cross section through a mark developed on card using 1,2-in-dandione, showing the depth of penetration of the amino acids into the card (positions of ridges shown by arrows).

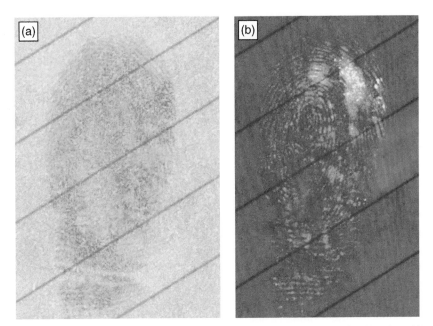

Figure 4.13 A fingermark on lined notebook paper enhanced using DMAC: (a) under white light, showing the distribution of the magenta reaction product formed with urea and (b) under fluorescence examination, showing the distribution of the fluorescent reaction product formed with amino acids. The urea has migrated to a greater extent and therefore the enhanced mark targeting this constituent is more diffused. Reproduced courtesy of the Home Office.

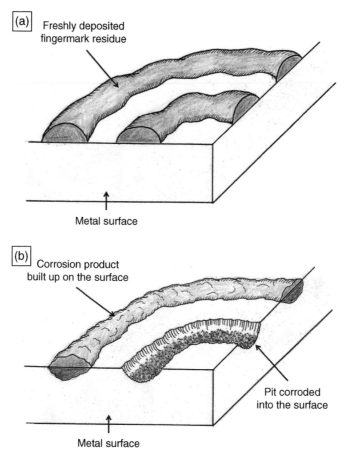

Figure 4.14 Schematic diagrams showing the changes in a fingermark deposited on a metal surface at different times after deposition: (a) immediately after deposition and (b) weeks after deposition.

either pits being etched into the surface or corrosion products building up on the surface (Figures 4.14 and 4.15).

In addition to individual chemical constituents in the mark that may react with the metal surface, the acidity or alkalinity of the environment provided by the finger-mark residue may influence how corrosion progresses. Kuno (1956) summarises studies of the pH of sweat and noted that in general pH is in the range 5.10–7.26 for palmar sweat, although values as high as 7.80 have been observed. For some subjects sweat becomes more acidic as sweating progresses, whereas for some other subjects sweat becomes progressively more alkaline. Eccrine sweat generally has lower pH than that from the apocrine glands.

The corrosion effect caused by the fingermark on the surface may be undetecta-ble by the eye and only revealed using specialist techniques. Such corrosion 'signa-tures' left on the surface may be of importance, as they can be used to reveal

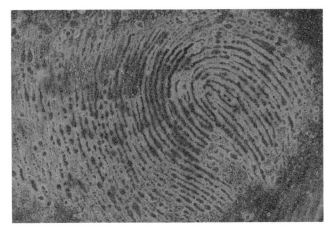

Figure 4.15 A fingermark revealed by the corrosion products formed between the constituents of the fingermark and a molybdenum metal foil sheet.

fingermarks in situations where none of the original fingermark residues remains, for example, where it has been removed by washing, heating or rubbing.

4.5.2 Interactions between fingermarks and the environment

It is principally the reactions that occur between the fingermark and the environment during the ageing period that determine whether the fingermark remains viable for enhancement at the time of initial examination. Because fingermarks may contain a wide range of chemical constituents, each constituent may be affected in different ways when exposed to different types of environment. This is equally true of the physical properties associated with the fingermark residues. Some of the interactions that may arise under different environmental conditions are described in the following text.

4.5.2.1 Heat

The thermal environment experienced by the fingermark may result in changes to the constituents within it. In general it is elevated temperatures that are most likely to cause these changes, low or sub-zero temperatures tending to delay any degradation of the fingermark constituents. Some of the effects that may be observed at elevated temperature include

- Accelerated drying of the fingermark (i.e. water loss)
- Crystallisation of salts within the deposit
- Evaporation of volatile constituents

- Melting and subsequent flow of low melting point constituents

- Oxidation of some constituents within the residue

- Chemical degradation of some compounds within the fingermark

The extent to which any of these effects occur will depend on both the temperature and the time for which the surface and fingermark are exposed. A very short exposure to a high temperature may be less damaging than a prolonged exposure to a lower temperature.

As discussed in Chapter 3, water is one of the principal constituents of fingermarks consisting of natural sweat deposits and on non-porous surfaces will be progressively lost from the mark by evaporation, resulting in a shrinking in the profile of the ridges (Thomas and Reynoldson, 1975). At elevated temperature, the rate of water loss and shrinkage of the ridge profile will be accelerated, and as water is driven off, any dissolved inorganic materials such as salts will recrystallise.

Water is not the only volatile substance within the fingermark residue, and other substances such as ketones and alcohols will also be driven off at an accelerated rate as temperature is increased. Olsen (1987) investigated the effect of exposing latent prints on glass slides to 90°C for periods of time between 30 min and 4 h and analysing the principal constituents of sebaceous sweat using thin-layer chromatography. It was observed that constituents disappeared from the fingermark over time, with free fatty acids, cholesterol and squalene being lost in that order. It was not established whether this loss in constituents arose from their degradation to other compounds or volatilisation.

In addition to volatile substances, fingermarks may also contain substances that can melt and flow as temperature is raised above the ambient. Many of the constituents of sebaceous sweat have melting points between ambient temperature and 150°C, some of which are summarised in Table 4.1.

The flow of these constituents across or into the surface the mark is deposited on may result in blurring and obscuring of the ridge detail. In addition to the physical flow of the fingermark constituents, exposure to elevated temperature in the presence of oxygen may also cause oxidative changes in composition.

Table 4.1   Melting points of typical constituents of sebaceous sweat.

Constituent	Type of compound	Melting point (°C)
Cholesterol	Cholesterol	148
Oleic acid	Unsaturated fatty acid	13
Lauric acid	Saturated fatty acid	43.2
Palmitic acid	Saturated fatty acid	63
Stearic acid	Saturated fatty acid	69.6
Trimyristin	Triglyceride	56–57
Tripalmitin	Triglyceride	67.4
Glycerol monostearate	Wax ester	58–59

The oxidation of squalene, which is abundant within fresh fingermarks, was investigated by Mountfort et al. (2007). Immediately after deposition of the mark, squalene, squalene epoxide and squalene monohydroperoxide were detected. The concentration of squalene progressively decreased until it was no longer detected after 7 days. In contrast, the quantity of squalene epoxide and squalene monohydroperoxide increased noticeably after 1 day and further increased in concentration for up to 5 days after mark deposition. However, neither of these substances was detected in the mark after 7 days. A progressive oxidation process was proposed through squalene dihydroperoxide (SQ-[OOH]2) and squalene trihydroperoxide (SQ-[OOH]3) and finally to squalene pentahydroperoxide (SQ-[OOH]5).

Oxidation and other thermal degradation mechanisms may also occur for the eccrine constituents of sweat. The thermal degradation of eccrine sweat constituents including amino acids, urea and lactic acid was investigated by De Paoli et al. (2010) using dilute solutions exposed to conditions designed to cause thermal and/or photodegradation. It was observed that amino acids, urea and lactic acid were all susceptible to thermal degradation, which began for exposure times of greater than 3 min at 100°C for both urea and amino acids. Richmond-Aylor et al. (2007) also studied the pyrolysis of certain amino acids and fingermark residues over the temperature range 50–500°C and characterised some of the products formed from thermal decomposition. These products included 2,5-furandione and maleimide, degradation products of aspartic acid and 3,6-dimethylpiperazine-2,5-dione, produced from decomposition of alanine.

It has also been noted that the products formed by thermal degradation of eccrine fingermark constituents on paper can be fluorescent (Brown et al., 2009; Dominick et al., 2010; Song et al., 2011). A range of thermal environments were found to produce fluorescence, with Brown et al. using hot air at approximately 300°C for 10–20 s and Dominick et al. observing optimum fluorescence after exposing marks to 150–160°C for 20 min. In both cases longer exposure times and/or higher temperatures resulted in the mark ceasing to be fluorescent and becoming visible as dark brown 'charred' ridges. Both Dominick et al. and Song et al. used amino acid spots deposited on paper to investigate if the fluorescence could be replicated for eccrine constituents and also studied alternative substrates to paper. Although Song et al. ascribed the fluorescence to accelerated oxidation of the cellulose in the paper caused by the presence of fingermark, Dominick et al. thought the fluorescence to be due to the formation of fluorescent degradation products of eccrine sweat. This was supported by observations that fluorescence was also observed from eccrine marks on ceramic tiles, where no cellulosic material was present in the substrate.

The changes in chemical composition, water content and so on that can be produced by the thermal environment can have a corresponding effect on other properties, such as electrical charge and adhesion. For example, a mark that has lost its water content and dried out will have considerably reduced adhesive properties.

4.5.2.2 Humidity

Water is the principal constituent of almost all uncontaminated fingermarks immediately after deposition, and therefore atmospheric humidity can play a part in determining what subsequently happens to those marks.

It may be assumed that at low humidity levels, drying of the residues may be accelerated and at high humidity levels, prolonged retention of water within the fingermark may occur. However, reported studies indicate that this may not be the case.

Barnett and Berger (1976) studied the effect of storage under different humidity conditions and times on the quality of marks developed using powders. The relative humidities used in the study were in the range 32–93% at a temperature of 20°C. It was concluded that under these conditions the relative humidity played a minimal role in determining the clarity of the developed mark, with the quality of the original mark being more important. This was supported by Thomas and Reynoldson (1975), who looked at the reduction in thickness of the fingermark residue when marks were held at constant relative humidities in the range 14–95% and found no direct relationship between rate of shrinkage and relative humidity. Thomas and Reynoldson noted that the mark dried out and shrank much more rapidly when placed in an outdoor location protected from rain. This indicates the additional drying effect of moving air (e.g. wind) across the surface.

High levels of humidity may play a more important role in promoting the migration of the water-soluble constituents in the fingermark, in particular those deposited on porous surfaces. As more moisture is absorbed into the surface, constituents such as urea and sodium chloride can migrate from their original location and lead to diffuse marks (Figures 4.11 and 4.13). When residues are exposed to the extremes of rain or water immersion, water-soluble constituents may redissolve and be washed entirely from the fingermark residues. The solubility of some of the eccrine constituents of marks is given in Table 4.2.

Table 4.2 Solubilities in water of typical constituents of eccrine sweat.

Constituent	Type of compound	Solubility in water at 25°C
Serine	Amino acid	250 mg/mL
Glycine	Amino acid	250 mg/mL
Alanine	Amino acid	167 mg/mL
Aspartic acid	Amino acid	4.5 mg/mL
Sodium chloride	Salt	360 mg/mL
Potassium chloride	Salt	340 mg/mL
Urea	Urea	480 mg/mL
Sodium lactate	Lactate	>1.5 g/mL

4.5.2.3 Ultraviolet radiation

Because ultraviolet radiation is emitted by the sun, fingermarks on exterior, outdoor surfaces will be most exposed to this type of environment. Standard window glass blocks most ultraviolet radiation, and therefore fingermarks deposited on surfaces indoors are less susceptible to any detrimental effects ultraviolet radiation may have.

Exposure to ultraviolet radiation may result in accelerated degradation of certain constituents within fingermarks. Archer et al. (2005) observed that squalene disappeared from fingermarks far more rapidly when marks were exposed to light. The action of ultraviolet radiation may be a significant contributor to this photodegradation of squalene. Studies by Dennis and Shibamoto (1989) and Yeo and Shibamoto (1992) showed that squalene decomposed to produce formaldehyde and malonaldehyde when exposed to ultraviolet radiation and that the rate of degradation was more rapid for the shorter wavelength UVB radiation than for long wavelength UVA.

The effect of ultraviolet radiation on the enhancement of both sebaceous sweat components and on fingermarks was studied by Gray (1978). In these studies, irradiation using both UVA and UVC radiation was seen to inhibit subsequent enhancement of marks with iodine, and results from spot tests showed that the effect of radiation was most detrimental on saturated compounds. Similar results were obtained by Goode et al. (1979), who used radioactive bromine to enhance marks after exposure to different environments including ultraviolet radiation.

De Paoli et al. (2010) also explored the effect or artificial sunlight on some of the eccrine constituents and found that although urea and amino acids were unaffected by photodegradation, the lactic acid constituent could degrade by a photochemical reaction.

4.5.2.4 Atmospheric pollutants

The types of atmospheric pollutant present will depend on the locality. In urban and industrial areas, there may be high levels of car exhaust fumes and combustion products present, whereas these will be less prevalent in rural environments. These atmospheric pollutants can have the following effects:

- Gases may be adsorbed into fingermarks and affect performance of enhancement processes.
- Gases may react with constituents of the fingermark.

It has been reported that sulphur dioxide gas can be preferentially adsorbed by, or react with, some of the constituents present in fingermarks (Spedding, 1971). It was suggested that SO_2 could react with the lipids present in fingermarks, in particular with oleic and linoleic acids.

The potential effects of other gases on fingermarks have not been extensively reported.

4.5.2.5 *Solid particulates*

A variety of solid particulates may be present in the atmosphere, including combustion products and fragments of fibres, skin and so on in the form of dust. The composition of the dust will again vary according to locality and whether the location is indoor or outdoor. These particles will progressively settle onto fingermark residues. In some cases these particles may act as preferential locations for fingermark enhancement techniques and mask reactions with fingermark constituents.

4.5.3 Interactions between the environment and the surface

The interactions between the environment and the surface will determine whether the original surface remains intact at the time of the initial examination. Where interactions occur that destroy the original surface (e.g. rusting), then the fingermark will no longer be present for enhancement. However, in general the surface will be more resistant than the fingermark to the effects of the environment, and it is more likely that a surface will withstand environmental exposure that removes or degrades the fingermark.

4.5.3.1 *Heat*

The temperature experienced by the surface may result in changes to its composition and physical state. In general it is elevated temperatures that are most likely to cause these changes. Some of the effects that may be observed at elevated temperature include

- Oxidation of the surface

- Deformation or melting

- Charring and burning

Elevated temperatures can increase the rates at which the oxidation of surfaces can occur and may also affect the nature of the oxidation products formed. Many metals can form stable oxide layers, as summarised in the section on surfaces earlier. If the oxide layer forms after the fingermark has been deposited, it may disrupt the deposits present. Alternatively, the presence of the fingermark deposits may protect the region of the surface beneath them from the effects of oxidation.

For some types of surface, elevated temperatures may bring about a change in state. Polymeric materials may deform or shrink as they are heated above their glass transition temperature; other surfaces such as waxes may melt if they are raised above their melting points.

Materials can also begin to chemically degrade due to the effect of heat. For example, paper starts to become brown, and char as hydrogen and oxygen are lost from the cellulose fibres leaving only the carbon. In extreme circumstances the surface can be destroyed by heat, for example, paper can ignite if the temperature is high enough, with auto-ignition temperatures in the range 218–246°C.

4.5.3.2 Humidity

Some surfaces can absorb water from the atmosphere. Porous surfaces can retain moisture in their structure, and where the relative humidity of the atmosphere is greater than that of the porous surface, there is the potential for additional water to be absorbed by the surface to equilibrate. This increase in moisture content may increase the chances of the diffusion of the eccrine constituents.

Water uptake may also occur for surfaces that are apparently non-porous in nature, for example, nylon polymers are hygroscopic and absorb moisture.

When surfaces are exposed to the extremes of rain or water immersion, damage may be caused to the surface by a range of processes. These may include initiation of corrosion on metal surfaces and dissolving of water-soluble additives from materials such as paper, potentially causing them to disintegrate.

4.5.3.3 Ultraviolet radiation

Long-term exposure to ultraviolet radiation can degrade certain types of surface.

Polymeric materials can be degraded by ultraviolet radiation, because either their structures contain species such as aromatic rings that can absorb ultraviolet or they have bonds that are susceptible to attack. LDPE is an example of a material that can be degraded by ultraviolet radiation. LDPE contains tertiary carbon bonds that break to form free radicals, which in turn form carbonyl groups in the main polymer chain via a further reaction with atmospheric oxygen. In some cases chemical species are deliberately added to plastics to accelerate their breakdown, for example, biodegradable polymers used to manufacture some types of plastic bags.

The 'yellowing' that is observed in some types of paper on prolonged exposure to light is another effect caused by ultraviolet radiation. In this case the effect is caused by ultraviolet initiated oxidative reactions that convert the colourless cellulose to a yellow/brown reaction product.

Ultraviolet radiation can also act as a bleaching agent on surfaces containing dyes to give them colour. Ultraviolet can convert water contained in the surface to hydrogen peroxide, which in turn can cause the bleaching of the dye. Ultraviolet radiation can also directly attack the bonds in the chromophore portion of some dye molecules, causing them to lose colour.

4.5.3.4 Atmospheric pollutants

As discussed previously, the types of atmospheric pollutant present will vary from locality to locality and can affect the surface in addition to the fingermark. Examples of interactions that may arise from interactions between the surface and atmospheric pollutants include the tarnishing of silver, where the reaction of silver with hydrogen sulphide gas or other organic sulphides results in the formation of black silver sulphide on the surface.

4.5.3.5 *Solid particulates*

Solid particulates from a variety of sources can progressively settle onto the surface, forming a loosely bonded layer.

4.6 Time

Time is a critical factor in determining the effects of the environment on the fingermark and the surface. In practice it is actually the combination of time and environmental exposure conditions that determines what changes occur to both fingermark and the surface. A knowledge of the approximate time that has elapsed since the deposition of the mark can be important. When this information is known or can be estimated, it can be used to the benefit of the investigation by assisting in selection of the most appropriate enhancement processes, for example, using processes known to remain effective on fingermarks several years old in cold case reviews.

However, there are many situations where marks are enhanced in a laboratory, and the timescale for the deposition of that mark becomes a point of debate in the subsequent prosecution of the case. The mere fact that someone's fingermark has been found at a crime scene does not necessarily imply that this person has anything to do with the crime committed; for example, the mark could have been deposited during an innocent visit to a location several months previously or is actually associated with a more recently committed crime. One of the general purposes of forensic investigations is the determination of the time frame in which an offence has taken place and as such determine if any traces found have a relation to this offence.

When the time window of the criminal act has been determined, it is of great importance that one can determine if any traces found fit in this window. Weyermann et al. (2011) proposed a framework for age estimation with three approaches. In respect to the ageing of fingermark, the following can be extracted from these suggested approaches: regardless of the effects of the surface the fingermark is deposited on, one can consider contextual tags that place boundaries on the timescales for deposition (e.g. a fingermark on a newspaper can't be older then the newspaper itself). The other approaches, ageing and chronology, very much depend on the surface and conservation conditions of the deposited fingermark.

With this in mind, many studies and reviews (Midkiff, 1993; Wertheim, 2003) have been conducted with the objective of developing methods of determining the age of latent fingermarks.

In studies conducted by Barnett and Berger (1976) and Schwabenland (1992), attempts were made to relate the quality of marks developed using powder to the time since deposition. However, it was recognised that the quality of the developed mark is strongly influenced by the initial composition of the fingermark residue, which may contain contaminants that persist for long periods of time. The lack of reliability associated with this approach is reinforced by documented case studies (Clements, 1986; Cohen et al., 2012) where marks have continued to develop strongly using powder over a year after they were deposited.

The changes in lipid composition identified by Olsen (1987) and Archer et al. (2005) have been proposed as a means of dating fingermarks. Although it is possible to map trends in the concentration of such constituents with time, a knowledge of the starting concentration of the constituent being measured and the conditions (e.g. light/dark/temperature) to which it has been exposed is necessary to accurately date fingermarks in this way. Refinements to this method have been investigated by Weyermann et al. (2011), who considered looking at the ageing of lipid constituents in combination to increase confidence in the estimate of age. Other researchers (van Dam et al., 2014) have explored the potential of fluorescence spectroscopy as a means of monitoring oxidation within fingermarks.

It has also been proposed by Watson et al. (2011) that the electric charge left on an insulating surface by the contact of a finger can be used to estimate the age of the mark. It is suggested that this charge decays with time and is donor independent, although further research would be required to investigate the influence of environment and surface on the charge decay characteristics.

There are also situations where marks are deposited that predominantly consist of a known contaminant, such as blood. The change in colour of blood from red to brown to dark brown/black over time is reasonably well researched, and the change in reflectivity of bloodstains and fingermarks in blood has been proposed as a means of dating such traces (Li et al., 2011, 2013).

The principal issue facing all models for the ageing of fingermarks is that the degradation mechanisms used for the dating process are influenced by temperature, light and a range of other environmental factors such as humidity. Although in indoor environments these may be known and may be relatively consistent, in outdoor environments these may not be known with any degree of certainty.

Cadd et al. (2015) and Girod et al. (2016) have presented a comprehensive overview of the existing literature, degradation mechanisms for fingermark constituents and suggestions for the use of methods for the age estimation of fingermarks. As described by Girod et al., the current standing of science with regards to age estimation (or determination) of fingermarks is insufficient for any form of reliable expression in a court of law, with none of the methods previously outlined having been validated. Known cases where expert testimony did include a statement regarding the age of a fingermark have seen an overturn of that statement in a higher court or a negative decision on whether the statement was admissible by a judge. In general professional societies concerned with scientific and legal standards in forensic science in general and fingerprints in particular are unanimous in their conclusion that at present, with current methods and technology, no reliable statement on the age of a fingermark can be made in a court of law.

References

Almog J, Azoury M, Elmaliah Y, Berenstein L, Zaban A, 'Fingerprints' third dimension: the depth and shape of fingerprints penetration into paper-cross section examination by fluorescence microscopy', J. Forensic Sci., vol 49(5), (2004), p 981–985.

Archer N E, Charles Y, Elliott J A, Jickells S, 'Changes in the lipid composition of latent fingerprint residue with time after deposition on a surface', Forensic Sci. Int., vol 154(2–3), (2005), p 224–239.

Barnett P D, Berger R A, 'The effects of temperature and humidity on the permanency of latent fingerprints', J. Forensic Sci. Soc., vol 16(3), (1976), p 249–254.

Bond J W, 'The thermodynamics of latent fingerprint corrosion of metal elements and alloys', J. Forensic Sci., vol 53(6), (2008), p 1344–1352.

Brown A G, Sommerville D, Reedy B J, Shimmon R G, Tahtouh M, 'Revisiting the thermal development of latent fingerprints on porous surfaces: new aspects and refinements', J. Forensic Sci., vol 54(1), (2009), p 114–121.

Brydson J, 'Plastics Materials' (7th edition), Butterworth Heinemann, Oxford, 1999.

Cadd S, Islam M, Manson P, Bleay S, 'Fingerprint composition and aging: a literature review', Sci. Justice, vol 55(4), (2015), p 219–238.

Champod C, Lennard C, Margot P, Stoilovic M, 'Fingerprints and Other Ridge Skin Impressions', CRC Press, Boca Raton, 2004, p 108–111.

Clements W W, 'Latent fingerprints – one year later', Identif. News, November 1986, p 13.

Cohen Y, Rozen E, Azoury M, Attias D, Gavrielli B, Levin Elad M, 'Survivability of latent fingerprints, part I: adhesion of latent fingerprints to smooth surfaces', J. Forensic Identif., vol 62(1), (2012), p 47–53.

van Dam A, Schwarz J C V, de Vos J, Siebes M, Sijen T, van Leeuwen T G, Aalders M C G, Lambrechts S A G, 'Oxidation monitoring by fluorescence spectroscopy reveals the age of fingermarks', Angew. Chem., vol 53(24), (2014), p 6272–6275.

De Paoli G, Lewis S A Sr, Schuette E L, Lewis L A, Connatser R M, Farkas T, 'Photo- and thermal-degradation studies of select eccrine fingerprint constituents', J. Forensic Sci., vol 55(4), (2010), p 962–969.

Dennis K J, Shibamoto T, 'Production of malonaldehyde from squalene, a major skin surface lipid, during UV-irradiation', Photochem. Photobiol., vol 49(5), (1989), p 711–716.

Dominick A J, NicDaeid N, Bleay S M, Sears V G, 'The recoverability of fingerprints on paper exposed to elevated temperatures, part 2: natural fluorescence', J. Forensic Identif., vol 59(3), (2010), p 340–355.

Fontana M G, 'Corrosion Engineering' (3rd edition), McGraw-Hill, New York, 1987.

Girod A, Spyratou A, Holmes D, Weyermann C, 'Aging of target lipid parameters in fingermark residue using GC/MS: effects of influence factors and perspectives for dating purposes', Sci. Justice, vol 56(3), (2016), p 165–180.

Goode G C, Morris J R, Wells J M, 'The application of radioactive bromine isotopes for the visualisation of latent fingerprints', J. Radioanal. Chem., vol 48, (1979), p 17–28.

Gray A C, 'Measurement of the Efficiency of Lipid Sensitive Fingerprint Reagents', SCS Report No. 520, AWRE Aldermaston, October 1978.

Kuno Y, 'Human Perspiration', Charles C Thomas, Springfield, IL, 1956.

Li B, Beveridge P, O'Hare W T, Islam M, 'The estimation of the age of a blood stain using reflectance spectroscopy with a microspectrophotometer, spectral pre-processing and linear discriminant analysis', Forensic Sci. Int., vol 212, (2011), p 198–204.

Li B, Beveridge P, O'Hare W T, Islam M, 'The age estimation of blood stains up to 30 days old using visible wavelength hyperspectral image analysis and linear discriminant analysis', Sci. Justice, vol 53(3), (2013), p 270–277.

Midkiff C, 'Lifetime of a latent print – How long? Can you tell?', J. Forensic Identif., vol 43(4), (1993), p 386–392.

Mountfort K A, Bronstein H, Archer N, Jickells S M, 'Identification of oxidation products of squalene in solution and in latent fingerprints by ESI-MS and LC/APCI-MS', Anal. Chem., vol 79(7), (2007), p 2650–2657.

Olsen R D Sr, 'Chemical dating techniques for latent fingerprints: a preliminary report', Identif. News, (4–5), February 1987, p 12.

Ramotowski R (Ed.) 'Lee and Gaensslen's Advances in Fingerprint Technology' (3rd edition), CRC Press, Boca Raton, 2013.

Richmond-Aylor A, Bell S, Callery P, Morris K, 'Thermal degradation analysis of amino acids in fingerprint residue by pyrolysis GC-MS to develop new latent fingerprint developing reagents', J. Forensic Sci., vol 52(2), (2007), p 380–382.

Roberts J C, 'The Chemistry of Paper', Royal Society of Chemistry, Cambridge, 1996.

Sampson W C, Sampson K L, Shonberger M F, 'Recovery of Latent Fingerprint Evidence from Human Skin: Causation, Isolation and Processing Techniques', KLS Forensics, 1997.

Schwabenland J F, 'Determining the evaporation rate of latent impressions on the exterior surfaces of aluminium beverage cans', J. Forensic Identif., vol 42(2), (1992), p 84–90.

Song D F, Sommerville D, Brown A G, Shimmon R G, Reedy B J, Tahtouh M, 'Thermal development of latent fingermarks on porous surfaces – further observations and refinements', Forensic Sci. Int., vol 204(1–3), (2011), p 97–110.

Spedding D J, 'Detection of latent fingerprints with $^{35}SO_2$', Nature, vol 229, (1971), p 123–124.

Thomas G L, Reynoldson T E, 'Some observations on fingerprint deposits', J. Phys. D Appl. Phys., vol 8, (1975), p 724–729.

Watson P, Prance R J, Beardsmore-Rust S T, Prance H, 'Imaging electrostatic fingerprints with implications for a forensic timeline', Forensic Sci. Int., vol 209(1–3), (2011), e41–e45.

Wertheim K, 'Fingerprint age determination: is there any hope?', J. Forensic Identif., vol 53(1), (2003), p 42–49.

Weyermann C, Roux C, Champod C, 'Initial results on the composition of fingerprints and its evolution as a function of time by GC/MS analysis', J. Forensic Sci., vol 56(1), (2011), p 102–108.

Wyatt O H, Dew-Hughes D, 'Metals, Ceramics and Polymers', Cambridge University Press, Cambridge, 1974.

Yeo H C, Shibamoto T, 'Formation of formaldehyde and malonaldehyde by photooxidation of squalene', Lipids, vol 27(1), (1992), p 50–53.

Young R J, 'Introduction to Polymers', Chapman and Hall, London, 1981.

5

Initial examination and the selection of fingermark enhancement processes

Stephen M. Bleay

Home Office Centre for Applied Science and Technology, Sandridge, UK

Key points

- A wide range of enhancement processes are available, targeting different properties and constituents of fingermarks and suited for use on different surfaces.

- An initial examination of the item should be conducted to obtain information about the surface, environment and fingermark before selection of the most appropriate enhancement process.

- The potential impact of the enhancement process on the surface should be considered as part of the selection process.

5.1 Introduction

The next stage of fingermark recovery is the point at which the article or surface is first examined by a person with an interest in locating fingermarks on it, generally the crime scene investigator. An initial examination of the surface should be conducted to obtain information that can assist in the selection of the most appropriate fingermark enhancement process(es) and also to locate any marks that may already

---

Fingerprint Development Techniques: Theory and Application, First Edition.
Stephen M. Bleay, Ruth S. Croxton and Marcel de Puit.
© 2018 John Wiley & Sons Ltd. Published 2018 by John Wiley & Sons Ltd.

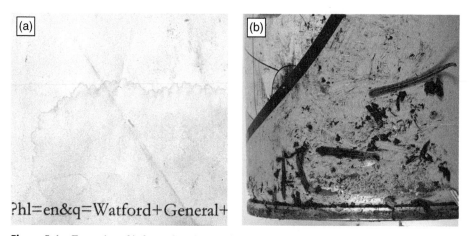

Figure 5.1 Examples of information that can be obtained during the initial examination of a surface: (a) evidence of water damage on paper and (b) grease contamination on an aerosol can. Reproduced courtesy of the Home Office.

be visible. The type of information that can be obtained in such an examination includes the nature of the surface type, its texture and colour and evidence of any exposure to particular environments (Figure 5.1). Building knowledge of any contaminants that may be present (e.g. grease or blood) will also impact upon the subsequent decision-making process.

5.2 Processing options

A basic knowledge of what situations individual enhancement processes may be most effective in is a requirement for process selection. There are significant differences between the mechanisms that can be used to enhance marks (Bleay et al., 2012; Bandey, 2014), and this can have an impact on which process(es) are ultimately selected. A summary of some of the commonly used fingermark enhancement processes and the constituents, properties and types of marks that they target is given in Table 5.1. The constituents are divided into the endogenous (eccrine and sebaceous sweat) and the exogenous materials in a fingermark that may be exploited for the visualisation of a fingermark.

How these differences in enhancement mode directly translate into differences in the effectiveness of the processes on eccrine, sebaceous and 'natural' marks can be observed directly in the examples illustrated in Figure 5.2. In this case the natural marks are those obtained from donors who have not washed their hands for at least 30 min and are likely to contain a mixture of eccrine and sebaceous sweat and any exogenous compounds/contaminants picked up from handled items.

Table 5.1 Some commonly used fingermark enhancement processes and the types of mark they can be used to enhance.

Process	Constituent/property targeted	Capable of developing marks of type		
		Eccrine	Sebaceous	Exogenous material or contaminant
Protein stains (acid dyes)	Proteins	X	X	✓ (blood)
Basic Violet 3	Lipids, epithelial cells	X	✓	✓ (grease)
Cyanoacrylate fuming	Combinations of water, salts, amino acids, lactate	✓	(✓)	X
DFO	Amino acids, amine-containing substances	✓	X	✓ (blood)
ESDA	Electric charge, dielectric constant	✓	✓	X
Fluorescence examination	Fluorescent constituents	(✓)	(✓)	✓
1,2-Indandione	Amino acids, amine-containing substances	✓	X	✓ (blood)
Iodine fuming	Squalene	X	✓	✓ (grease)
Ninhydrin	Amino acids, amine-containing substances	✓	X	✓ (blood)
Multi-metal deposition	Proteins, combinations of eccrine constituents in water-insoluble matrix	✓	✓	X
Oil Red O	Lipids	X	✓	✓ (grease)
Peroxidase reagents	Haem	X	X	✓ (blood)
Physical developer	Combinations of eccrine constituents in water-insoluble matrix	✓	✓	X
Powders	Adhesive properties	✓ (water content)	✓	✓ (grease)
Powder suspensions	Combinations of eccrine constituents in water-insoluble matrix	✓	✓	✓ (blood)
Silver nitrate	Chlorides	✓	X	X
Small particle reagent	Lipids	X	✓	X
Solvent Black 3	Lipids	X	✓	✓ (grease)
Ultraviolet reflection	Topography, UV absorption	✓	✓	✓
Visual examination	Optical properties	✓	✓	✓
Vacuum metal deposition	Differences in surface properties	✓	✓	✓

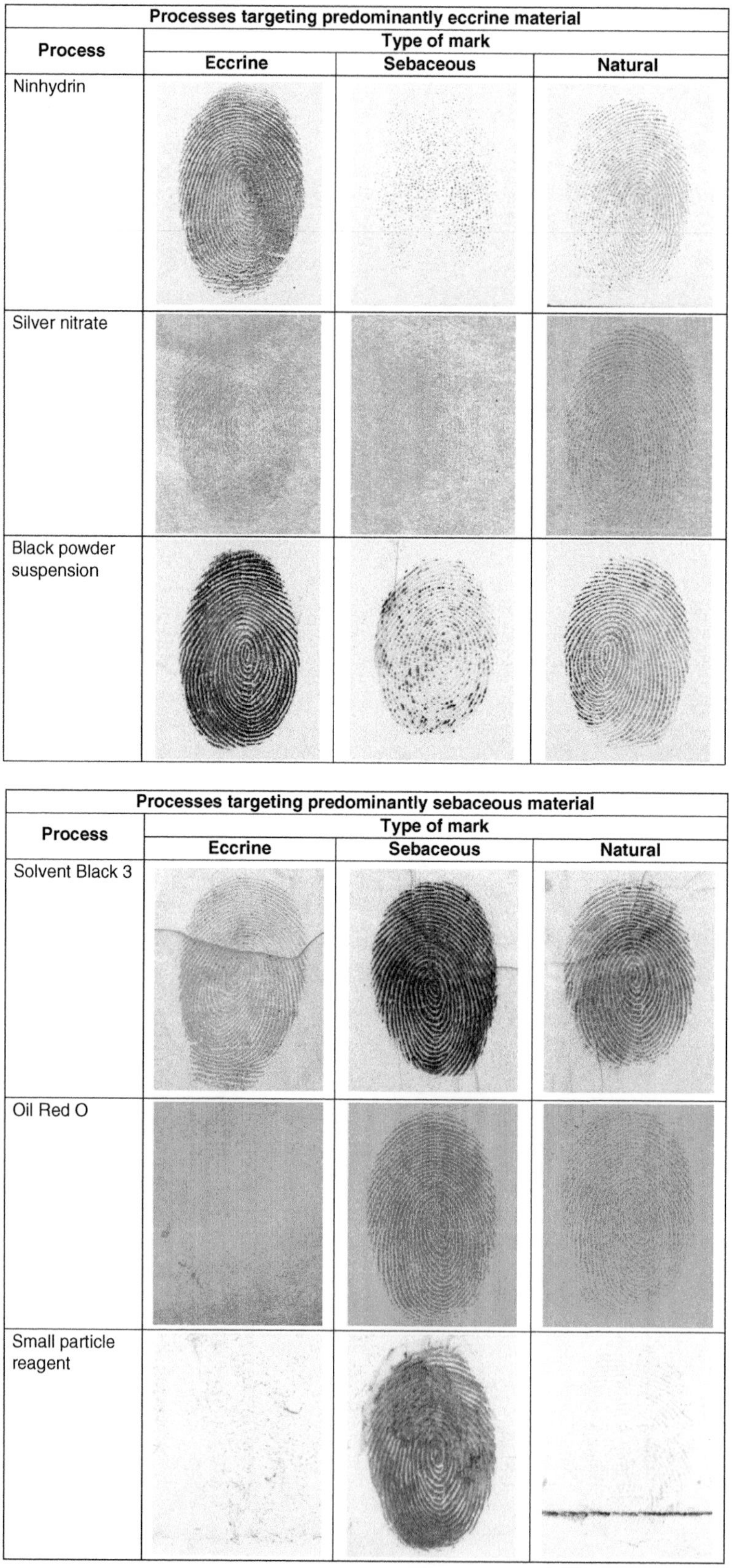

Processes targeting predominantly eccrine material		
Process	**Type of mark**		
	Eccrine	**Sebaceous**	**Natural**
Ninhydrin			
Silver nitrate			
Black powder suspension			

Processes targeting predominantly sebaceous material		
Process	**Type of mark**		
	Eccrine	**Sebaceous**	**Natural**
Solvent Black 3			
Oil Red O			
Small particle reagent			

Figure 5.2 A summary of various enhancement processes and their relative effectiveness on marks of different types. Reproduced courtesy of the Home Office.

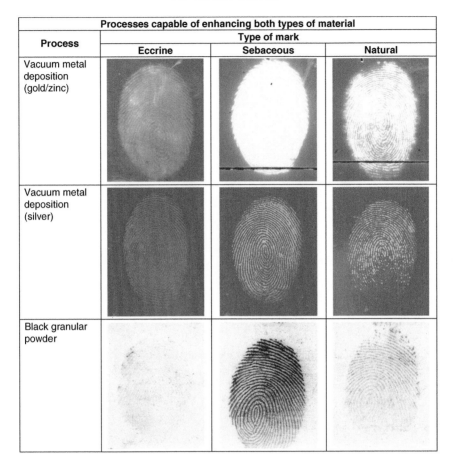

Processes capable of enhancing both types of material			
Process	**Type of mark**		
	Eccrine	**Sebaceous**	**Natural**
Vacuum metal deposition (gold/zinc)			
Vacuum metal deposition (silver)			
Black granular powder			

Figure 5.2   (Continued)

5.3   Process selection

The triangle of interaction described in Chapter 4 is a useful tool to assist in understanding what may have occurred since deposition of the mark and to assist with the identification of the optimum fingermark enhancement process(es) for a particular scenario. When using the triangle of interaction to inform decision-making about process selection, as much information as possible should be obtained about each of three elements of the triangle during initial examination, and the interactions that could progressively occur during the ageing interval should be taken into consideration.

Some of the questions that should be posed during process selection associated with the three elements of the triangle of interaction include the following.

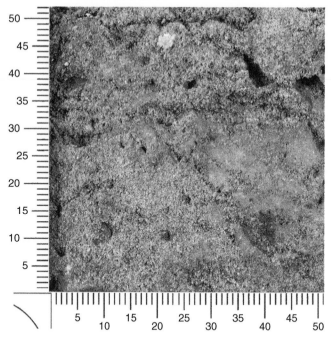

Figure 5.3   A rough brick surface that appears too textured to retain fingermark ridge detail. Reproduced courtesy of the Home Office.

5.3.1 Surface

How textured is the surface? Some surfaces may be too rough to make fingermark recovery likely (Figure 5.3). The reasons for this have already been described in Chapter 2.

Even in this situation, skin cells may be sloughed from the finger by the rough surface, and the use of fingermark enhancement processes may enable the location of an area where contact has occurred to target DNA swabbing.

What colour is the surface? It will be important to select an enhancement process that produces an enhanced mark of contrasting colour to the surface; otherwise some fingermarks present may not be located.

5.3.2 Fingermark

Have any fingermarks been located during the initial examination? Images of these marks should be captured before proceeding with any further enhancement processes, which may necessitate the use of more specialist lighting methods to obtain the optimum image.

Is there any evidence that the mark may be deposited in a contaminant? If there is no evidence that contaminants are present, it is generally assumed that the principal constituents are eccrine and sebaceous sweat and process selection made on that basis. If the initial examination gives indications of contaminants being present, then the selection can be modified to include processes targeting these substances. This initial information may be supplemented with the results of any presumptive testing carried out, for example, a Kastle–Meyer test conducted on a red-brown stain to indicate the presence of blood. Table 5.1 provides a reference guide to which processes may be appropriate for different types of contaminant.

5.3.3   Environment

Is there any evidence of exposure to particular environments? If it can be established that the surface and fingermark have been exposed to water, or high temperature, then the likely effect of these environments on fingermark and the surface (as outlined in Chapter 4) should be assessed and fed back into process selection. For example, if the article has been wetted, then it is extremely unlikely that processes targeting water-soluble constituents such as amino acids and salts will continue to be effective and should therefore be excluded from the process selection.

5.4   The processing environment

The triangle of interaction can also be utilised when considering the interactions that can occur during application of the fingermark enhancement process. In this situation the process itself becomes the 'environment' element of the triangle. The purpose of applying the process is to produce an interaction with the fingermark that makes it become sufficiently visible, but the potential interactions between the process and the surface also need to be carefully considered. This is because there are situations where the nature of the surface may preclude the use of a particular process, examples being as follows:

- The processing environment involves temperatures likely to cause damage to the surface (melting, deformation, etc.).

- The surface texture may retain excessive amounts of the processing substance.

- Adverse reactions may occur between the surface and the chemicals used in the enhancement process.

Particular cases where each of these may be a consideration are expanded upon in the succeeding text.

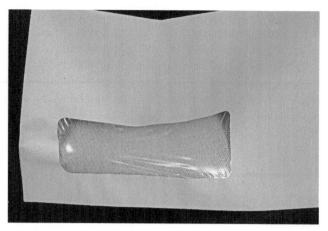

Figure 5.4   Polymer window of an envelope showing shrinkage and distortion caused by excessive heating.

5.4.1   Excessive heating

Excessive heating can arise in more than one way. One example is where the glass transition temperature or melting point of the surface is exceeded by the processing environment. An example of this is where paper labels on plastic bottles or paper envelopes with polymeric windows are processed using DFO, which requires heating in an oven at 100°C for 20 min. This combination of high temperature for an extended period of time may cause significant shrinkage and deformation of the polymers (Figure 5.4), and to avoid this from occurring, either the paper could be separated from the polymer prior to processing or an alternative process that does not require high temperatures could be selected instead.

Excessive heating may also occur in situations where the ambient temperature is not obviously high enough to cause damage. An example of this is where high intensity light sources such as lasers are used to examine dark surfaces containing fillers that can absorb energy of the wavelengths used. The absorbed energy may result in the surface being raised above its melting point or to a temperature where charring or ignition may occur.

5.4.2   Retention by surface texture

On smooth surfaces there are few, if any, physical features to inhibit the functioning of any enhancement processes. However, on textured surfaces the surface topography can influence the way in which fingermark enhancement occurs. If, for example, a fine powder (such as aluminium flake) is used to develop a fingermark on a rough textured surface, the small particles in the powder may become trapped by the

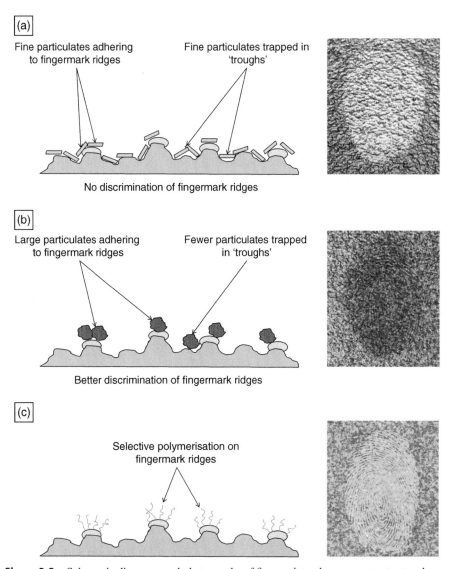

Figure 5.5 Schematic diagrams and photographs of fingerprint enhancement on textured surfaces: (a) aluminium powder, (b) black magnetic powder and (c) cyanoacrylate fuming. Photographs reproduced courtesy of the Home Office.

depressions in the surface, which can result in uniform deposition of powder over the surface and poor discrimination of fingerprint ridges (Figure 5.5). This can be addressed by using a powder with a larger particle size (e.g. black magnetic powder) where the larger particles are not retained by the textured surface and ridge detail can be discriminated. Alternatively, liquid or gas phase processes that selectively deposit on fingermark residues (such as powder suspensions or cyanoacrylate fuming) may be used. More detailed descriptions of all of these development processes will be given in Chapters 6–15.

5.4.3   Chemical incompatibility

Chemical incompatibility is most likely to be an issue when the surface is chemically reactive, as is the case for some types of metal, for example, brass. A theoretical example of where chemical incompatibility could occur is in the selection of a process to enhance marks in the blood on a brass surface. Processes that could be used in this scenario are the acid dyes, which stain the proteins present in the blood, or the peroxidase reagents, which react with the haem constituent in the blood to give a coloured reaction product. However, the peroxidase reagents utilise hydrogen peroxide in their formulation to catalyse the reaction, which can also attack the surface, producing gaseous products that can disrupt the ridge detail. The results of using a peroxidase reagent (Leuco Crystal Violet) and an acid dye (Acid Black 1) to develop a mark in the blood on a brass surface are illustrated in Figure 5.6.

If the nature of the surface is uncertain and it is unknown how it may interact with the processing environment, preliminary 'spot tests' can occasionally be applied to small areas away from the region of operational importance to evaluate how a surface will respond to individual enhancement processes.

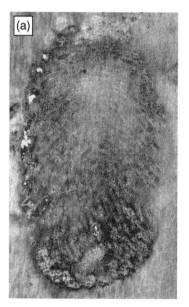 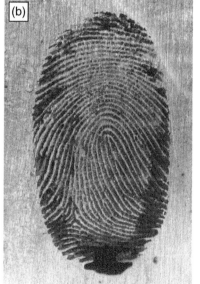

Figure 5.6   Fingermarks in the blood enhanced on a brass surface using (a) Leuco Crystal Violet and (b) Acid Black 1, showing the degradation to the ridge detail caused by the reaction between hydrogen peroxide and the brass. Reproduced courtesy of the Home Office.

References

Bandey H (ed.), Fingermark Visualisation Manual, Home Office, London, 2014, ISBN 978-1-78246-234-7.

Bleay S M, Sears V G, Bandey H L, Gibson A P, Bowman V J, Downham R, Fitzgerald L, Ciuksza T, Ramadani J, Selway C, Home Office Fingerprint Source Book, 6 June 2012 (https://www.gov.uk/government/publications/fingerprint-source-book, accessed 16 October 2017).

6

Optical detection and enhancement techniques

Stephen M. Bleay

Home Office Centre for Applied Science and Technology, Sandridge, UK

Key points

- Optical processes are non-contact and generally non-destructive and can therefore be used at the beginning of processing sequences. They can also be used to enhance marks developed using other processes.

- Optical processes utilise a range of interactions between electromagnetic radiation, the surface and the fingermark to produce contrast, such interactions including reflection, absorption and transmission.

- The interactions utilised are not confined to the visible region of the spectrum and both ultraviolet and infrared radiation can be utilised for fingermark detection and enhancement.

6.1 Introduction

The first processes that should be considered for fingermark detection and enhancement, in particular where sequential treatments are being used, are the group of 'optical' processes. This term describes processes that essentially utilise the differences between the response of the fingermark and the surface to electromagnetic radiation in the ultraviolet (UV), visible and near-infrared (IR) regions of the spectrum to visualise the mark. Such processes can be used in two ways: to detect fingermarks in a mostly non-destructive way without the need to apply any

---

Fingerprint Development Techniques: Theory and Application, First Edition.
Stephen M. Bleay, Ruth S. Croxton and Marcel de Puit.

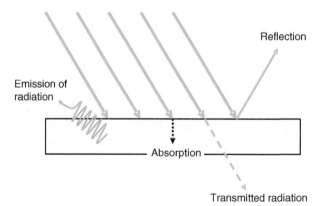

Figure 6.1 Schematic diagram of the interactions between electromagnetic radiation and a surface.

chemical or physical treatment or to enhance the contrast between a fingermark already developed by another process and the surface it has been deposited on.

Before proceeding to more specific descriptions of the optical techniques that are used in mark enhancement, it is necessary to have an understanding of the interactions that can occur between light/radiation and the surfaces it is incident on. These are outlined in Figure 6.1.

The three principal interactions that occur between the surface (and the mark) and the incident light/radiation are reflection, absorption and transmission.

Different types of reflection will occur depending on the nature of the surface. If the surface is smooth, opaque and highly reflective, specular reflections are most likely to occur. Specular reflection is where the radiation is reflected from the surface at the same angle that it is incident on it. Where surfaces are textured, opaque and reflective, or covered with irregularly shaped contaminants such as dust particles, radiation can be strongly scattered, that is, reflected in multiple directions unrelated to the original angle of incidence. On surfaces with greasy contamination, reflection may be diffused and of lower intensity over a wide range of angles (Figure 6.2).

In absorption, the incident radiation is absorbed by the surface and may be converted to other forms of energy such as heat. In some circumstances this absorption of radiation may be sufficient to promote emission of radiation of a different wavelength from the mark and/or the surface, such as visible fluorescence or X-ray emission.

Finally, the surface may be transparent to the wavelengths of radiation incident on it, in which case the radiation may be transmitted (e.g. as observed with visible radiation and window glass). Radiation passing through the material may be refracted at the interface between air and the surface or diffracted by any nanometre-scale particles present. The level of refraction and diffraction may differ between the pristine regions of the surface and those where the fingermark is present.

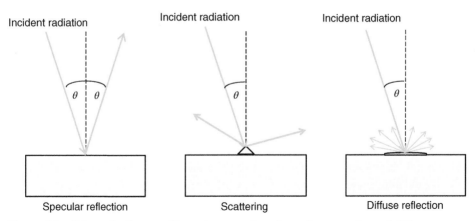

Figure 6.2   Schematic diagrams illustrating examples of specular, scattering and diffuse reflection.

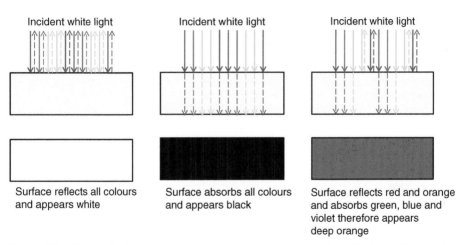

Figure 6.3   Schematic diagrams showing how colour results from the reflection and absorption of different wavelengths of light.

The response of the surface and fingermark to incident radiation is not constant across all wavelengths, and some attributes of the surface and/or fingermark arise from a combination of both reflection and absorption over a wavelength range. The visible colour of a surface is defined by which colours are absorbed and which are reflected (Figure 6.3).

In some scenarios the difference in response between the fingermark and the surface may be sufficient for the mark to be revealed, which is the case during the 'visual examination' process. In other scenarios it may be necessary to use a filter to magnify the difference in response between the fingermark and surface to the extent that it may be easily seen, which is the case in the fluorescence examination process.

A summary of the principal optical processes, the type of interaction or property that they target and whether they are used to detect latent fingermarks and/or enhance marks developed by other processes is given in Table 6.1.

'Visual examination' is a general term describing the examination of an item under a range of (usually white) lighting conditions. Although this may seem a simplistic approach, it can be very effective, and by varying lighting angles many different types of fingermark may be detected. Most marks found in the early days of fingerprint identification were located by means of some form of visual examination (Beavan, 2002). Many specialised lighting techniques were adapted for revealing and photographing fingermarks in the first half of the 20th century (Cherrill, 1954), and almost all of these are still in use today.

Table 6.1 Summary of the mode of operation and principal applications of optical processes.

Process	Interaction/properties utilised	Detection of latent marks	Enhancement of developed marks
Visual examination (oblique lighting)	Scattering, topography	✓	✓
Visual examination (specular lighting)	Specular reflection, absorption, diffuse reflection	✓	✓
Visual examination (diffuse lighting)	Diffuse reflection, absorption	✓	✓
Visual examination (dark-field reflection)	Scattering, refraction	✗	✓
Visual examination (bright-field transmission)	Scattering, refraction, diffraction	✗	✓
Visual examination (dark-field transmission)	Scattering, refraction	✓	✓
Visual examination (cross polarisation)	Specular reflection, absorption, diffuse reflection	✗	✓
Fluorescence examination	Fluorescence, absorption	✓	✓
Ultraviolet reflection	(Ultraviolet) absorption, (ultraviolet) reflection	✓	✓
Colour filtration/ monochromatic illumination	Colour (i.e. reflection + absorption)	✗	✓
Infrared reflection	(Infrared) absorption, (infrared) reflection	✗	✓
Multispectral imaging	Colour (i.e. reflection + absorption) Fluorescence	✗	✓

The first reported use of fluorescence examination for fingermark detection was in the 1930s, using powders that fluoresced under UV radiation to first develop the fingermark (Brose, 1934). This technique required the subsequent use of specialist lighting and filters to photograph the developed mark. For many years this was the only method of fluorescence examination used for fingermark detection and enhancement until the trials with the UV-excited amino acid reagents fluorescamine and *o*-phthalaldehyde in the mid-1970s (Benson and Hare, 1975). Later that decade it was observed that lasers could be used to promote fluorescence in untreated latent marks (Dalrymple et al., 1977), and this prompted subsequent research into lasers and the development of filtered high intensity light sources. Research effort was also directed towards fluorescent dyes and reagents that could be used in conjunction with these light sources to optimise fingermark recovery.

In the early 1970s, it was also observed that certain fingermark constituents would absorb short-wave UV radiation (Ohki, 1970), and this could be used to detect untreated fingermarks on porous surfaces. Later research (Creer, 1995; Fraval et al., 1995; Qiang, 1995) demonstrated that the scattering of short-wave UV radiation by fingermarks on non-porous surfaces could also be used as a means of directly imaging untreated marks, and portable imaging equipment based on image intensifiers was developed to enable searching for fingermarks at scenes (German, 1995).

IR reflection began to be explored for forensic applications as early as the 1930s, with uses in footwear imaging and location of blood stains being reported (Bloch, 1932; Martin, 1933). These early applications required IR-sensitive film (von Bremen, 1967), and photography was speculative, based on an assumption that evidence was present to capture. The use of IR reflection for the detection of fingermarks was first reported in the 1940s (Clark, 1946), and with the advent of live viewing vidicon devices, it became used for document examination from the 1950s onwards (Hilton, 1962; Ellen and Creer, 1970). However, it was not until the 1970s that its use in enhancing developed fingermarks was revived (Wilkinson, 1979). It was in use for this purpose in some specialist laboratories in the mid-1980s (Creer and Brennan, 1987), but never widely adopted. The wider introduction of 'live' and 'semi-live' view digital imaging systems with IR sensitivity led to a re-evaluation of the process in the mid-2000s (Bleay and Kent, 2005). This demonstrated that IR reflection was an effective technique in suppressing background patterns when metallic or inorganic development reagents (e.g. vacuum metal deposition, powders, powder suspensions and physical developer) were used.

The principles of colour filtration are long understood, and the use of coloured filters of contrasting or similar colour to the background to enhance fingermarks during photography was described in the early 1900s (Home Office, 1940). Monochromatic illumination is essentially an adaptation of colour filtration, utilising a tunable linear filter – slit combination to give more control of the colour of light incident on the surface. Systems with an integral linear filter that could be fitted to high intensity light sources and used for fingermark enhancement became available in the late 1980s/early 1990s.

Multispectral imaging is a technology originally developed for aerial photography and describes a system capable of simultaneously capturing spectral as well as spatial information. The spectral information can be used to distinguish between areas of nominally similar appearance, for example, identifying different types of crop or vegetation by the differences between their reflected light spectra. The potential of the technique for forensic applications became recognised in the late 1990s, and in 2003 it was demonstrated that chemically treated fingerprints could be imaged in both absorption and fluorescence modes using multispectral imaging systems and that the improved spectral resolution obtained revealed more ridge detail than conventional imaging routes (Exline et al., 2003; Payne et al., 2005). Faint ninhydrin marks in particular could be significantly enhanced by this method.

6.2   Current operational use

Because of their non-contact, generally non-destructive nature, optical processes can be used both at the beginning of any processing sequence to visualise marks and should also be considered as a means of enhancing the contrast of any marks that have been visualised by other chemical and physical processes.

Visual examination is a simple process to implement and has been demonstrated to detect a small but appreciable proportion of marks that will not be subsequently developed by any chemical process. However, it is not as widely used as perhaps it should be, possibly because marks are easily detected but less easily imaged. Obtaining optimum results from visual examination requires a skilled operator with expertise in lighting and imaging techniques. The fundamental techniques used in visual examination have changed little over time, and it is not anticipated that any major advances in the technique will emerge.

Colour filtration may be used in conjunction with visual examination to increase the contrast between fingermarks and the surface. The most commonly used colour filtration technique used is the use of a green filter to enhance the contrast of the purple marks developed using ninhydrin, although the physical use of coloured filters is reducing because the same effect can now be readily obtained by adjustments to the red–green–blue (RGB) colour channels of the captured image using imaging software such as Adobe Photoshop.

Fluorescence examination is routinely used in laboratories for the enhancement of chemically treated marks and to a lesser extent for the detection of latent marks, which may fluoresce due to the presence of contaminants and certain constituents of eccrine sweat. The use of fluorescence examination for the detection of latent fingermarks at scenes is increasing with the introduction of scene-portable, high intensity light sources. Lasers with output powers of up to 8 W are available at a size and weight that makes them usable by a single person, and 1 W lasers of certain wavelengths are even available as handheld devices. The use of such high power sources makes detection of very small amounts of fingermark residues possible.

Improvements in light-emitting diode (LED) technology have resulted in the introduction of handheld light sources that are routinely carried to a scene, and hence light source examination is made both easier and more likely.

Although specialist equipment for UV reflection is commercially available, it is not a process that is routinely used for examination of exhibits or scenes, and operationally its use tends to be confined to specialist units. Its main application is in the detection of latent fingermarks on smooth, non-porous surfaces and glossy porous and semi-porous surfaces, although it is also highly effective in enhancing marks developed using cyanoacrylate fuming. This is because of the raised topography of these marks that strongly scatters the short wavelengths of UV radiation. UV reflection has an advantage over fluorescence examination in that it can be carried out in daylight. It may also detect marks not found by fluorescence examination (and vice versa). The health and safety implications of the use of short-wave UV radiation and the damage that it may cause to DNA (Anderson and Bramble, 1997) make it less widely used than fluorescence examination. However, provided that personnel are suitably trained in both UV safety and fluorescence examination and appropriate precautions are taken in terms of eye and skin protection, UV reflection can be used safely both in a laboratory and at a scene.

IR reflection does not generally reveal fingermarks in its own right but can aid the visualisation of marks developed using other processes, in particular physical developer. It is used occasionally as a specialist imaging technique to suppress the interfering effect of multicoloured, patterned backgrounds, but with the introduction of digital SLR cameras and other live-view imaging systems adapted for IR imaging, the use of IR reflection may become more widespread.

Both multispectral imaging and monochromatic illumination are specialist techniques, and their use tends to be confined to laboratories that have access to the equipment required. Both processes can be used to discriminate coloured, developed marks from patterned, multicoloured surfaces. Multispectral imaging is also particularly useful in enhancing faint coloured marks such as those developed using ninhydrin.

All optical processes have the potential to detect and enhance fingermarks on dry and wetted surfaces. Provided that sufficient fingermark residue survives the wetting process and its optical properties continue to provide contrast with those of the surface, marks may still be found.

6.3 Visual examination

6.3.1 Outline history of the process

1880: Faulds suggested visual examination for detection of several types of fingermarks.

1902: Fingermark impressions in paint were used in the first UK conviction based on fingerprint evidence.

1940: Home Office publication 'Notes on Fingerprints and Palmprints' lists several methods of visual examination for detecting and enhancing fingermarks, subsequently expanded upon in Cherrill's, 1954 publication 'The Finger Print System at Scotland Yard'.

6.3.2 Theory

The principle of visual examination is to utilise lighting in such a way to provide as much contrast as possible between the fingermark ridges and the surface, if possible suppressing any interference from any background patterns or textures. For the initial detection of marks, this is performed by investigating different lighting angles and different types of light source. Some of these are described in the succeeding text, together with a description of the situations that they are most appropriate for. The processes outlined in the succeeding text are not exhaustive, and many other specialist lighting techniques (Langford, 1980; Hunter et al., 2011; Bandey, 2014) can be used as part of a visual examination.

6.3.2.1 *Oblique lighting*

In oblique lighting, the light source is located so that the light beam is almost parallel to the surface and the detection system (the eye or camera) is situated perpendicular to it. With this geometry, if the surface is perfectly smooth with no contaminants present, no light will be reflected back to the camera and the surface will appear dark.

In cases where, for example, a layer of dust is present on the surface, the dust particles can strongly scatter the light, and some of this will be scattered back towards the camera, making the dust appear lighter than the surface beneath it. For this reason, oblique lighting is an effective method for detecting negative marks in dust, because the regions where the ridges on the fingertip have removed dust remain dark (Figure 6.4).

The reverse effect can be observed if the developed mark on the surface has a topography that makes the ridges stand out above the surface. In this case, the ridges scatter the light strongly, and they therefore appear lighter than the surface. This effect is particularly useful in enhancing marks developed using cyanoacrylate fuming, especially where it is not possible to apply fluorescent dyes to the surface.

Oblique lighting can also detect impressions left in soft surfaces such as wax, wet paint or putty. In this case the light passing across the surface casts shadows in the depressions left in the surface, increasing the contrast between the fingermark and the surface (Figure 6.5).

Imaging system

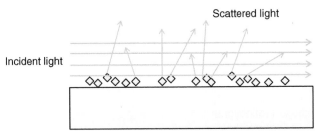

Figure 6.4   Schematic diagram of oblique lighting used to reveal negative marks in dust.

Imaging system

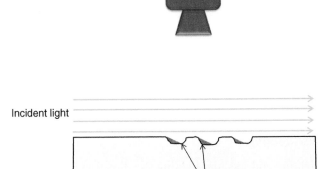

Figure 6.5   Schematic diagram of oblique lighting used to reveal impressions in the substrate.

6.3.2.2   *Specular lighting*

Specular lighting can be used for latent marks or marks with contaminant on smooth, reflective surfaces. It is essentially the opposite of oblique lighting, with the light source being placed at a high illumination angle in close proximity to the eye or detection system. Where light falls upon a reflective region of background, it is

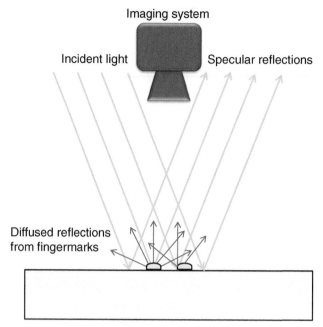

Figure 6.6   Schematic diagram of specular lighting.

specularly reflected at an angle where the reflected light does not reach the eye/ detector. Where light falls upon fingermark ridges, it is either scattered or diffusely reflected, resulting in some light being reflected to the eye (Figure 6.6). The ridges will therefore appear lighter than the background.

6.3.2.3   *Diffuse lighting*

Both oblique lighting and specular lighting use directional light beams to produce the desired effect. In other cases, the use of diffuse lighting may give better results. In diffuse lighting, the light source (e.g. a ball light) emits soft light in all directions. The light source is positioned so that a soft, diffused pool of light falls onto the surface, with the eye or detection system located so that it captures the reflection of the pool of light. Fingermarks in contaminants may absorb some of the incident light (Figure 6.7) and therefore be visible as dark ridges against a light background.

6.3.2.4   *Dark-field reflection*

Dark-field reflection is particularly suited to the examination and imaging of marks on transparent surfaces, in particular marks developed using processes that deposit reflective material on the fingermark ridges. It has been used for many years in the

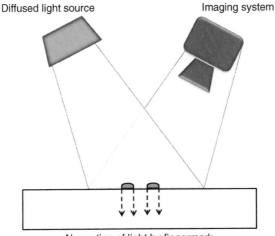

Figure 6.7   Schematic diagram of diffuse lighting used to reveal marks in absorbing contaminant on a reflective surface.

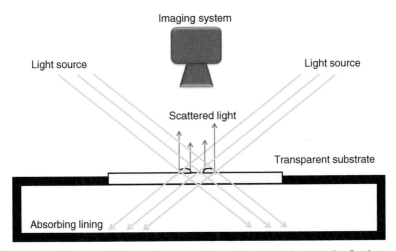

Figure 6.8   Schematic diagram of dark-field reflected lighting used to reveal reflective marks on a transparent substrate.

imaging of lifted marks developed using aluminium and other light-coloured powders. In dark-field reflection, the transparent substrate bearing the marks is placed over a cavity lined with dark, light-absorbing material. Incident light is angled so that if nothing is present on the substrate, it will be transmitted through it and be absorbed by the lined cavity (Figure 6.8). Where reflective particles are present on the surface, they scatter the incident light, and some will be reflected back to the imaging system, resulting in light ridges against a dark background.

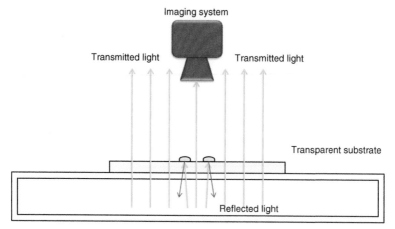

Figure 6.9   Schematic diagram of bright-field transmitted lighting used to reveal opaque marks on a transparent substrate.

6.3.2.5   Bright-field transmission

Bright-field transmission is a very simple technique that is used on transparent or translucent surfaces where marks have been developed using materials that are optically opaque, such as powders or powder suspensions. The process is also useful for visualising the zinc coatings produced by vacuum metal deposition. The substrate to be examined is placed on a light box and light passes through it. Where opaque material has been deposited on the surface, this reflects or absorbs the light (Figure 6.9), and fingermarks are seen as darker ridges against a light background. In the case of silver vacuum metal deposition, the coating consists of nanometre-scale silver clusters, and diffraction may be a major contributing factor to providing the different colours that give contrast between ridges and background.

6.3.2.6   Dark-field transmission

Dark-field transmission is suited to cases where fingermarks in sweat, oil or grease are present on transparent substrates such as glass or plastic packaging. The sample is illuminated from underneath at oblique angles. In regions with no fingermark deposit present, light is transmitted and does not reach the eye. Where there is a fingermark present, the light is scattered and/or refracted, some of it reaching the eye/imaging system (Figure 6.10). This results in light fingermark ridges against a dark background.

6.3.2.7   Cross polarisation

Cross polarisation can be used to reveal both latent and developed fingermarks on highly reflective surfaces such as metals. It requires the use of two linear polarised filters, oriented in cross-polarised mode. The light emitted by the light source passes

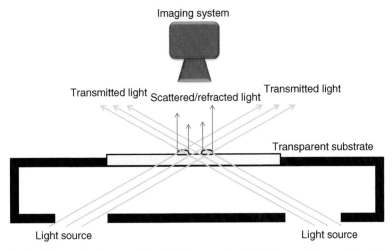

Figure 6.10 Schematic diagram of dark-field transmitted lighting used to reveal marks on a transparent substrate.

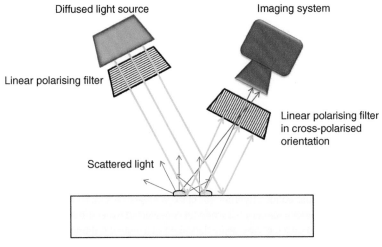

Figure 6.11 Schematic diagram of cross-polarised lighting used to reveal marks on a reflective substrate.

through the first linear polarising filter where it becomes polarised in a single direction. Incident light that hits the reflective surface is specularly reflected, without any change in the polarisation of the light. Light that hits the fingermark may be scattered or diffusely reflected, with a corresponding change in its polarisation state. When the light reflected from the surface reaches the cross-polarised linear filter in front of the imaging system, the specularly reflected light is blocked by the filter and the scattered/diffusely reflected light passes through it (Figure 6.11), producing light ridges against a dark background.

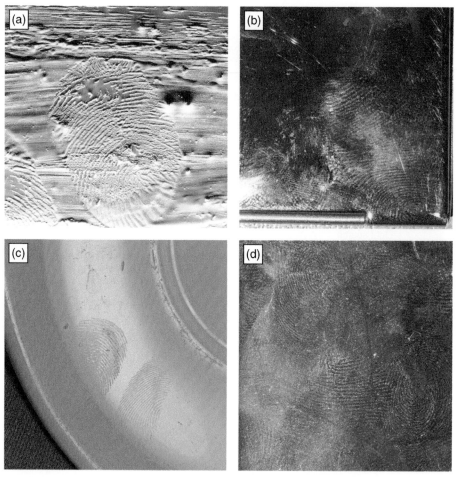

Figure 6.12   Different types of marks that may be detected by visual examination: (a) mark in wet paint detected using oblique lighting, (b) mark in grease on a metal tin detected using specular lighting, (c) marks in butter on a white saucer detected using diffuse lighting and (d) latent marks detected on a CD case using dark-field transmitted lighting.

Examples of marks visualised using some of the processes described previously are illustrated in Figure 6.12.

6.3.3   The visual examination process

The process recommended for visual examination consists of an initial examination under natural light, turning the article so that illumination falls on it from different angles. This should be followed by an examination using an even, white light source, again altering the angle of illumination from perpendicular to the exhibit to oblique and changing the proximity of the light source to the surface.

If there are indications of fingermarks after this initial examination, the practitioner should utilise a range of more specialised light sources to provide the lighting conditions outlined previously. These may include linear arrays to produce even, oblique illumination across a large area and ball lights to provide diffused lighting conditions.

6.4 Fluorescence examination

6.4.1 Outline history of the process

1930s: Use of UV-excited fluorescent/phosphorescent fingerprint powders proposed for fingermark development by Brose.

1970: Ohki identified UV-excited fluorescent compounds in fingermark constituents.

Mid-1970s: Research into fluorescamine and *o*-phthalaldehyde as amino acid reagents (Benson and Hare, 1975), producing UV-excited fluorescent reaction products.

1977: Dalrymple, Duff and Menzel reported detection of fluorescence in latent fingermarks using an argon ion laser (principal line 514.5 nm).

1980: Menzel published *Fingerprint Detection with Lasers*, the first comprehensive work into detection of fingermarks using high intensity light sources.

Early 1980s: Research in the United Kingdom, Australia and Canada into production of filtered high intensity white light sources as lower cost alternatives to lasers.

1982: Zinc toning process introduced for producing fluorescence in marks developed using ninhydrin (Herod and Menzel, 1982) and increasing the sensitivity of the ninhydrin process.

1983: Menzel et al. proposed Basic Red 1 (Rhodamine 6G) as a fluorescent dye solution for staining marks developed using cyanoacrylate fuming, increasing the number of marks detected.

1989: Grigg and co-workers developed DFO as a highly sensitive amino acid reagent giving fluorescent reaction products and detecting greater numbers of fingermarks than ninhydrin (Grigg et al., 1990).

1990: The first comprehensive guidance on the use of fluorescence examination for detecting different types of fluorescent marks and selection of appropriate light source/filter combinations was published (Hardwick et al., 1990).

Early 2000s: First LED-based light sources were developed for forensic applications.

Mid-2000s: Scene portable green (532 nm) lasers with high output powers became widely available.

2008: Scene portable yellow (577 nm) laser with high output power became commercially available.

2009: Scene portable blue (460 nm) laser with high output power became commercially available.

6.4.2 Theory

Fluorescence is one of a number of mechanisms by which materials can emit light upon the application of an external stimulus, which can be described by the general term 'luminescence'. The individual means by which light is generated is described by more specific terms, including triboluminescence, where light is emitted as a result of a material being rubbed, broken or abraded, and chemiluminescence, where light is emitted as a result of a chemical reaction (as utilised in the haem reagent luminol). When this light-generating chemical reaction occurs in living organisms, such as fireflies or glow-worms, it is described as bioluminescence.

Fluorescence is one of two processes described by the term photoluminescence, where light is generated in response to illumination. In most cases the light emitted is of a different wavelength range to that used in illumination. In fluorescence, the emission of light ceases almost instantaneously (nanoseconds to microseconds) after removal of the illumination. In the other related process, phosphorescence, energy is absorbed and re-emitted over a much longer timescale, with emission continuing for minutes and sometimes hours after removal of the illumination.

Fluorescence examination relies on either the fingermark or the surface containing fluorescent chemicals that can emit light when illuminated with light of appropriate wavelengths. Fluorescent chemicals have a series of discrete energy levels where electrons associated with them can exist. Normally, these electrons exist in a 'ground state' and will remain in this state unless additional energy is provided via another source (e.g. light, heat, friction). In fluorescence examination, the energy is provided by the incident light. If the wavelength of the incident light provides sufficient energy, electrons can be promoted from the ground state to an excited state, that is, one of a series of higher energy levels that are not normally occupied by electrons. The energy of these excited electrons rapidly decays so that they drop into lowest available excited state, and then over a longer time period (but still within nanoseconds), the electron falls back to the ground state by emitting the remaining additional energy as a photon of longer wavelength than the original illumination. The mechanism of fluorescence is shown schematically in Figure 6.13.

Because the energy levels at which electrons can exist have discrete values, there are only specific wavelengths of light that can be absorbed, and the emission of light will also occur over a specific wavelength range. In fluorescence, shorter

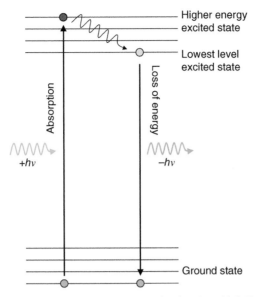

Figure 6.13 Schematic diagram showing the mechanism by which fluorescence occurs.

wavelengths of light are absorbed, and some of this absorbed energy is subsequently emitted as light of a different colour and longer wavelength.

There are in practice several excited states to which electrons can be promoted and several ground states to which they can return, so that absorption and emission actually occur over ranges of the electromagnetic spectrum rather than at single-wavelength values. Figure 6.14 provides a schematic illustration of a representative emission and absorption spectrum and the corresponding excited states.

It can also be seen in Figure 6.14 that there are wavelengths of light where the energy does not correspond to a discrete gap in energy levels, and as a result no absorption occurs at these wavelengths. The peaks in the excitation spectrum correspond to where energy is absorbed by the chemical in promoting electrons to excited states. The peak in the emission spectrum corresponds to the wavelengths where energy is emitted as electrons return to the ground state.

Typically, the longer wavelengths of light (UV, violet, blue, green or yellow) are used to illuminate the surface during fluorescence examination, and the corresponding fluorescence is emitted in the yellow, orange, red or IR regions of the electromagnetic spectrum. Most of the illuminating light is not absorbed but scattered or reflected from the surface being examined. The intensity of the reflected light is significantly greater than that emitted as fluorescence, and therefore under normal circumstances the fluorescence will not be seen. In order to view only the emitted fluorescence, filters that transmit the wavelengths of the fluorescence and block those of the illuminating light are placed in front of the eye and/or image capture device. This is shown schematically in Figure 6.15 for a case where fluorescent fingermarks are present on a non-fluorescing surface.

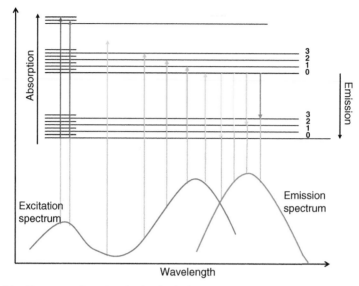

Figure 6.14   Representation of excitation/emission spectra of a chemical with corresponding transitions between excited and ground states.

The scenario illustrated in Figure 6.15 is one means by which fluorescence examination can reveal fingermarks. However, fluorescence examination can also be useful where the surface fluoresces and the fingermark absorbs the illuminating wavelengths (Figures 6.16 and 6.17). An appropriate viewing filter is also required to block the illuminating wavelengths.

Mention should also be made of 'anti-Stokes' fluorescence, a property exhibited by a very limited number of substances, which is now beginning to be exploited for fingermark enhancement. Such materials are also described as 'up-converters'. In 'anti-Stokes' fluorescence, the electrons in the material absorb energy from two photons of lower energy (higher wavelength) to become excited to the higher energy level, and they emit a single higher energy (lower wavelength) photon of light to return to the lower energy level. The most commonly used anti-Stokes materials are excited by IR radiation and fluoresce in the red, green or blue regions of the spectrum. A main application of such materials is in security markings.

Although anti-Stokes fluorescence is a less efficient process than conventional fluorescence, its principal advantage is that very few naturally occurring materials exhibit this behaviour and interfering background fluorescence can potentially be eliminated. A variety of means including filtered flash guns and IR lasers have been considered to promote anti-Stokes fluorescence, and fingerprint powders with anti-Stokes properties have been reported (Ma et al., 2011; Drabarek et al., 2012). Such materials will not be described further in this book.

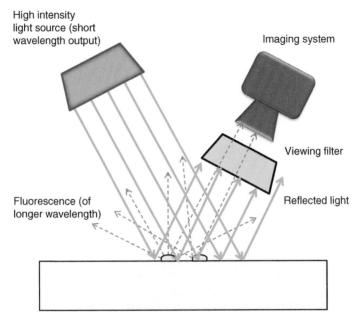

High intensity
light source (short
wavelength output)

Imaging system

Viewing filter

Fluorescence (of
longer wavelength)

Reflected light

Figure 6.15 Schematic diagram illustrating the viewing of fluorescence from fingermark ridges containing a fluorescent species.

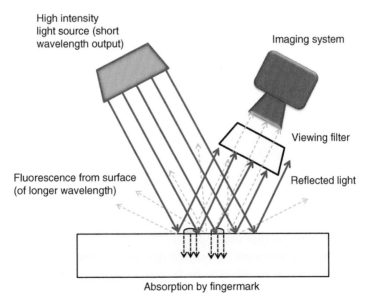

High intensity
light source (short
wavelength output)

Imaging system

Viewing filter

Fluorescence from surface
(of longer wavelength)

Reflected light

Absorption by fingermark

Figure 6.16 Schematic diagram illustrating the viewing of fluorescence for fingermark ridges containing an absorbing species against a fluorescing background.

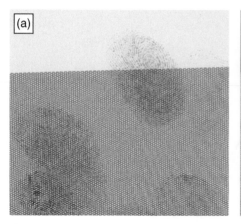 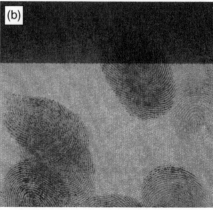

Figure 6.17 Images showing marks deposited on a coloured background and developed using ninhydrin, (a) viewed under white light and (b) fluorescence examination under green light, viewing the absorbing marks and fluorescing background through an orange filter.

6.4.3   The fluorescence examination process

Fluorescence examination is essentially a non-destructive process and may be used as the initial stage in a sequential processing regime. To optimise the results obtained from fluorescence examination, there are four factors that need to be taken into consideration:

1. The light source used for illumination

2. The fluorescent properties of the fingermark

3. The viewing filter used

4. The fluorescent properties of the surface

A range of light sources are available for fluorescence examination, differing in terms of their output wavelengths and output power. These include high output power, single-wavelength systems such as lasers, filtered white light sources and LEDs. The different generic types of output spectra for these types of light source are illustrated in Figure 6.18.

Fingermarks may fluoresce for a number of reasons: they may contain naturally fluorescent substances or fluorescent contaminants, they may have been enhanced using a chemical process that either produces a fluorescent reaction product or stains the mark with a fluorescent dye, or they may have degraded to form a fluorescent product due to the action of heat. In the case of untreated marks that contain fluorescent contaminants or have been developed by heat, the excitation and emission spectra associated with the mark will not be known. However, in the case of chemically developed marks, the excitation and emission spectra have been

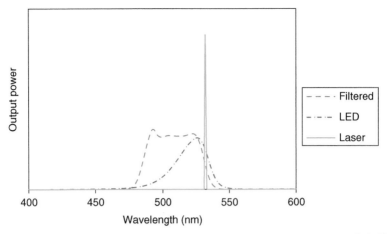

Figure 6.18 Output spectra for three types of light source used to produce green light illumination, a green laser with output at 532 nm, a green LED and a white high intensity arc lamp with a green excitation filter combination.

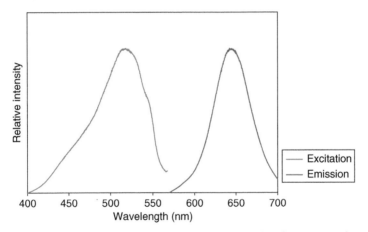

Figure 6.19 Excitation and emission spectra for a theoretical fluorescent substance.

measured and are known. These spectra are reproduced in the appropriate sections of this book. Excitation and emission spectra for a theoretical substance are illustrated in Figure 6.19 and will be used to illustrate the principles of optimising the fluorescence examination process.

Two generic types of filter are used for viewing fluorescence, long-pass filters and bandpass filters. Long-pass filters block all wavelengths of light below a 'cut-on' value, and band pass filters only pass a narrow range of wavelengths about a single peak value.

Background fluorescence is generally an unknown quantity during fluorescence examination. It may be advantageous, increasing contrast with absorbing finger-marks, or detrimental, obscuring fluorescence from the fingermark.

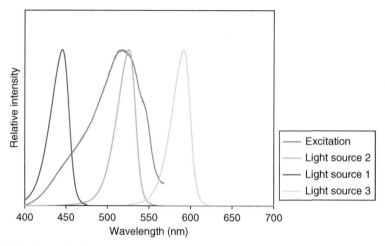

Figure 6.20   An excitation spectrum for a theoretical fluorescent substance and output spectra from three different LED light sources.

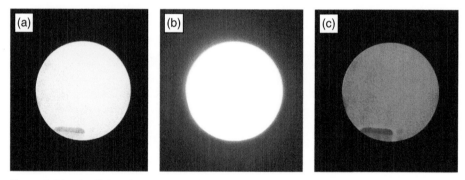

Figure 6.21   An illustration of the relative levels of fluorescence obtained by using light sources with output wavelengths corresponding to light sources 1, 2 and 3 in Figure 6.20. Reproduced courtesy of the Home Office.

The effectiveness of the fluorescence examination process is optimised by selecting the most appropriate combination of light source and filter for the particular fluorescent chemicals present. The rules are as follows:

Rule 1: The output spectrum of the light source used to excite fluorescence needs to be selected to be as close to the peak of the dye's excitation spectrum as possible or to overlap with a large proportion of the excitation curve (Figures 6.20 and 6.21).

In the aforementioned example, the output of light source 1 has some overlap with the excitation spectrum of the chemical, and although fluorescence is observed, it is of low intensity. Light source 2 has an output that corresponds closely to the peak excitation wavelengths, and the resultant fluorescence is very intense. Light source 3 has output wavelengths higher than the excitation range, and

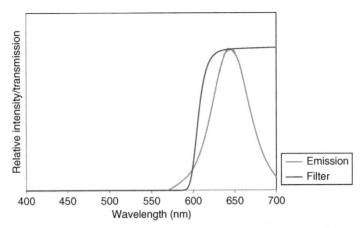

Figure 6.22 An emission spectrum for a theoretical fluorescent substance and the transmission spectrum for a generic long-pass filter.

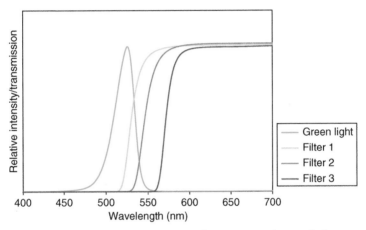

Figure 6.23 An output spectrum for a green LED light source and transmission spectra from three different long-pass filters.

very little fluorescence is observed. The intensity of fluorescence can also be increased by increasing the output power of the illuminating light source used.

Rule 2: The viewing filter selected must transmit as much of the emission spectrum of the fluorescent chemical as possible, ideally including the emission maximum (Figure 6.22).

Rule 3: The combination of light source and viewing filter should then be considered. It is necessary to select a viewing filter that does not transmit any of the output spectrum of the light source, but does transmit wavelengths above it so that the emitted fluorescence can be seen (as described in 2). The results obtained from different light source/filter combinations are shown in Figures 6.23 and 6.24.

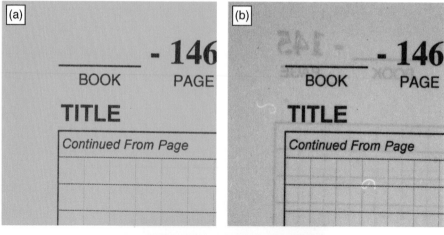

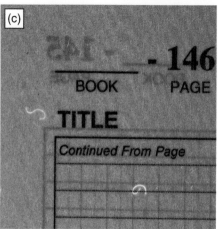

Figure 6.24 An illustration of the relative levels of light leakage obtained by using long-pass filters with transmission spectra corresponding to filters 1, 2 and 3 in Figure 6.23. Reproduced courtesy of the Home Office.

Filter 1 allows a significant proportion of the output from the light source to pass through it, and as a consequence only reflected green light is seen. Filter 2 allows much less of the output wavelengths to pass through, and hence the green colouration of the background is considerably reduced to the extent that some fluorescent fibres are seen, but faint fluorescence may still be obscured. Filter 3 is the optimum filter for use with this light source, because it blocks all of the output wavelengths, and thus the background remains darker, with the fluorescent fibres being clearly defined.

An example of where light source and filter selection can be closely matched to the excitation and emission spectra of the chemical present is shown in Figure 6.25.

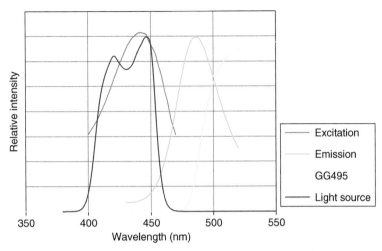

Figure 6.25 Emission and excitation spectra for Basic Yellow 40, with the output spectrum of a blue/violet light source and the transmission spectrum of a yellow viewing filter overlaid.

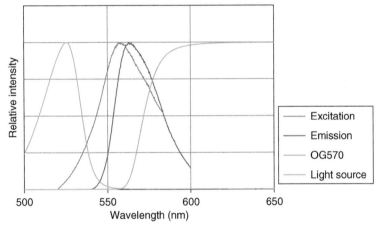

Figure 6.26 Emission and excitation spectra for DFO, with the output spectrum of a green light source and the transmission spectrum of an orange viewing filter overlaid.

In this particular example, the blue/violet output of a filtered arc lamp overlaps almost all of the excitation spectrum of the Basic Yellow 40 cyanoacrylate dye, maximising the emission output. The Schott yellow glass GG495 filter has no overlap with the output of the light source and transmits a significant proportion of the emitted fluorescence.

The proximity between the excitation and emission peaks for many fluorescent substances means that rules 1, 2 and 3 cannot always be satisfied in this way and the combination of light source and filter is more often a compromise, as shown for DFO in Figure 6.26.

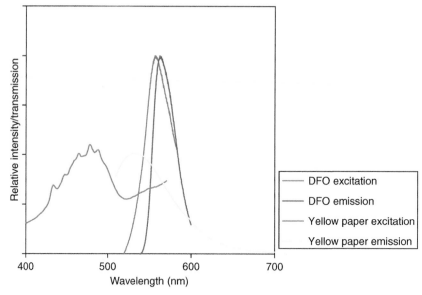

Figure 6.27   Emission and excitation spectra for DFO and for a yellow paper substrate.

The selection of light source and filter combinations may need to be modified to account for the presence of any background fluorescence that may occur. Figure 6.27 illustrates the emission and excitation spectra of DFO and a yellow paper substrate that the fingermark is present.

It can be seen that the excitation and emission peaks for the yellow paper substrate occur at lower wavelengths than the corresponding peaks for DFO, but that emission from the paper occurs over a broader range of wavelengths. The detrimental effect of background fluorescence can therefore be reduced by one or more of the following methods:

1. Using a light source with a higher excitation wavelength range, so that it is further from the excitation peak for the yellow paper

2. Using a transmission filter with a higher cut-on wavelength, so that it is further from the emission maximum of the yellow paper

3. Using a bandpass filter instead of a long-pass filter, reducing the contribution from the higher wavelength emission from the yellow paper

The practical effect of applying these measures to reduce background fluorescence can be seen in Figure 6.28.

There are many light sources and filters available for fluorescence examination, and it is not possible to describe all of these in great detail. Some of the approximate excitation and viewing conditions that are used and their operational applications are summarised in Tables 6.2 and 6.3.

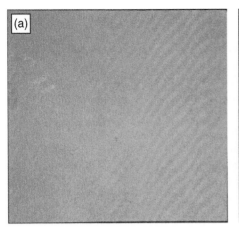 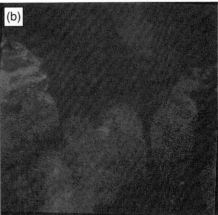

Figure 6.28 A fingermark developed using DFO on a yellow paper substrate, illuminated using (a) a green light source and viewed through an orange filter and (b) a yellow light source and viewed through a red filter.

Table 6.2 An overview of the types of light source used for location of untreated marks during initial fluorescence examination.

Application	Excitation colour	Viewing filter colour
Enhancement of fingermarks in absorbing materials, for example, blood, where background fluorescence may improve contrast	Violet/blue	Yellow
Detection of marks in fluorescent contaminants on all surfaces. Background fluorescence may obscure some fingermarks	Blue	Yellow
As aforementioned, but with reduced background fluorescence	Blue/green	Orange
Detection of latent fingermarks on polythene packaging and other surfaces including painted walls	Green	Orange
As aforementioned, but with reduced background fluorescence	Yellow	Red

Table 6.3 An overview of the types of light source used for enhancement of marks developed using other processes using fluorescence examination.

Application	Excitation colour	Viewing filter colour
Absorbing treatments, for example, ninhydrin, Acid Black 1, Acid Violet 17, powders (on surfaces where background fluorescence is present)	Violet	Yellow
Cyanoacrylate dyed with Basic Yellow 40	Blue/violet	Yellow
Acid Yellow 7	Blue	Yellow
Ninhydrin toned with zinc salts	Blue/green	Orange
DFO or 1,2-indandione for maximum contrast on most types of paper	Green	Orange
Cyanoacrylate dyed with Basic Red 14	Green	Orange
DFO or 1,2-indandione for maximum contrast on paper with background fluorescence	Yellow	Red

Examples of fluorescent fingermarks produced by individual development processes are illustrated within the appropriate chapters.

Fluorescence examination can be carried out both in a laboratory and at a scene, provided that appropriate health and safety precautions associated with the use of high intensity light sources are taken. Wherever possible, fluorescence examination should be carried out in a darkened room free of highly fluorescent items and surfaces, and users should allow themselves to become dark adapted before commencing examination. All safety precautions appropriate to the light source being used should be taken to ensure the safety of both the operator and others in the vicinity. The light source should be passed slowly over the article to be examined, taking care to minimise exposure time on articles that may be damaged by the heat associated with some high power light sources. Handling of the article during examination should be minimised to avoid damage to any marks present on the surface. Any marks detected should be photographed using an imaging system fitted with an appropriate viewing filter.

6.5 Ultraviolet reflection

6.5.1 Outline history of the process

1801: 'Discovery' of UV radiation.

By 1930s: Use of UV examination for document examination, analysis of glass fragments, detection of body fluids, enhancement of marks developed using fluorescent powder (Rhodes, 1931; Radley and Grant, 1954).

1970: Ohki observed absorption of short-wave UV by latent fingermarks and corresponding fluorescence at higher wavelengths.

1972: First use of image intensifiers for real-time viewing of latent fingermarks exposed to UV radiation (Saito and Arai, 1972).

1995: Development of scene portable reflected UV imaging systems (RUVIS) (German, 1995).

6.5.2 Theory

The theory associated with the UV reflection process is closely related to how reflected light is used in visual examination. The principal difference is in the wavelength of the radiation used. The short-wave (UVC) radiation used for fingermark enhancement usually has a principal output at 254 nm.

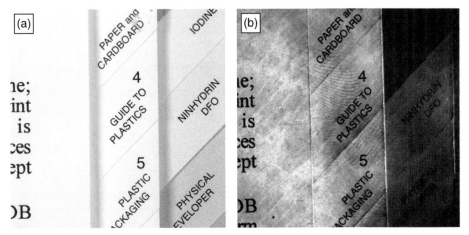

Figure 6.29 Latent fingermarks detected on glossy paper by short-wave UV reflection: (a) appearance under visible light, (b) appearance under reflected UVC radiation.

On glossy paper, the principal mechanism used to produce contrast is absorption by the fingermark and reflection by the smooth paper surface (Figure 6.29). Fingermark residues can absorb UV strongly, with an absorption maximum occurring at 277 nm (Ohki, 1970). This is primarily due to absorption by fatty acids. Detection rates are greater on smooth papers where there is less scattering from the texture of the surface.

On smooth, non-porous surfaces, reflected UV provides contrast between the fingermark and the background because of a greater degree of reflection or scatter from the fingermark ridges than that from the background. This contrast may be enhanced by the fact that the background absorbs UV more strongly than the fingermark (as is the case with many types of glass) or by the fingermark having a more textured topography than the background and scattering more UV radiation towards the detection system. This effect is more pronounced in the UV region of the spectrum than in the visible region because the wavelength of the radiation is of a similar scale to the height of the fingermark ridges and hence is scattered more strongly. This preferential scattering by the mark is shown schematically in Figure 6.30.

An example of how short-wave UV reflection can reveal untreated fingermarks on smooth, non-porous surfaces is given in Figure 6.31.

6.5.3 The ultraviolet reflection process

Because UV radiation is not visible to the eye, specialist imaging systems are required to visualise marks. UV reflection requires a detection system that is either

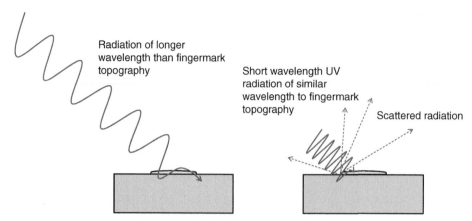

Figure 6.30 Schematic diagram showing how longer wavelength radiation is unaffected by the presence of the fingermark on the surface, whereas UV radiation of similar wavelength to the fingermark topography is scattered strongly.

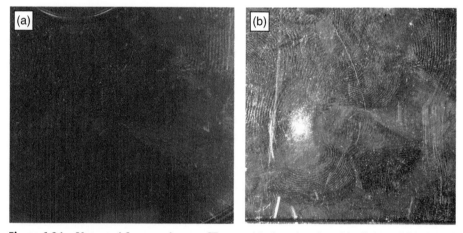

Figure 6.31 Untreated fingermarks on a CD case: (a) viewed under white light and (b) viewed under reflected UV radiation.

directly sensitive to UV radiation (e.g. a back-thinned sensor) or can convert UV radiation to visible output (e.g. an image intensifier). It also requires optics that can transmit short-wave UV radiation. Conventional glass optics are not suitable because they absorb UV radiation wavelengths below approximately 320 nm, so quartz or calcium fluoride are used for this purpose instead.

The effectiveness of UV reflection is influenced by a number of factors:

• The wavelength of radiation

• The angle of irradiation

- The properties of the surface in the UV region of the spectrum

- The filter used with the imaging system

The shorter the wavelength of radiation used, the more effective the process will be. In most cases, mercury vapour lamps with principal output at 254 nm are used in UV reflection. Mid-wave or long-wave UV radiation can also be used, but the longer wavelengths are further from the absorption peak of fingermark constituents, and are not as strongly scattered by fingermark residues.

As is the case for visual examination, the angle of irradiation can be important in the detection of fingermarks. Lighting from oblique angles up to 45° to the surface is best in maximising the scattering from fingermarks on smooth non-porous surfaces. Detection of absorbing fingermarks on smooth, porous surfaces is less influenced by the angle of incidence, although uniform lighting is preferred.

The properties of the surface may also influence detection of the mark. Some materials such as glass may absorb UV radiation, providing a dark background that provides better contrast with the scattering from the marks. Other materials such as printing inks that have different colours in the visible region of the spectrum may reflect UV in the same way, and therefore UV reflection may reduce the interfering effect of patterned backgrounds.

A short-wave UV bandpass filter is generally used in front of the detection system to block any fluorescence from the surface and any reflected radiation of other wavelengths that is emitted by the radiation source.

Because UV radiation can cause damage to both eyes and skin, it is essential that appropriate health and safety precautions are taken when using the process. Prolonged exposure to UV radiation can also degrade DNA, and therefore the process should be used with caution when recovery of DNA may also be a consideration.

6.6   Infrared reflection

6.6.1   Outline history of the process

1800: William Herschel proposed the existence of 'calorific rays'.

1930s: Use of IR reflection reported for forensic applications including visualisation of blood and footwear imaging, utilising IR-sensitive film.

1940s: Development of the first 'live view' IR imaging devices (vidicons).

1940s: First reported use of IR reflection for imaging of fingermarks.

1950s: First forensic applications of IR reflection in document examination.

1979: Wilkinson reported the use of IR reflection for the enhancement of a powdered mark on a dark bottle.

1984: Pearson, Creer, et al. described the use of IR reflection in enhancing marks developed using processes such as physical developer.

2005: Bleay and Kent reported the use of semi-live image capture systems for enhancing a range of marks using IR reflection.

6.6.2   Theory

In the near-IR (700–1100 nm) region of the electromagnetic spectrum, the mechanisms used for fingermark enhancement are essentially the same as those used in the visible and UV regions, namely, absorption/reflection. Fluorescence may also occur but this is little utilised for fingermark enhancement at present. The principal difference from the visible region is that many of the organic pigments used in printing inks are IR transparent and surfaces that appear highly patterned and/or coloured under white light may appear devoid of printing when viewed using IR reflection (Figure 6.32).

An application of IR reflection to remove interference from background patterns and text is illustrated in Figure 6.33.

6.6.3   The infrared reflection process

The IR reflection process requires three elements:

- An IR-sensitive imaging system

- A light source outputting IR radiation in the 700–1100 nm range

- An IR transmitting filter that blocks visible wavelengths of light

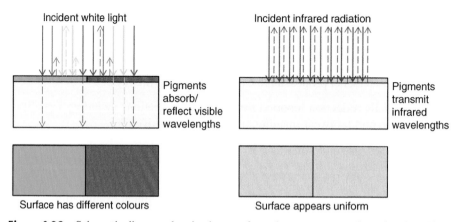

Figure 6.32   Schematic diagram showing how surfaces that can appear coloured under white light may appear uniform when viewed using infrared reflection.

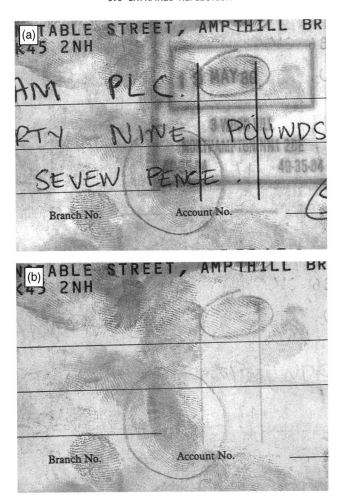

Figure 6.33 Images of fingerprint developed using physical developer on a patterned background: (a) imaged under tungsten illumination and (b) imaged under tungsten illumination using an infrared long-pass filter (Schott glass RG830).

IR radiation is not visible to the eye and specialist imaging systems are required to detect it. Although the sensors used in most digital imaging systems are sensitive to IR radiation, UV/IR blocking filters are generally bonded to the sensor to improve the response in the visible region, and this must be removed before the system can be used for IR reflection.

Light sources that output IR radiation are also required. Fluorescent tubes and white LEDs are not suitable because they have no IR output, and incandescent tungsten lamps or LEDs should be used instead.

To view the reflected IR radiation and block the visible region of the spectrum, long-pass filters with a cut-on wavelength in the IR region of the spectrum are used in front of the imaging system. A range of glass filters are available giving cut-on wavelengths between 645 and 1000 nm. Although the lower wavelength filters do have some use in document examination, those of most use in suppression of patterned/coloured backgrounds during fingermark enhancement include Schott glass filters RG715, RG780, RG850 and RG1000.

To date, it does not seem that latent fingermarks can be detected by IR reflection and applications are restricted to enhancement of developed marks. Marks developed using deposition processes using inorganic or metallic materials including vacuum metal deposition, powders and powder suspensions either absorb or scatter IR radiation more than the background, and thus developed marks remain visible when imaged in the IR. Many organic reagents and dyes including ninhydrin, Solvent Black 3 and cyanoacrylate are transparent in the near-IR region, and marks developed using these processes are not detected during IR reflection.

6.7 Colour filtration and monochromatic illumination

6.7.1 Outline history of the process

1940: Home Office publication 'Notes on Fingerprints and Palmprints' listed several methods of colour filtration for detecting and enhancing fingermarks.

1954: Cherrill's 1954 publication 'The Finger Print System at Scotland Yard' expanded on the use of colour filtration for fingermark imaging.

1980s: UK Home Office developed the Quaserchrome system, allowing monochromatic illumination to be performed using high intensity arc lamp systems.

6.7.2 Theory

The fundamental concept used during colour filtration and monochromatic illumination is the colour wheel, a representation of which is illustrated in Figure 6.34.

This displays the colours of the visible region of the spectrum as a circle, although 'purples' are added to the colours seen in the true spectrum to represent a combination of the violets and reds at the extreme ends of visible light.

In this representation, it can be seen that there are primary colours and secondary colours formed by the combination of pairs of primary colours (e.g. orange = red + yellow). Each colour on the wheel has its own complementary colour.

Colour filtration uses these colour relationships to enhance the visibility of the fingermark ridges against the background, and there are several ways in which it can be applied. The principal methods employed are to increase the contrast between the fingermark ridges and the background and to suppress the interfering effects of a patterned background. The success of the process relies on the fingermark ridges and/or the background being coloured.

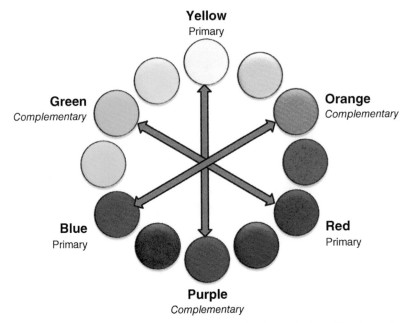

Figure 6.34   The concept of the colour wheel, used as the basis of colour filtration and monochromatic illumination.

For situations where coloured fingermark ridges are present against a light background, colour filtration can be used to increase the contrast of the ridges by using
a filter of the complementary colour to the ridges (Figure 6.35).

In this scenario, the purple-red ridges absorb green light and reflect blue and red,
and the surface reflects all colours. The coloured filter blocks the blue and red light,
so the imaging system detects reflected green light from the surface (which appears
light) but very little from the fingermark (which has absorbed the green light). As a
consequence, the fingermark appears darker in relation to the surface than it would
do under white light.

A similar effect can be utilised if light-coloured fingermarks are present on a
coloured surface. In this case the contrast can be increased by selecting a filter of a
complementary colour to the surface (Figure 6.36).

In this case the background is darkened in relation to the background, increasing
the contrast with the white ridges.

The other way in which colour filtration can be used is to enhance fingermarks in
situations where they have been deposited on patterned backgrounds with printing
of a single colour. In these cases the filter is chosen to match the printed background
as closely as possible, effectively cancelling out the background colour and allowing the flow of the ridges to be distinguished (Figure 6.37).

Colour filtration will only be effective if a filter can be selected that either matches
or complements the colours present in the mark and/or background. A limited range
of coloured filters are available and therefore this approach is not always possible.

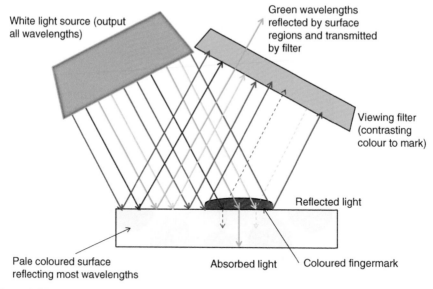

Figure 6.35 A schematic diagram showing how colour filtration can be used to increase the contrast of coloured ridges against a light background, by selecting a filter of complementary colour to the fingermark ridges.

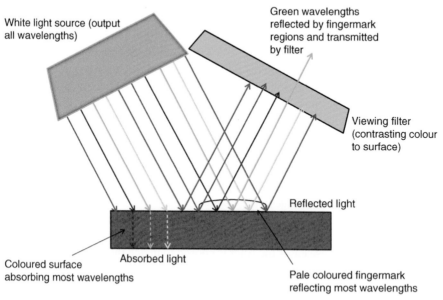

Figure 6.36 A schematic diagram showing how colour filtration can be used to increase the contrast of white ridges against a coloured background, by selecting a filter of complementary colour to the background.

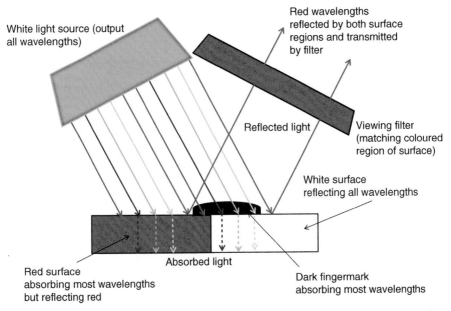

Figure 6.37 A schematic diagram showing how colour filtration can be used to suppress the interfering effect of coloured, patterned backgrounds, by selecting a coloured filter to match the coloured background.

Colour filtration can also be applied in a more discriminating, dynamic way using the monochromatic illumination process.

Monochromatic illumination utilises a linear filter in combination with a narrow slit and a high intensity white light source to select a small region (typically ~25 nm) of the visible spectrum that is used to illuminate the surface (Figure 6.38).

By varying the position of the linear filter in front of the slit, it is possible to tune the colour of illumination that falls on the surface and to match or contrast the colours much more closely than is achievable with simple colour filtration. The use of monochromatic illumination to produce contrast and to match background colours is shown in Figure 6.39.

6.7.3 The colour filtration/monochromatic illumination process

The colour filtration process requires a set of coloured filters and a white light source or a set of light sources with different coloured outputs. The colour of filter (or light source) is selected to provide contrast with or cancel the colours present in the mark or surface, as shown in the Theory section earlier. If the range of filters or light sources does not sufficiently match or contrast with the colours present, monochromatic illumination can be used to provide finer control over the illumination conditions used and greater discrimination between colours that are very close in

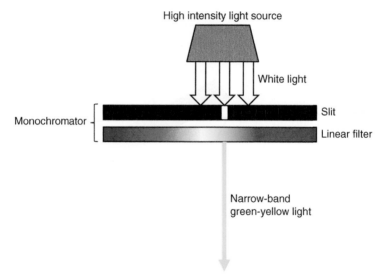

Figure 6.38 Schematic diagram illustrating how monochromatic illumination is produced from a linear filter – slit combination and a high intensity light source.

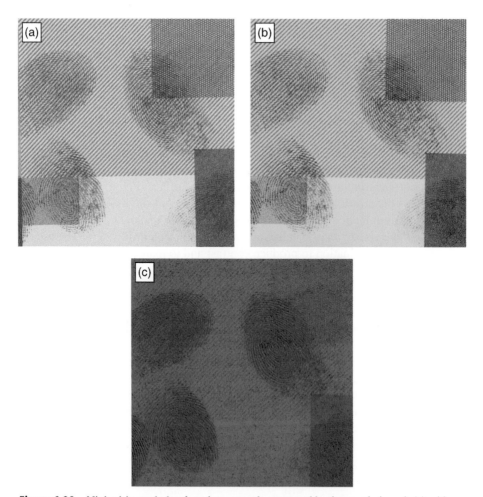

Figure 6.39 Ninhydrin mark developed on a purple patterned background viewed: (a) with white light illumination, (b) with green monochromatic illumination and (c) with red monochromatic illumination.

spectral output. However, monochromatic illumination is not capable of contrasting or cancelling backgrounds in circumstances where multiple colours are present, where processes such as multispectral imaging may be of more use.

6.8 Multispectral imaging

6.8.1 Outline history of the process

Late 1990s: The first multispectral imaging systems specifically for forensic application became commercially available.

2003: Exline et al. demonstrated that chemically treated fingerprints can be imaged in both absorption and fluorescence modes using multispectral imaging systems, the improved spectral resolution obtained revealing more ridge detail than conventional imaging routes.

2005: Tahtouh et al. demonstrated that multispectral imaging in the IR region of the spectrum can also be utilised for enhancement of marks developed using other processes.

6.8.2 Theory

Multispectral imaging describes a range of techniques that all ultimately result in the capture of a digital image providing both spatial and spectral information, with each pixel having a reflectivity or fluorescence spectrum associated with it.

The approach most commonly used for multispectral imaging in the visible to near-IR region is to use a monochrome sensor array in combination with a tunable filter or a series of light sources. Different tunable filter technologies are available, including liquid crystal and acousto-optical, but both types operate in essentially the same way. The tunable filter is a narrow bandwidth bandpass filter (typically with bandwidth in the range 2–20 nm) for which the central wavelength of the bandpass can be controlled within the selected wavelength range. When carrying out multispectral imaging, the surface and fingermark are illuminated with an appropriate light source and the tunable filter programmed to capture monochrome images at set wavelength intervals over the selected wavelength range. Alternatively, an equivalent set of images may be obtained by illuminating the surface and fingermark with a series of light sources with different wavelength outputs. The series of monochrome images thus collected are known as an 'image cube' (or 'image stack') and can be interpreted by software to give an RGB (i.e. colour) representation of the surface, as shown schematically in Figure 6.40.

Once the 'image cube' has been obtained, a range of processing techniques can be applied to the spatial and spectral information to extract the desired information.

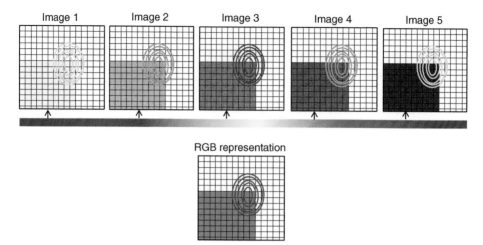

Figure 6.40 A schematic illustration of how a series of images are collected by a multispectral imager to form an 'image cube' and the corresponding RGB representation.

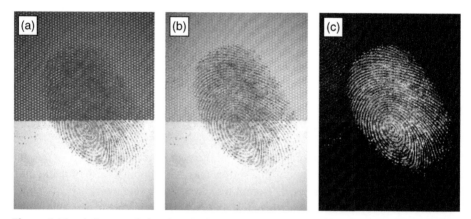

Figure 6.41 A fingermark developed using ninhydrin over a purple printed pattern: (a) RGB representation of the image cube collected by a multispectral imaging system, (b) a false colour, unmixed image and (c) an image showing the distribution of the ninhydrin colour spectrum only.

In the simplest form of analysis, regions with the desired spectrum (e.g. ninhydrin) can be identified, as can the spectra associated with regions of unwanted background colour/pattern. These can be assigned false colours and the image unmixed to show the fingermark in greater contrast. Alternatively, the regions corresponding to each colour channel can be viewed individually to see if any of these show the fingermark more clearly than the unmixed image (Figure 6.41).

For images where there are multiple colours in the background and the developed fingermark crossing several colour boundaries, other approaches such as principal component analysis can be adopted to separate out the major spectral responses from the image or a pure spectrum can be calculated from a subtraction from regions of background and mixed background/fingermark spectrum.

6.8.3   The multispectral imaging process

The multispectral imaging process requires specialist equipment to capture the set of images that form the image cube.

For multispectral imaging systems that utilise a tunable filter for image collection, it is essential that a white light source with an even beam and an output that is consistent across the visible and near-IR regions of the spectrum is used. Illumination sources such as fluorescent tubes that have gaps in their output are not suitable for multispectral imaging because useful images will not be collected at wavelengths corresponding to the gaps in output.

For multispectral imaging systems that utilise a series of light sources during image collection, the surface being imaged should be situated so that the only light incident on it comes from the coloured light source and not from any stray ambient light.

References

Anderson J, Bramble S, 'The effects of fingermark enhancement light sources on subsequent PCR-STR DNA analysis of fresh bloodstains', J Forensic Sci, vol 42(2), (1997), p 303–306.

Bandey, H (ed.), 'Fingermark Visualisation Manual', Home Office, London, 2014, ISBN 978-1-78246-234-7.

Beavan C, 'Fingerprints', Fourth Estate, London, 2002, ISBN 1-84115-739-2.

Benson J R, Hare P E, 'o-Phthalaldehyde: fluorogenic detection of primary amines in the picomole range. Comparison with fluorescamine and ninhydrin', Proc Natl Acad Sci U S A, vol 72(2), (1975), p 619–622.

Bleay S M, Kent T, 'The use of infra-red filters to remove background patterns in fingerprint imaging', Fingerprint World, vol 31(122), (2005), p 225–238.

Bloch O, 'Developments in infra-red photography', Phot J, vol 72, (1932), p 324–340.

Brose H L, 'Finger-print detection', Analyst, vol 59, (1934), p 25–27.

Cherrill F R, 'The Finger Print System at Scotland Yard', HMSO, London, 1954.

Clark W, 'Photography by Infrared: Its Principles and Applications', 2nd edition, John Wiley & Sons, Inc, London, 1946, ISBN1406744867.

Creer K E, 'The detection and enhancement of latent marks using specialised lighting and imaging techniques', Proceedings of the International Symposium on Fingerprint Detection and Identification, 26–30 June 1995, Ne'urim, Israel.

Creer K E, Brennan J S, 'The work of the serious crime unit', Proceedings of the International Forensic Symposium on Latent Prints, 7–10 July 1987, FBI Academy, Quantico, VA, p 91–99.

Dalrymple B E, Duff J M, Menzel E R, 'Inherent fingerprint luminescence – detection by laser', J Forensic Sci, vol 22(1), (1977), p 106–115.

Drabarek B, Siejca A, Moszczyński J, Konior B, 'Applying anti-stokes phosphors in development of fingerprints on surfaces characterized by strong luminescence', J Forensic Identif, vol 62(1), (2012), p 28–35.

Ellen D M, Creer K, 'Infra-red luminescence in examination of documents', J Forensic Sci Soc, vol 10, (1970), p 159–164.

Exline D L, Wallace C, Roux C, Lennard C, Nelson M P, Treado P J, 'Forensic applications of chemical imaging: latent fingerprint detection using visible absorption and luminescence', J Forensic Sci, vol 48, (2003), p 1047–1053.

Faulds H, 'On the skin-furrows of the hand', Nature, vol 22, (1880), p 605.

Fraval H, Bennett A, Springer E, 'UV detection of untreated latent fingerprints', Proceedings of the International Symposium on Fingerprint Detection and Identification, 26–30 June 1995, Ne'urim, Israel.

German E R, 'Reflected ultraviolet imaging system applications', Proceedings of the International Symposium on Fingerprint Detection and Identification, 26–30 June 1995, Ne'urim, Israel.

Grigg R, Mongkolaussavaratana T, Pounds C A, Sivagnanam S, '1,8-Diazafluorenone and related compounds: a new reagent for the detection of α-amino acids and latent fingerprints', Tetrahedron Lett, vol 31(49), (1990), p 7215–7218.

Hardwick S A, Kent T, Sears V G, 'Fingerprint Detection by Fluorescence Examination – A Guide to Operational Implementation', PSDB Publication No. 3/90, 1990.

Herod D W, Menzel E R, 'Laser detection of latent fingerprints: ninhydrin followed by zinc chloride', J Forensic Sci, vol 27(3), (1982), p 513–518.

Hilton O, 'Traced forgery and infra red photography', Int Crim Police Rev, vol 159, (1962), p 195–197.

Home Office, 'Notes on Fingerprints and Palmprints Left at Scenes of Crime, With Suggestions as to Their Detection and Preservation, and Notes on Photography', HMSO, London, 1940.

Hunter F, Biver S, Fuqua P, 'Light Science and Magic: An Introduction to Photographic Lighting', 4th edition, Focal Press, London, 2011.

Langford M J, 'Advanced Photography', 4th edition, Focal Press Ltd, London, 1980, ISBN 0-240-51029-1.

Ma R, Bullock E, Maynard P, Reedy B, Shimmon R, Lennard C, Roux C, McDonagh A, 'Fingermark detection on non-porous and semi-porous surfaces using NaYF4:Er,Yb up-converter particles', Forensic Sci Int, vol 207(1–3), (2011), p 145–149.

Martin F W, 'Infra-red rays in criminal investigation', Br Med J, vol 1, (1933), p 1025–1026.

Menzel E R, 'Fingerprint Detection with Lasers', Marcel Dekker, New York, 1980.

Menzel E R, Burt J A, Sinor T W, Tubach-Ley W B, Jordan K J, 'Laser detection of latent fingerprints: treatment with glue containing ester', J Forensic Sci, vol 28(2), (1983), p 307–317.

Ohki H, 'Physio-chemical study of latent fingerprint: 1, ultraviolet absorption and fluorescence of human epidermal secretion', Rep Natl Res Inst Police Sci (Jpn), vol 23(1), (1970), p 33–40.

Payne G, Reedy B, Lennard C, Comber B, Exline D, Roux C, 'A further study to investigate the detection and enhancement of latent fingerprints using visible absorption and luminescence chemical imaging', Forensic Sci Int, vol 150(1), (2005), p 33–51.

Qiang W G, 'Detecting and enhancing latent fingerprints with short wave UV reflection photography', Proceedings of the International Symposium on Fingerprint Detection and Identification, 26–30 June 1995, Ne'urim, Israel.

Radley J A, Grant J, 'Fluorescence Analysis in Ultra-Violet Light', 4th edition, D Van Nostrand Company Inc., New York, 1954.

Rhodes H T F, 'Some Persons Unknown', John Murray, London, 1931.

Saito N, Arai S, 'The detection of fingerprint by ultraviolet ray television', Rep Natl Res Inst Police Sci (Jpn), vol 25(1), (1972), p 57–58.

Tahtouh M, Kalman J R, Roux C, Lennard C, Reedy B J, 'The detection and enhancement of latent fingermarks using infrared chemical imaging', J Forensic Sci, vol 50(1), (2005), p 1–9.

Von Bremen U, 'Systematic application of specialised photographic techniques', J Crim Law Criminol Police Sci, vol 58(3), (1967), p 410–413.

Wilkinson R D, 'The use of infrared microscopy in detecting latent fingerprints', Identif News, August 1979, p 10–11.

Further reading

Akiba N, Saitoh N, Kuroki K, 'Fluorescence spectra and images of latent fingerprints excited with a tunable laser in the ultraviolet region', J Forensic Sci, vol 52(5), (2007), p 1103–1106.

Bandey H, Bleay S, Bowman V, Fitzgerald L, Gibson A, Hart A, Sears V, 'Fingerprint imaging across EM spectrum', Imaging Sci J, vol 54, (2006), p 211–219.

Bramble S K, Creer K E, Qiang W G, Sheard B, 'Ultraviolet luminescence from latent fingerprints', Forensic Sci Int, vol 59, (1993), p 3–14.

Dalrymple B E, 'Use of narrow band-pass filters to enhance detail in latent fingerprint photography by laser', J Forensic Sci, vol 27(4), (1982), p 801–804.

Herod D W, Menzel E R, 'Spatially resolved fluorescence spectroscopy: application to latent fingerprint development', J Forensic Sci, vol 28(3), (1983), p 615–622.

Keith L V, Runion W, 'Short-wave UV imaging casework applications', J Forensic Identif, vol 48(5), (1998), p 563–569.

Marsh N, 'Forensic Photography: A Practitioner's Guide', Wiley-Blackwell, London, 2014, ISBN 978-1119975823.

Menzel E R, 'Laser detection of latent fingerprints – treatment with phosphorescers', J Forensic Sci, vol 24(3), (1979), p 582–585.

Menzel E R, 'Detection of latent fingerprints by laser-excited luminescence', Anal Chem, vol 61(8), (1989), p 557–561.

Menzel E R, 'Lanthanide-based fingerprint detection', Fingerprint World, vol 23(88), (1997), p 45–51.

Menzel E R, 'Fingerprint Detection with Lasers', 2nd edition, CRC Press, Boca Raton, FL, 1999.

Menzel E R, Duff J M, 'Laser detection of latent fingerprints – treatment with fluorescers', J Forensic Sci, vol 24(1), (1979), p 96–100.

Nissim B Y, Almog J, Frank A, Springer E, Cantu A, 'Short UV luminescence for forensic applications: design of a real time observation system for detection of latent fingerprints and body fluids', J Forensic Sci, vol 43(2), (1998), p 299–304.

Pearson E F, Creer K, Brennan J S, Newson N E, Pounds C A, 'An advanced technology unit for the detection of fingerprints', Proceedings of the E.E.C International Fingerprint Conference, 27–30 November 1984, London.

Pfister R, 'The optical revelation of latent fingerprints', Fingerprint Whorld, vol 10(39), (1985), p 64–70.

Saferstein R, Graf S, 'Evaluation of a reflected UV imaging system for fingerprint detection', J Forensic Identif, vol 51(4), (2001), p 385–393.

Tahtouh M, Despland P, Shimmon R, Kalman J R, Reedy B J, 'The application of infrared chemical imaging to the detection and enhancement of latent fingerprints: method optimisation and further findings', J Forensic Sci, vol 52(5), (2007), p 1089–1096.

7

Vapour phase techniques

Stephen M. Bleay[1] and Marcel de Puit[2]

[1] Home Office Centre for Applied Science and Technology, Sandridge, UK

[2] Ministerie van Veiligheid en Justitie, Nederlands Forensisch Instituut, Digitale Technologie en Biometrie, The Hague, The Netherlands

---

Key points

- There are a wide range of vapour phase processes available for fingermark enhancement, and these utilise a number of different mechanisms.

- The processes that are most widely used operate by selective deposition and growth of material on the surface or by selective absorption of the vapour into the fingermark.

- These processes generally have low impact on the item being treated and are used towards the beginning of processing sequences.

7.1 Introduction

The principal advantage of vapour phase techniques is that they are generally low impact to the surface being treated and do not react with constituents within the mark, meaning that other processes can generally be used after them.

The use of vapour phase techniques dates back to the 1860s, when fumes of iodine were observed to detect traces of fingermarks on paper (Quinche and Margot, 2010). Vapour phase techniques including iodine and osmium tetroxide were amongst the earliest chemical development processes, being proposed for fingermark development in the 1920s (Mitchell, 1920).

The next vapour phase techniques to be proposed for fingermark enhancement were vacuum metal deposition and radioactive sulphur dioxide, both first reported

---

Fingerprint Development Techniques: Theory and Application, First Edition.
Stephen M. Bleay, Ruth S. Croxton and Marcel de Puit.
© 2018 John Wiley & Sons Ltd. Published 2018 by John Wiley & Sons Ltd.

in the 1960s (Grant et al., 1963a; Theys et al., 1968) and developed for operational work from the 1970s onwards. The vacuum metal deposition process involved selective deposition of metals from a vapour phase onto a surface held within a vacuum chamber, and radioactive sulphur dioxide utilised radioactively labelled sulphur dioxide gas, which was selectively absorbed by the fingermark. The mark could then be subsequently visualised by placing the article between sheets of photographic paper, which were locally developed by the radioactive particles emitted from the ridges.

The most significant vapour phase process is superglue/cyanoacrylate fuming, which was first noted in the late 1970s (Haines, 1982; Wood, 1991) and utilised as an operational technique from the early 1980s onwards. The ease of use and high effectiveness of the process has seen it become the primary development technique for non-porous surfaces in many laboratories, and the number of marks detected can be increased further by the use of fluorescent dyes.

There are a range of other rarely used techniques that utilise the vapour phase, utilising a range of different mechanisms to visualise fingerprints. A summary of these is given at the end of this chapter.

7.2   Current operational use

The most widely used of all of the vapour phase processes is superglue, or cyanoacrylate fuming. Cyanoacrylate fuming is one of the most effective processes for development of fingermarks on most non-porous surfaces and is in regular use around the world. It is simple to carry out and can be applied using improvised equipment as well as in specialist processing cabinets. The technique can also be used at crime scenes and on vehicles, and a range of equipment has been developed for this purpose.

The versatility of the process is matched by the number of ways in which marks can be enhanced post development, including ultraviolet reflection, powdering, vacuum metal deposition and the use of fluorescent dyes in a range of solvents. The recent introduction of effective one-step cyanoacrylate fuming processes (Prete et al., 2013; Groeneveld et al., 2014) that produce inherently fluorescent marks has made the process useful for a wider range of surface types, including semi-porous surfaces where it was not possible to use solvent-based fluorescent dyes to enhance developed marks.

Cyanoacrylate fuming is anticipated to remain one of the principal techniques available for fingermark development, although there are some applications for which powder suspensions (see Chapter 12) may supersede it, especially where the environmental exposure of the exhibit is unknown. The ability of powder suspensions to continue to develop marks on surfaces that have been wetted is an advantage over cyanoacrylate fuming in this respect.

Because of the specialist nature and the high cost of the equipment used to carry out vacuum metal deposition, its use has always been confined to specialist laboratories. Vacuum metal deposition was until recently recommended as the primary process for development of fingermarks on polymeric bags and wrappings. Although still effective in this role, it is no longer as effective as alternative processes such as cyanoacrylate fuming and powder suspensions (Downham et al., 2012), possibly because of the increased recycled content of these materials and the presence of recycling additives in the surface layers that can inhibit metal deposition.

Vacuum metal deposition can be used on nearly all types of non-porous surface and is one of the more effective techniques on 'semi-porous' surfaces such as glossy magazines and wrapping paper. There is much overlap between the types of item that can be treated with vacuum metal deposition and those that are treated using cyanoacrylate fuming. In many cases, the deciding factor in which technique is to be used is whether the article has been wetted, because vacuum metal deposition remains effective on wetted items whereas cyanoacrylate fuming is generally not. In practice it is possible to use the two processes in sequence, and more marks may be detected in this way because the two processes work on different fingermark constituents. Vacuum metal deposition is one of a very limited number of processes that are capable of developing fingermarks on fabrics (Hambley, 1972; Fraser et al., 2011; Knighting et al., 2013), and it is also an important process for enhancing marks on polymeric banknotes, which are growing in usage worldwide.

Iodine fuming is still used in several countries and has the advantage that it is generally non-destructive to non-metallic articles such as paper documents. The developed marks will gradually disappear if they are not fixed, and this can also be an advantage when treating high value items that cannot be immersed in liquids or left with permanent signs of treatment. It is also a cheap process to carry out and requires little in the way of equipment or chemicals. It is however significantly less effective than amino acid reagents on porous surfaces, and its effectiveness falls rapidly as the age of the mark increases because the constituent it principally targets (squalene) decomposes rapidly with time. Iodine is not generally used when amino acid reagents are available.

Radioactive sulphur dioxide was used for nearly 30 years in certain specialist laboratories as a method for treating fabrics and adhesive tapes. Due to some early successes in casework in the early 1970s (Godsell, 1972), it became a treatment that was routinely requested in high profile cases, particularly those related to terrorism (Smith, 1981). However, the complexity of the equipment and the issues associated with the handling of radioactive substances meant that use of the technique declined and since 2005 there has been no laboratory in the United Kingdom able to carry out the technique. It is included in this book to give an indication of the range of fingermark enhancement processes that can be utilised and because it has not been fully described in any previous publication of this type.

Most of the other vapour phase processes summarised in Section 7.7 are not widely used because they are either less effective than other techniques or there are health and safety issues associated with their use. In particular there are concerns about the fuming of concentrated acids because they are highly corrosive. In general, all vapour phase processes need to be well contained and carried out in areas with good ventilation.

7.3 Superglue/cyanoacrylate fuming

7.3.1 Outline history of the process

1940s: Cyanoacrylate-based adhesive formulated by researchers developing an acrylic polymer to produce gun sights for the aircraft industry.

1950s: Coover and Joyner formulated the first commercial polycyanoacrylate adhesive, Eastman #910, which is first marketed in 1958.

Late 1970s: Exposure to superglue vapour reported apparently independently in Japan, North America and the United Kingdom as a possible method for the development of latent fingermarks.

Early 1980s: Research into mechanisms for initiation of cyanoacrylate fuming, including heating the glue to accelerate the process (Besonen, 1983; Olenik, 1984) and the use of other accelerating agents including sodium hydroxide (Kendall and Rehn, 1983) and sodium carbonate (Martindale, 1983).

Early 1980s: Commercial, purpose-built cyanoacrylate fuming chambers began to be manufactured. These cabinets are fitted with a heat and a separate humidity source (cotton doped in water for example) and a ventilator. The ventilator provides circulation of the air in the cabinet, so that the evaporated cyanoacrylate is distributed throughout the cabinet.

1983: Menzel et al. proposed the use of Rhodamine 6G (Basic Red 1) as a fluorescent stain for marks developed using cyanoacrylate fuming, either applied as a stain or by evaporation. Other fluorescent dye stains such as Ardrox (Olsen, 1984) and Basic Yellow 40 (Kent, 1986) were subsequently introduced.

Mid-1980s: Research by the UK Home Office demonstrated that for optimum development on most surfaces, the relative humidity within the treatment chamber should be maintained at $80 \pm 2\%$. A controlled humidity, rapid superglue treatment chamber was developed to provide these conditions.

1993: Weaver described initial attempts to develop a one-step fluorescent cyanoacrylate fuming process.

Mid-1990s: Introduction of the vacuum cyanoacrylate fuming process as an alternative to processing at ambient temperature and pressure at elevated humidity (Watkin et al., 1994; Hebrand et al., 1995).

2000s: Fundamental studies into fingermark constituents responsible for cyanoacrylate polymerisation (Lewis et al., 2001; Wargacki et al., 2007).

2010: McLaren et al. proposed methylamine as a pretreatment for reintroducing moisture to dehydrated marks and increasing process effectiveness for older fingermarks.

Early 2010s: Introduction of one-step fluorescent cyanoacrylate fuming processes with significantly improved effectiveness.

7.3.2 Theory

Marks developed by superglue become visible because white deposits are preferentially formed on fingermark ridges during treatment. These deposits are structures of polycyanoacrylate, formed by the polymerisation of a cyanoacrylate monomer. Figure 7.1 shows the molecular structure of ethyl cyanoacrylate, the most commonly used monomer for fingermark enhancement. Other esters, such as methyl cyanoacrylate or butyl cyanoacrylate, may also be used for the polymerisation reaction. It was found however in very early studies that the ethyl ester gave the best results for the visualisation of latent fingermarks, and this was supported by a recent study (Casault et al., 2016) that compared various alkyl cyanoacrylates (methyl, ethyl, *n*-butyl and 2-octyl) and found that ethyl and butyl polymers formed polymer microstructures that scattered light more effectively than methyl and octyl polymers.

In this section the general principles behind the polymerisation will be explained. Organic reactions, including polymerisation, take place by a transfer of electrons from one molecule to the other. The polymerisation reaction of cyanoacrylate, which can be regarded as a very good electrophile, needs to be initiated by a nucleophile. In general terms of organic synthetic chemistry, an electrophile accepts electrons dominated by a nucleophile. This means that any entity in a fingermark carrying a free electron pair can initiate the polymerisation.

A prime example of the simplicity of the reaction was shown by Thiburce et al. (2011) who demonstrated a solution of sodium hydroxide could be used as a form of a positive control test in a cyanoacrylate fuming cabinet to check that it is functioning properly. By leaving a small amount of this strong nucleophile in the cabinet where the evidential material is being treated, the hydroxide will act as an initiator of the polymerisation. Therefore the white polymer will appear on the drop of the sodium hydroxide solution whilst simultaneously generating a contrast between the latent fingermark and the substrate it has been deposited on.

In general a polymerisation reaction follows three distinct steps:

- Initiation

- Propagation

- Termination

In Figure 7.2 the initiation reaction and first propagation reaction of the polymerisation are shown. A nucleophile, here shown as Nu⁻, will donate its electrons to

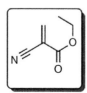

Figure 7.1   The molecular structure of ethyl cyanoacrylate.

an electrophilic centre. An arrow represents the movement of the electrons from the nucleophile to the CH$_2$ side group of the ethyl cyanoacrylate. The double carbon–carbon bond will open up and leave a single carbon–carbon bond that is now attached to the nucleophile. At the same time the electrons involved in this process will be pushed further into the cyanoacrylate, and an intramolecular cascade of electronic movements takes place. Ultimately, when the carbon–oxygen double bond is broken, the electrons will attach to a proton (H$^+$), and a new oxygen–hydrogen bond is formed. After the formation of this stable ketal intermediate, the generated hydroxide (OH$^-$) can act as a base to pull the proton of the ketal intermediate. That particular step can be the trigger for the propagation reaction, which results in a new intermolecular cascade of electron movements, involving a second cyanoacrylate monomer. This propagation reaction goes through a negatively charged intermediate, shown in the box in Figure 7.2.

This intermediate is one of the reasons that the polymerisation of cyanoacrylate is so successful. The negative charge can be located on the tertiary carbon, and this intermediate is stable as the negative charge can be distributed over the cyano group (the carbon–nitrogen triple bond) and the ester group, as shown in Figure 7.3.

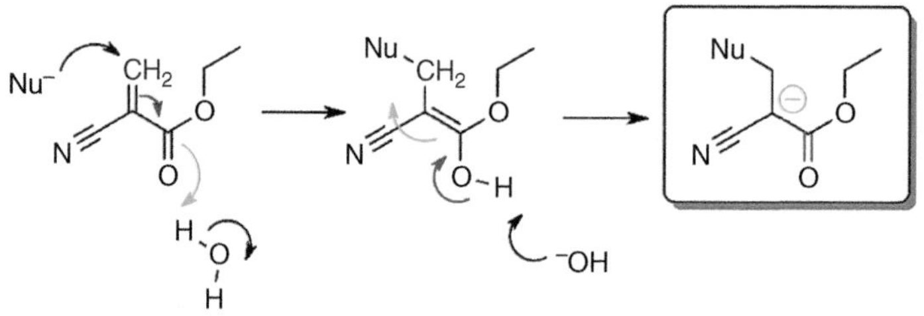

Figure 7.2   Initiation and first propagation of the polymerisation of ethyl cyanoacrylate.

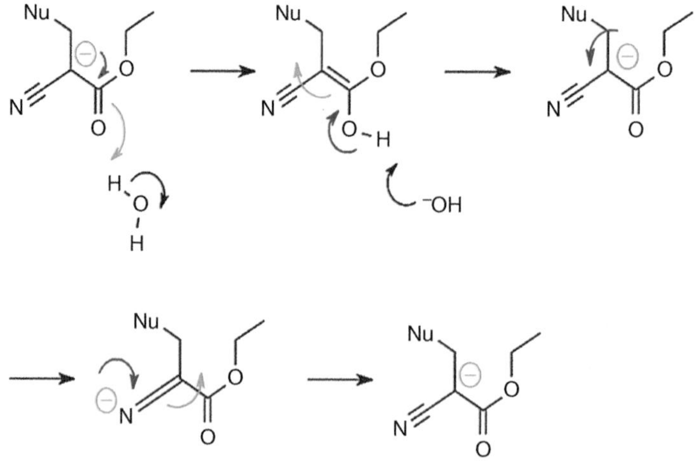

Figure 7.3   Delocalisation of the negative charge, stabilising the reaction intermediate.

After the initiation reaction (Figure 7.2), a propagation reaction follows to leave another stable intermediate, which is shown in Figure 7.4. The hydroxide produced in the initiation reaction can act as a base, accepting the proton of the stable intermediate (which in this case acts as an acid) in the same fashion as shown in Figure 7.2, only in this case to produce a nucleophilic attack on another monomeric form of ethyl cyanoacrylate.

The resulting intermediate of the propagation reaction, shown on the right-hand side in Figure 7.4, can undergo the same acid–base reaction as shown on the left-hand side in Figure 7.4. This process is still a part of the propagation step of the polymerisation, and the duration of this part is very much related to the ultimate length of the polymer. Ultimately the polymer will cease to grow, and the polymerisation is terminated by accepting a proton as shown in Figure 7.5.

The generic polymerisation reaction for all the types of cyanoacrylate monomers that can be used in the cyanoacrylate fuming process is shown in Figure 7.6.

Because cyanoacrylate polymerisation is base initiated, even weak bases such as water will initiate the polymerisation reaction described previously, and it was long thought that this was the primary constituent in fingermarks responsible for polymerisation. The importance of moisture in the fingermark prior to fuming was confirmed by Lewis and co-workers (2001), who observed that for eccrine marks the quality of the developed mark reduced as the mark dried out and moisture was

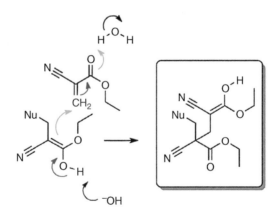

Figure 7.4 Propagation step in the polymerisation process.

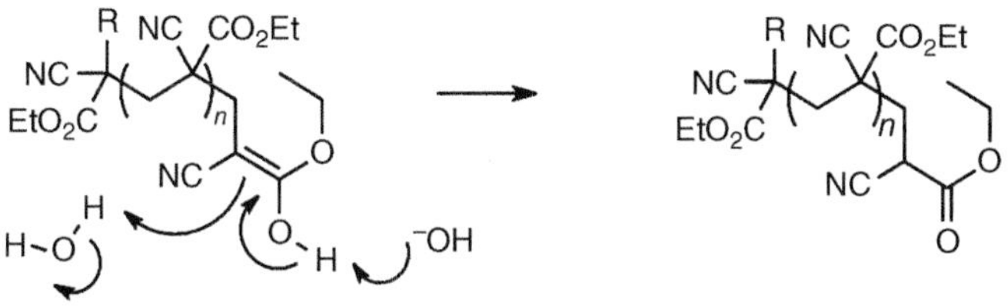

Figure 7.5 Termination of the polymerisation reaction.

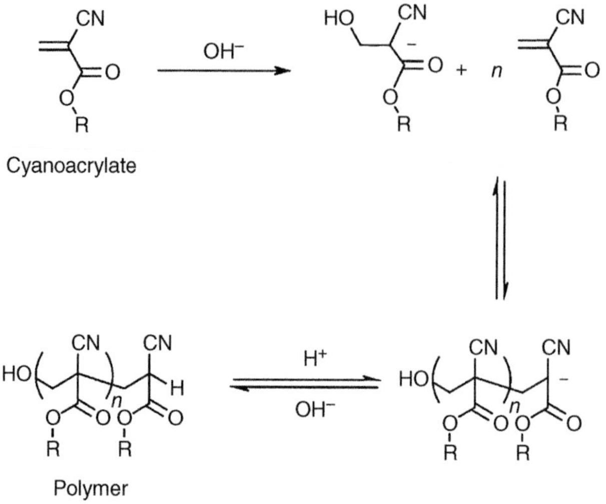

Figure 7.6 Generic polymerisation reaction for cyanoacrylate monomers (the -R group representing the different carbon chain lengths).

lost. Sebaceous marks were thought to retain moisture better and did not exhibit the same age dependence, although sebaceous constituents did not, in themselves, contribute to initiation of polymerisation.

However, there have been further studies to explore whether any other individual fingermark constituents could contribute to initiate of the polymerisation reaction. Lewis et al. (2001) thought that fingermarks contained multiple bases in addition to water that could initiate polymerisation. Wargacki et al. (2007) found that the polymerisation reaction could also be initiated by the lactate and alanine constituents of eccrine sweat, in both cases initiation occurring via the carboxylate functional group. There was no evidence that the amine functional group in alanine played any role in polymerisation. Wargacki et al. (2008) also proposed that the degradation of the lactate constituent under exposure to ultraviolet light was another contributing factor to the reduction in the quality of development for aged marks.

The presence of sodium chloride in the fingermark is thought to be important in the polymerisation process, but it is not believed to play a role in initiation of polymerisation itself. The role of sodium chloride can be best seen when cyanoacrylate fuming is conducted at different levels of relative humidity. It is believed that elevating the relative humidity to above 75% causes sodium chloride crystals in the latent fingermark to absorb water from the environment around it, which in turn aids in initiating the polymerisation reaction. It can be seen that the fingermark environment is a complex one, and it is possible that combinations of constituents are required for optimum polymerisation to occur, rather than any individual constituent in isolation.

What is known is that if the polymerisation conditions are changed, the microstructure of the resultant polycyanoacrylate deposits can change significantly, and this may be influenced by what constituents are responsible for initiation. Fundamental studies by Mankidy et al. (2008) have illustrated how a range of polymer structures can be obtained by altering initiation conditions. This is supported by observations by other researchers (Paine et al., 2011) looking at the development observed on fingermarks of different donors.

In the optimum range of relative humidity for fingermark development (75–90%), the fingermarks can reabsorb water from the environment, and electron microscopy shows that long, fibrous polymer deposits form on the fingermark (Figure 7.7), which make it more visible to the eye. This 'noodle-like' structure is also effective in retaining the fluorescent dyes subsequently used to enhance the marks.

Below 75% relative humidity developed fingermarks often appear to be 'patchy' and underdeveloped, and microscopy reveals the polymer structure to be much flatter in morphology (Figure 7.8).

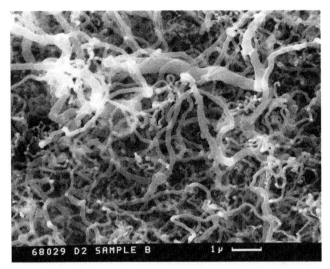

Figure 7.7 Electron micrograph of the fibrous deposits formed by cyanoacrylate fuming at a relative humidity of approximately 80%. Reproduced courtesy of the Home Office.

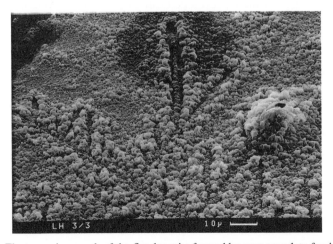

Figure 7.8 Electron micrograph of the flat deposits formed by cyanoacrylate fuming at a relative humidity of approximately 40%. Reproduced courtesy of the Home Office.

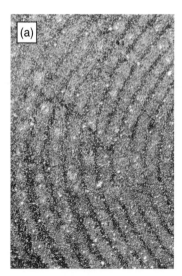 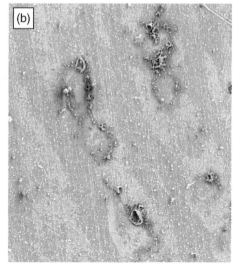

Figure 7.9 A fingermark developed at a relative humidity of approximately 100%: (a) high magnification photograph showing poor definition between ridges and furrows and (b) electron micrograph showing flat polymer structure. Reproduced courtesy of the Home Office (a) and London South Bank University (b).

Development at relative humidity levels above 90% causes an increased background development and reduced definition of the developed mark (Figure 7.9), possibly due to condensation beginning to occur on the surface that produces multiple initiation sites between the ridges. Electron microscopy shows a predominantly flat morphology with some raised features (Figure 7.9).

The microstructure of purely sebaceous marks developed at 80% relative humidity was found to differ considerably from eccrine and 'normal' marks, suggesting a different mode of polymer growth, Figure 7.10.

The microstructure of marks developed using cyanoacrylate fuming in a vacuum is different again, exhibiting a series of isolated droplets of polycyanoacrylate that are less visible by eye and also less receptive to subsequent dye staining (Figure 7.11).

In recent years there has been increased emphasis on the development of so-called one-step fluorescent cyanoacrylates, which successful commercial products beginning to emerge. Tahtouh et al. (2007) reported preparation of derivatives of alkyl 2-cyanoacrylates, which showed an increased IR activity, via a Knoevenagel and Diels–Alder/retro-Diels–Alder route. The exact synthetic route can be found in Tahtouh's full article. Although not in itself fluorescent, the preparation of these derivatives demonstrated that it was possible to produce one-step systems with increased functionality.

Almog and Gabay (1986) described a novel alternative to the liquid cyanoacrylate monomer and instead proposed the use of polycyanoacrylate for the fuming of latent fingermarks, which involved pyrolysis and subsequent polymerisation of the

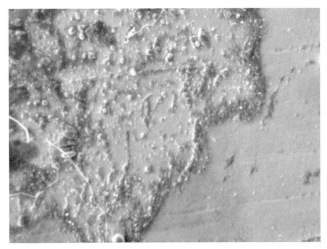

Figure 7.10   Scanning electron micrograph of the edge of a ridge of a sebaceous fingermark developed at 80% relative humidity (×1700 magnification). Reproduced courtesy of London South Bank University.

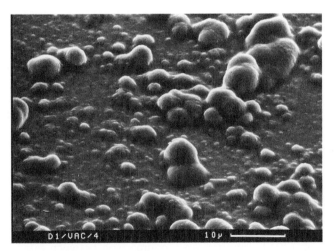

Figure 7.11   Scanning electron micrograph of a fingermark developed under vacuum conditions. Reproduced courtesy of the Home Office.

monomer thus created. One of the main benefits of this route for development was the use of an easy-to-handle powder, rather than the very reactive liquid monomer.

Bentolila et al. (2013) reported on the synthesis of ester derivatives of cyanoacrylate via a similar route, where the alkyl units in the monomer are replaced by fluorescent aryl entities. The cyanoacrylate monomeric derivatives obtained can be used in the same way as the alkyl-cyanoacrylate equivalents.

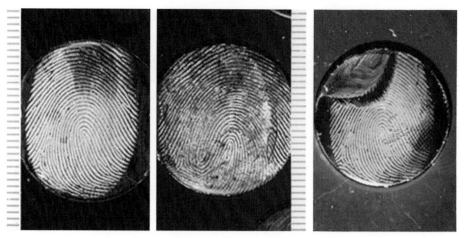

Figure 7.12 Examples of fingermarks developed using different initiators: (left) fingermark developed with DMAB-initiated polycyanoacrylate, producing blue fluorescence; (middle) fingermark developed using DMAC-initiated polycyanoacrylate, producing yellow fluorescence; and (right) fingermark developed with dansyl-initiated polycyanoacrylate, producing green fluorescence.

These developments lead to the insight that the use of polymeric entities, with predefined fluorescent initiators, could be used to visualise fingerprints. Groeneveld et al. (2014) described the use of commonly used fluorescent compounds for the initialisation of the polymerisation of cyanoacrylate. Typical images of fingermarks visualised with these reagents are shown in Figure 7.12.

Other approaches for the one-step development of latent fingermarks with cyanoacrylate, with the aim to introduce fluorescence in the visualised fingermark, have been described by adding a readily evaporated fluorophore (such as dimethylaminobenzaldehyde (DMAB)) to mono-cyanoacrylate before fuming the monomer. Several commercial formulations have been put on the market, with variable results.

Farrugia et al. (2014) reported on a comparison between one of these reagents, Lumicyano, and the conventional cyanoacrylate treatment with a Basic Yellow 40 post-treatment. The treatment of latent fingermarks deposited on LDPE, HDPE and cellulose carrier bags with Lumicyano showed similar results in terms of 'marks found fit for individualisation purposes' as the conventional cyanoacrylate treatment with a Basic Yellow 40 post-treatment. However, if the deposited fingermarks that were initially treated with Lumicyano underwent a post-treatment with Basic Yellow 40, additional marks suitable for individualisation were detected.

A comparison between several one-step luminescent fuming reagents and formulations was conducted by Khuu et al. (2016). In this study the following (commercially) available one-step fuming materials were compared to two-step processing with cyanoacrylate fuming followed by a post- treatment with the fluorescent dye Rhodamine 6G:

- CN Yellow Crystals (Aneval Inc.)
- PolyCyano UV (Foster + Freeman Ltd.)
- PECA Fluor Extra (BVDA)
- PECA Multiband (BVDA)
- Lumikit (Crime Scene Technology)

Although the two-step process generally gave better results on most of the surfaces examined, there were some surfaces such as polystyrene where the results produced with one-step systems were superior.

7.3.3 The cyanoacrylate fuming process

The chemicals and processing parameters used in situations where cyanoacrylate fuming is conducted in humidity-controlled processing cabinets are as follows:

Monomer:

Unthickened ethyl cyanoacrylate

Fuming initiation:

Hot plate heated to approximately 120°C

Humidity conditions:

80% relative humidity at approximately 20°C

The bases for the selection of these chemicals and processing parameters are described as follows:

Unthickened ethyl cyanoacrylate	The use of low viscosity (unthickened) ethyl cyanoacrylate is thought to give better results than those including thickeners, which may leave residual deposits in the aluminium pot. Methyl cyanoacrylate is thought to give similar results to the ethyl system, but other monomers are not generally recommended.
120°C hot plate temperature	This temperature is sufficiently hot to enable evaporation of the ethyl cyanoacrylate in a reasonable time frame, but not high enough to cause toxic degradation products such as hydrogen cyanide to be formed.
	One-step fluorescent cyanoacrylate systems utilising polycyanoacrylate powders require a higher hot plate temperature of ~230°C to degrade and evaporate the polymer. This is still low enough to avoid formation of unsafe levels of toxic gases.

80% relative humidity

The relative humidity level of 80% is required for some of the rehumidification processes outlined in Section 7.3.2 to occur. It is also important in controlling the microstructure of the polycyanoacrylate deposit that forms on the fingermark ridges (see Figures 7.7, 7.8 and 7.9). The noodle-like structure formed at 80% relative humidity is the optimum for subsequent fluorescent dye staining.

Constant temperature of ~20°C

Obtaining a constant temperature within the closed treatment chamber is essential in order to maintain a constant relative humidity because of the relationship between the two variables in a situation where air currents and fans carry air around a closed system (Figure 7.13). Small fluctuations in temperature can have appreciable effects on the local relative humidity, and it is therefore essential to ensure that the temperature profile within the treatment chamber is as even as possible.

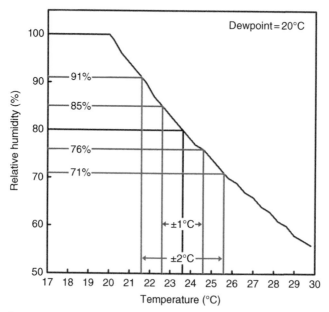

Figure 7.13 Relationship between temperature and humidity in a closed system, shown using a theoretical plot derived from a known mass of water contained in air at 80% relative humidity and 20°C. Reproduced courtesy of the Home Office.

In the cyanoacrylate fuming process, the items to be treated are suspended or placed on shelves within the cabinet, ensuring sufficient space between them for circulation of the vapours and exposure of all surfaces of interest. Ideally, similar items should be treated together in batches as development may take place at different rates on dissimilar surfaces. Liquid cyanoacrylate is then dispensed into an aluminium foil pot that is placed onto a heater block within the chamber and the door closed. The amount of cyanoacrylate used varies between different types of chamber depending on capacity but is selected to give a sufficient concentration of cyanoacrylate vapour in the atmosphere to allow the polymerisation reaction to proceed to the extent that marks are visible. The quantity actually used should be optimised for a particular cabinet configuration by observing the quantity of residue left in the aluminium pot and adjusting it to ensure very little excess remains at the end of the cycle.

The humidity in the treatment chamber is first raised to 80% relative humidity, and then the hot plate is heated to approximately 120°C to evaporate cyanoacrylate from the aluminium pot. It is best practice for the operator to watch development on the samples and halt the cycle if it looks as if overdevelopment of marks is beginning to occur. The cabinet is then placed through a purge cycle to remove fumes of cyanoacrylate vapour before the cabinet is opened and articles are removed. Articles with underdeveloped marks can be replaced into the cabinet and redeveloped. Larger cabinets allow several items to be treated in a single run, unlike some processes such as vacuum metal deposition where it may only be possible to treat one item at a time.

It is recommended that initial photography of any visible marks be carried out after cyanoacrylate fuming and prior to proceeding to treatment with a fluorescent dye stain. This is because some marks may be degraded or destroyed by the dye process, and to maximise evidence recovery all marks should be recorded before dyeing. Other enhancement processes such as powdering and vacuum metal deposition can also be considered at this stage.

The number of marks detected by cyanoacrylate fuming can often be significantly increased by fluorescent dye staining followed by fluorescence examination. If an item is to be dyed, it is immersed in a tank containing dye solution (which may be either solvent (usually ethanol) or water based) and then removed to a second tank containing running water until excess dye has been removed. The dyeing time for an ethanol-based dye is approximately 1 min, but longer dyeing times (~2 min) may be required when water-based dyes are used. The article is then allowed to dry at room temperature. For larger items, the fluorescent dye solution may be applied from a wash bottle, and the dye washed off using a wash bottle, hose or running tap water.

In the United Kingdom two fluorescent dyes (Basic Yellow 40 and Basic Red 14) are used and can be interchanged in the fluorescent dye formulation as follows:

- 2 g fluorescent dye
- 1 L ethanol

The roles of these constituents are as follows:

Basic dyes (Basic Yellow 40, Basic Red 14)	Most of the dyes used for staining polycyanoacrylate are basic in nature. It is suggested that the success of these dyes may be due to the fact that they form van der Waals bonds with the polycyanoacrylate fibres, with weak binding occurring between the dye cations and the anions associated with the CN^- groups in the polymer fibres. Both dyes are highly fluorescent, but with different excitation and emission characteristics
Ethanol	Ethanol is selected because it has lower toxicity than earlier dye formulations based on methanol and has been shown to be effective in delivering the dye into the polymer deposits

There are cases where the flammable ethanol-based formulations cannot be used (e.g. a laboratory has insufficient extraction, the dye is being applied at a scene, ethanol is causing some printed inks to run, or there is excessive dye take-up by the substrate) and a water-based Basic Yellow 40 formulation is recommended as an alternative.

The excitation and emission spectra for Basic Yellow 40 and Basic Red 14 are shown in Figures 7.14 and 7.15, respectively.

It can be seen that Basic Yellow 40 is excited by violet and blue light sources, with fluorescence in the blue-green region of the spectrum. These excitation wavelengths can sometimes cause significant background fluorescence in some materials, and Basic Red 14 can be used as an alternative. This dye has an excitation in the green region of the spectrum, where background fluorescence is generally lower, and emission in the orange-red region.

The recent introduction of one-step fluorescent cyanoacrylate fuming systems eliminates the need for solvent-based dyes and makes cyanoacrylate fuming more applicable to semi-porous surfaces that would otherwise be damaged by, or strongly absorb, the liquid dyes (Figure 7.16).

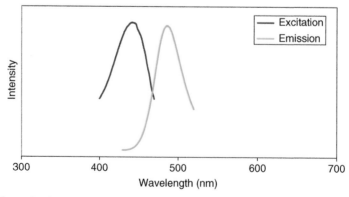

Figure 7.14 Measured excitation and emission spectra for Basic Yellow 40.

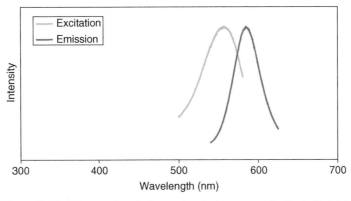

Figure 7.15 Measured excitation and emission spectra for Basic Red 14.

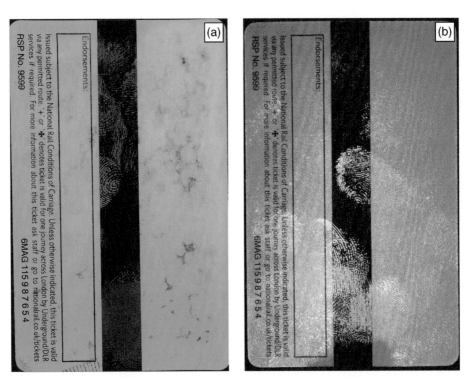

Figure 7.16 A semi-porous surface treated using (a) cyanoacrylate fuming followed by a liquid dye and (b) by one-step fluorescent cyanoacrylate fuming.

7.4 Vacuum metal deposition

7.4.1 Outline history of the process

1964: Tolansky, whilst working on the manufacture of interference filters, noted that the deposition of silver in a vacuum system developed unwanted fingermarks on glass optical components (Hambley, 1972). This is reported to the UK Home Office but not pursued further.

1968: Theys et al. reported that vacuum metal deposition from a mixture of zinc, antimony and copper powder can be used to develop latent marks on paper.

1972: Hambley completed a PhD programme under the supervision of Tolansky, investigating different metal combinations for developing fingermarks on paper and fabrics. He concluded that the best results are obtained by the use of a combination of metals, typically gold (or silver), followed by cadmium (or zinc).

1975: Kent et al. demonstrated the use of converted industrial vacuum metal coaters for fingermark development on polythene, and the process is subsequently introduced for operational work (Kent et al., 1976).

Late 1970s: Use of cadmium ceases due to its toxicity and the preferred metal combination became gold followed by zinc.

2007: Philipson and Bleay reported the use of silver deposition process as a method for enhancing marks on heavily plasticised substrates such as cling film.

2007: Guraratne et al. reported the use of aluminium as an alternative single-metal deposition process.

2011: Yu et al. reported that the evaporation of the inorganic compound zinc oxide (ZnO) in a vacuum can be used develop fingermarks on polymer surfaces.

7.4.2 Theory

The theory of vacuum metal deposition in its application for fingermark enhancement is associated with the condensation characteristics of metals on surfaces. In industrial applications of vacuum metal deposition, surfaces are generally clean and smooth, and uniform metal films are deposited. In forensic applications, the surfaces encountered are nonideal, and there are many characteristics of the surface that can influence the condensation characteristics of metal from the vapour phase, including:

- Presence of thin films of grease
- Local differences in chemical composition

- Local differences in oxidation state

- Abrasion of the surface

A fingermark can be enhanced if the surface properties of the regions occupied by the fingermark differ sufficiently from those of the regions where no deposit is present. When a metal condenses onto the surface, the surface properties influence the way in which metal nuclei are formed and nuclei of different sizes and distributions can be deposited in each region. This can be considered as analogous to breathing on a mirror, where the fingermarks or greasy deposits are revealed because the water droplets that condense on them differ from the fine mist that forms on the clean regions of the mirror.

The process most often used for vacuum metal deposition is to use a metal combination, depositing a small amount of gold followed by a deposition of a much thicker film of zinc.

When gold is evaporated, it can deposit across the entire surface and begins to form nuclei, the size and distribution of which depends on the nature of the surface (as outlined previously). The resultant gold coating is very thin (several nanometres only) and discontinuous. If the fingermark contains appreciable amounts of fatty material, any gold nuclei that have formed may also diffuse into the fats instead of remaining on the surface (Stroud, 1971, 1972). The fingermark will not be visible at this stage.

Zinc is used to produce a thicker, visible layer that enables the fingermark to be seen. It is chosen for this purpose because it will not condense on areas of grease, such as the sebaceous constituents of fingermarks or foodstuffs, even when these substances are only present as a monolayer. However, zinc can deposit and grow on small nuclei of metal. As a consequence, when zinc is deposited, it will condense on the regions where gold nuclei are available (i.e. the background substrate), but not on the regions of the fatty deposit (i.e. the fingermark ridges).

Zinc deposition may be inhibited by the presence of many different types of greasy contaminant and constituents of natural sweat. Tests carried out to determine which constituents of latent marks could affect zinc deposition identified several fatty substances (stearic acid, palmitic acid, cholesterol oleate, glycerol trioleate) and some amino acids (L-arginine monohydrochloride, L-leucine and DL-threonine) as having strong influences on deposition behaviour. Most of these substances are non-water-soluble, long-chain fats or acids with low vapour pressure. This means that they are likely to be stable and remain *in situ* under the high vacuum conditions used during vacuum metal deposition.

This theory of metal deposition where zinc deposition occurs on the background but not on the fingermark ridges has been described by researchers (Jones et al., 2001a) as 'normal development', and this process is depicted schematically in Figure 7.17.

The appearance of a mark revealed by 'normal development' during vacuum metal deposition is illustrated in Figure 7.18.

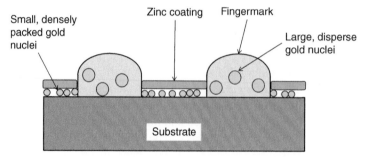

Figure 7.17 Schematic diagram of normal development, showing zinc depositing where gold nuclei are available on the surface.

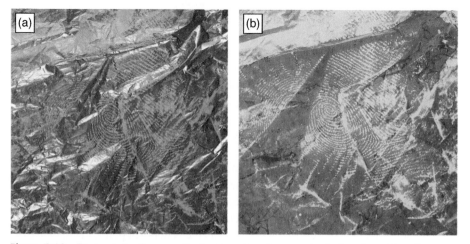

Figure 7.18 Photograph of a normally developed mark on a polyethylene bag, (a) under reflected white light and (b) viewed using bright-field transmitted light.

Figure 7.18a clearly shows the thick metallic zinc film that has been deposited on the surface, and 7.18b reveals the fact that deposition has not occurred on the ridges, making the mark clearly visible using transmitted light.

The theory of 'normal development' does not account for the fact that many marks encountered in operational work have the reverse appearance, that is, the zinc film is deposited more rapidly on the fingermark ridges than it is on the background. This form of enhancement has been described as 'reverse development' (Jones et al., 2001a), and there are several theories about how this arises.

Kent et al. (1976) attribute reverse development to the substrate not being truly non-porous and being able to absorb some of the mobile species of the fingermark, leaving a solid, primarily inorganic residue on the surface that acts as a preferential nucleation site for the zinc. The fact that the surface may not be truly non-porous means that more gold could diffuse into the polymer substrate than can penetrate the solid residue; hence zinc deposits on the ridges first. A closely related theory is that reverse development occurs because the fingermark becomes dried out or contains a contaminant, inhibiting the diffusion of the gold nuclei into the fingermark residue. Because the gold nuclei in the region of the ridges are larger and are now available of the surface of the mark, zinc deposition occurs at a faster rate in these regions. This is illustrated schematically in Figure 7.19.

Figure 7.20 shows a 'reverse developed' mark on a low density polyethylene bag, where this type of mark is most commonly encountered.

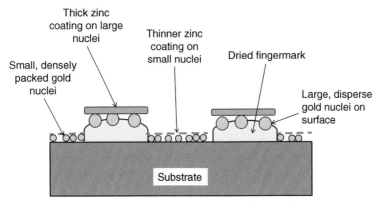

Figure 7.19   Schematic diagram of reverse development, showing different rates of zinc deposition according to size of gold nuclei available on the surface.

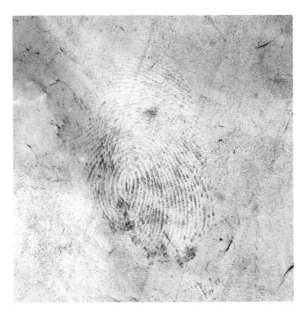

Figure 7.20   A 'reverse developed' mark on a low density polyethylene bag.

Most recently, Jones et al. (2001a, 2001b, 2001c) have proposed an alternative theory related to the types of gold nuclei formed. In this theory the gold nuclei being deposited on the fingermark ridges are postulated to form at a different rate to those growing on the substrate and in the furrows; hence a regime exists where the gold film on the background has reached a state where zinc cannot nucleate, but on the ridges the nuclei are a suitable size for zinc to deposit. This theory closely relates the type of mark that is developed to the amount of gold deposited initially and proposes that the mode of development can be controlled by adjusting the amount of gold deposited. Jones et al. also propose that under this model there are situations where excessive amounts of gold are used, large gold nuclei grow on both ridge and background and 'overdevelopment' occurs because a uniform zinc film deposits and the fingermark cannot be easily discriminated.

None of the theories earlier has been categorically proven, and in some cases reverse and normal development may be observed on the same substrate. The fact that the type of development is controlled both by the amount of gold deposited and the type of substrate present can be illustrated in Figure 7.21, where a single mark has been deposited across two different types of polyethylene and developed in the same processing cycle of a vacuum metal deposition chamber.

It is recognised that the gold/zinc vacuum metal deposition process does not work well (or at all) on substrates that are heavily plasticised (e.g. cling film, plasticised

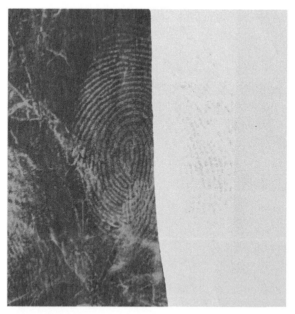

Figure 7.21 A single fingermark crossing a boundary between dissimilar materials, processed using a single gold/zinc vacuum metal deposition run. Left-hand side: high density polyethylene, showing 'normal' development. Right hand side: low density polyethylene, showing 'reverse' development. Reproduced courtesy of the Home Office.

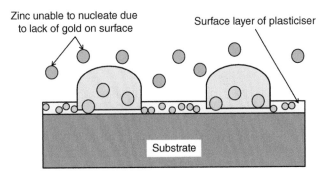

Figure 7.22 Schematic diagram of a case where no development occurs, showing zinc unable to find gold nuclei on surface.

polyvinyl chloride) where additives may migrate to form a layer on the surface or on materials that have surface release films or oily contamination present. This is attributed to the fact that the gold nuclei formed may diffuse into the surface layer on the substrate as well as into the fingermark residue with the result that there are no nuclei on the surface of zinc to deposit on, as is illustrated schematically in Figure 7.22.

This effect may also be observed on a localised basis where marks with high contents of sebaceous sweat or oily contaminants are deposited on certain types of polymer and monolayers of grease can spread to fill the furrows between the ridges. In these cases gold/zinc vacuum metal deposition may not be able to define the ridge detail within the perimeter of the contact area, and an 'empty' mark results.

For all of the circumstances described earlier, a single-metal vacuum metal deposition process has been proposed. The most effective single metal for the majority of surfaces encountered has been found to be silver (Philipson and Bleay, 2007). The silver deposition process is thought to work because silver, like gold, deposits uniformly across the surface. The type of silver nuclei that are formed are influenced by the surface properties in the same way as gold nuclei are and vary in size and distribution between the fingermark ridges and the background. This difference in nuclei size translates to a difference in colour between the two regions, either due to diffraction or interference effects. The silver metal deposition process is shown schematically in Figure 7.23, and example of a developed mark is illustrated in Figure 7.24.

7.4.3 The vacuum metal deposition process

The vacuum metal deposition process described hereafter is that included in the Home Office Fingermark Visualisation Manual (Bandey, 2014) and involves the use of a high vacuum chamber. The materials and processing parameters used in

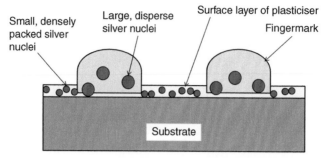

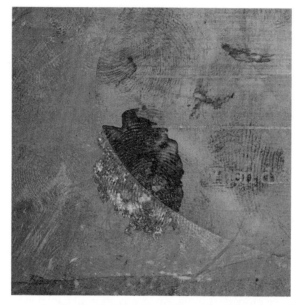

Figure 7.23 Schematic diagram of silver vacuum metal deposition on a plasticised surface, showing the different sizes of silver nuclei formed in the ridges and on the surface.

Figure 7.24 An example of marks developed on a clear polyethylene bag using silver vacuum metal deposition, showing developed ridges both lighter and darker than the background.

the two-stage gold/zinc process are as follows. Quantities of metals given are typical of those for a 750–900 mm diameter vacuum chamber:

Approximately 2 mg of gold is evaporated at a pressure of 3×10^{-4} mbar or lower.

Zinc is evaporated at a pressure between 3 and 5×10^{-4} mbar until a suitable coating is formed and fingermarks become visible.

These steps can be repeated until the desired level of coating and fingermark development has been obtained.

The reason for choosing these particular materials and processing conditions can be expanded as follows:

Gold	The role of gold in the vacuum metal deposition process is to act as the 'primer' for subsequent zinc deposition. Gold is not selective in that it will deposit across the entire surface, but the size and dispersion of the gold nuclei formed will be determined by the surface properties. Any differences between the nuclei formed in the regions of the fingermark ridges and the background will be magnified during subsequent zinc deposition. Gold is also used as the initial deposition metal because it is inert and does not react with fingermark residues or atmospheric pollutants.
	The low deposition pressure is used so that gold atoms can travel from the evaporation vessel to the surface without colliding with a significant number of air molecules in the chamber, giving an even coating.
Zinc	Zinc is used to delineate the fingermark, primarily by the difference between the growth rate of zinc on the nuclei present on the fingermark ridges and the growth rate on those present on the background. Zinc is highly effective for this purpose because it easily re-evaporates from the surface unless there is a suitable nucleation site present; thus the type of gold nuclei formed controls the way in which zinc layers subsequently form.
	The chamber pressure used during evaporation of zinc is higher than that for gold, and this is to allow the user more control over the zinc deposition process. Allowing more air into the chamber makes the deposition of zinc more uniform across the area of the exhibit, but the pressure needs to be kept low enough to prevent oxidation of the zinc film formed.

In the single-metal silver vacuum metal deposition process, silver is deposited using the same conditions as for gold in the gold/zinc process described earlier. The optimum amount of silver to use for most surfaces has been identified as 30 mg (Philipson and Bleay, 2007). If less silver is used, development is too faint. If much more silver is used, on some surfaces, ridges start to become filled in and detail can be lost. The role of silver is expanded upon in the following text:

Silver	Silver is used because it condenses on surfaces in a similar way to gold, and the size and dispersion of the nuclei formed are influenced by the surface properties. A sufficient quantity of silver is used so that the deposited film is visible to the eye, and the difference in nuclei size is manifested as a colour difference that enables the mark to be visualised.
	As for gold, a low deposition pressure is used so that silver can be deposited directly onto the surface without colliding with a significant number of molecules in the chamber, giving an even coating.

The equipment used for vacuum metal deposition may vary according to manufacturer, but the essential elements of the system are the same. The equipment consists of a vacuum chamber capable of being pumped down to high levels of vacuum

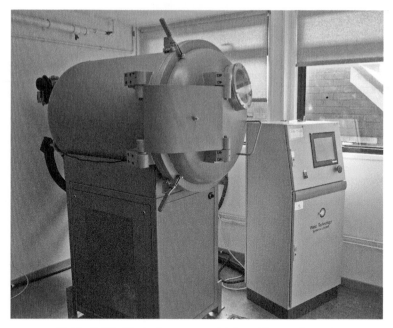

Figure 7.25   Typical vacuum metal deposition equipment.

($<3 \times 10^{-4}$ mbar), high melting point metal vessels for evaporation of gold, silver and zinc and a viewing window so that the progress of the deposition process can be monitored. The chamber may also contain a 'cold finger', chilled to low temperature to aid condensation of water vapour and other contaminants extracted from the item by the vacuum and to reduce pump-down times.

A typical system is illustrated in Figure 7.25.

Items to be coated are attached to the perimeter of the vacuum chamber, above the evaporation vessels. The chamber is then sealed and pumped down to a high level of vacuum. Once the desired level of vacuum has been achieved, metal contained within high melting point metal vessels is evaporated by passing a current through them.

The evaporation vessels are typically formed from thin sheets of molybdenum, which can withstand the high temperatures used to evaporate the metals used without melting itself.

The gold evaporation vessel usually consists of a shallow dimple in a thin strip of molybdenum. This is because the quantity of gold used is very small (~2–3 mg), and it is important that all the gold reaches the substrate. If deeper containers are used, 'shadowing' may occur where there is no direct line of sight from the base of the evaporation vessel and to the sample holder, resulting in some regions of the item not receiving a coating. During gold deposition the current to the evaporation vessel is increased until it reaches a yellow/white heat. Deposition of gold should be complete within 10 s, but if any residue is observed on the filament as the current is reduced, the temperature should be increased again until all gold has been evaporated.

Once gold deposition is completed, a small amount of air is admitted to the chamber to raise the pressure and the current to the zinc evaporation vessel(s) is turned on. The zinc evaporation vessels are larger and significantly deeper than the gold filament, and the quantity of zinc added is larger, typically 1 g per run. The zinc used is in the form of foil, shot or powder. For zinc deposition, the current is increased until the evaporation vessel glows a cherry red/dull orange colour. Once this occurs, the operator should turn on the interior chamber lights and observe the deposition process through the viewing window, ceasing deposition as soon as marks become visible on the substrate. After zinc deposition, the gold evaporation vessel should be briefly heated to yellow/white heat to burn off any residual zinc contamination.

There is a great variability in the speed at which different substrates coat, and it may take over 10 min to obtain a suitable coating on some types of material. In some cases it may be necessary to carry out multiple deposition runs in order to obtain satisfactory results or to develop all the marks present. The presence of surface contamination, release agents or plasticisers may mean that it is not possible to obtain a zinc coating at all, and in these circumstances the deposition of 30 mg of silver using the same deposition conditions for gold may yield additional marks.

7.5 Iodine fuming

7.5.1 Outline history of the process

1863: Coulier made the observation that iodine fumes could be used to both detect handwriting alterations and develop latent fingermarks (Quinche and Margot, 2010). It was noted that fumes of iodine directed onto paper produced a yellow colour where the iodine was absorbed by the fingermark residues, similarly to the marks illustrated in Figure 7.26. However, this staining was only transitory, fading in minutes.

1935: A method using moist paper carrying rice starch was proposed for transferring and fixing developed marks from surfaces (Morris, 1974).

1961: McLaughlin published an alternative means of 'lifting' developed marks by means of a silver foil, the iodine selectively reacting with the surface to form silver iodide, which then darkened when exposed to strong light.

1962: Larsen described a refinement to the starch fixing process, involving brushing the mark with finely ground starch powder, blowing to remove the excess and then exposing the mark to gentle steam for 1–2 s.

1975: Trowell investigated 'tetrabase' (4,4-bis(dimethylamino)diphenylmethane) both as a fixing solution and as an additive in uncured silicone rubber mixes that could be moulded over a developed mark to fix it without recourse to solvent dipping or spraying.

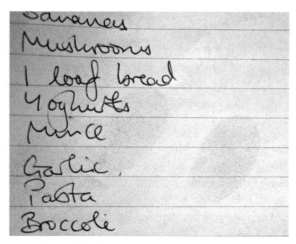

Figure 7.26   Fingermarks on white lined notepaper developed by iodine fuming. Reproduced courtesy of the Home Office.

1977: Mashiko and Ishizaki suggested α-naphthoflavone as an alternative fixing agent to starch.

1979: Almog et al. proposed simultaneous fuming of iodine and steaming as a means of improving the sensitivity of iodine fuming on paper and also of improving the performance of the reagent on older marks.

7.5.2   Theory

Iodine is capable of a range of interactions with different fingermark constituents. One suggestion is that iodine can undergo a reversible addition reaction across the carbon double bonds in the unsaturated fatty acid components of the fingermark residue (Olsen, 1975). This is supported by studies on individual constituents associated with sebaceous sweat (Chu, 2011) that show strong absorption of iodine by the unsaturated squalene constituent and considerably less interaction with the saturated fatty acids (Figure 7.27).

The fading of marks over time is attributed to the reversible nature of the addition reaction. It was subsequently suggested (Almog et al., 1979) that other interactions must also be occurring, because free iodine must be present for the observed fixing reactions to take place. If all iodine had reacted across the double bonds, fixing of the marks would not be possible. Almog et al. proposed that the principal interaction taking place is a dipole-induced dipole interaction between iodine and water molecules. In this interaction a temporary dipole can be induced in the iodine molecule by the permanent dipole in the water molecules present in the fingermark residue. Iodine may also act as a Lewis acid and the oxygen end of the water molecule as a

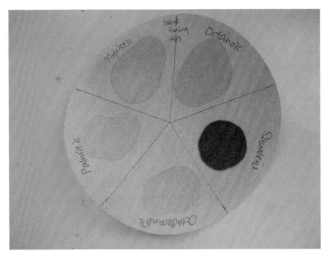

Figure 7.27 Spots of sebaceous fingermark constituents (octadecanoic acid, palmitic acid, myristic acid, octanoic acid, squalene) on filter paper processed using iodine fuming, showing strong reaction with the unsaturated squalene. Reproduced courtesy of Loughborough University.

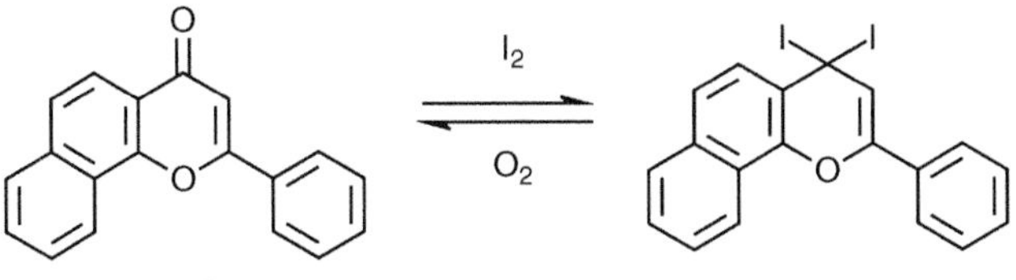

Figure 7.28 Proposed fixing mechanism for iodine using α-naphthoflavone.

Lewis base, resulting in the formation of a loosely bound Lewis-type charge transfer complex, in which there is a partial transfer of electrons from the water to the iodine. The formation of the complex is responsible for changing the wavelengths of light absorbed so that the enhanced fingermark appears yellow/brown instead of the violet colour of iodine observed in non-polar solvents.

The observed drop in effectiveness of iodine fuming on older marks is attributed to the relatively rapid evaporation of water and degradation of squalene, meaning that two of the principal constituents that iodine interacts with are no longer available for these interactions to occur.

Fixing of the marks can be achieved using starch, where the triiodide ions present in the fingermark form a blue-black complex with the amylose constituent of starch by trapping iodine ions in the coiled amylose chains. The mechanism of the fixing reaction with α-naphthoflavone has not been extensively studied, although a reversible reaction between iodine and α-naphthoflavone has been proposed by Sears (1987). This reaction is illustrated in Figure 7.28, and the reversible nature of the reaction accounts for the observed fading of marks over time, even after fixing has occurred.

7.5.3 The iodine fuming process

The iodine fuming process is a simple one, and the only chemical that is required to develop marks is iodine in solid crystalline form.

Iodine is used because it can begin to sublime at ambient temperature to produce vapours that are readily and selectively absorbed by fingermarks, as described in Section 7.5.2.

In the fuming process, the item to be treated is supported or suspended within a small chamber, 1 g of iodine placed onto a glass dish at the base of the chamber and the chamber sealed. The iodine is then allowed to sublime (or can be gently heated to 50°C to increase the sublimation rate), producing a violet/brown vapour that fills the chamber and begins to interact with the item and the fingermark (Figure 7.29).

The development of fingermarks is monitored by direct observation, and when it is considered that maximum contrast has been reached between ridges and the background, the chamber is opened to allow excess iodine vapour to be vented and the item removed for photography.

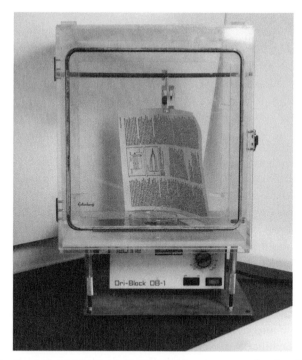

Figure 7.29 An item being treated by iodine fuming in a treatment chamber. Reproduced courtesy of the Home Office.

If required, fingermarks may then be fixed by spraying them with a fixing solution. A formulation previously suggested for this application is:

α-Naphthoflavone	1 g
Acetic acid	50 mL
Trichlorotrifluoroethane (CFC113)	300 mL

The CFC113 component would require replacement by a non-ozone-depleting solvent such as HFE7100 if the solution were in routine operational use.

Fuming can also be carried out on larger items or at scenes of crime using portable glass pipes with heated compartments to start iodine fuming and desiccant crystals to dry the fumes. Because of the toxic and corrosive nature of iodine vapour, this should only be carried out in well-ventilated and/or extracted areas by operators with the appropriate protective equipment.

7.6 Radioactive sulphur dioxide

7.6.1 Outline history of the process

1963: The potential application of radioactive sulphur dioxide ($^{35}SO_2$) for the development of latent fingermarks was reported (Grant et al., 1963a, 1963b) during the course of investigations into the resistance of paper to attack by atmospheric pollution.

1971: Spedding reported refinements to the radioactive sulphur dioxide process and suggested that SO_2 reacts with the lipids present in fingermarks, in particular oleic and linoleic acids. Spedding also showed that marks could be developed on paper that had been wetted.

Early 1970s: Godsell and co-workers (Godsell, 1972; Godsell and Vincent, 1973) demonstrated the practical application of radioactive sulphur dioxide to a range of substrates including paper, banknotes and adhesive tapes. The process is implemented for operational use.

1984: A study by Albinson confirmed that radioactive sulphur dioxide is the most sensitive process available for enhancement of fingermarks on fabrics (Albinson, Unpublished).

2005: The last fully operational radioactive sulphur dioxide cabinet in the United Kingdom was decommissioned.

Examples of marks developed using radioactive sulphur dioxide on different types of paper substrate are shown in Figure 7.30.

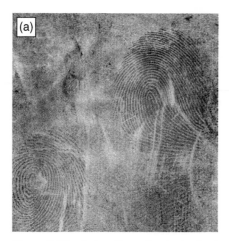 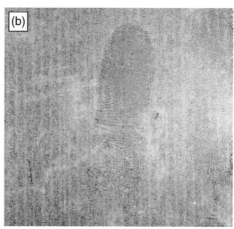

Figure 7.30 Autoradiographs obtained using the radioactive sulphur dioxide process: (a) from a 1970s Bank of England £5 note and (b) from brown wrapping paper. Reproduced courtesy of the Home Office.

7.6.2 Theory

Wells (1975) conducted the most comprehensive reported study of the radioactive SO_2 process and suggested that several reactions could occur between the sulphur dioxide gas and fingermarks. It was proposed that a complex combination of these reactions contributed to the fingermark development process. The mechanisms proposed by Wells included the following:

- Sulphur dioxide being converted to SO_4^{2-} ions and fixed in the water present in the fingermark. The water present originates both from natural sweat deposits and from water absorbed from the atmosphere due to the hygroscopic nature of the deposit.
- Contact from the fingermark ridges causing local sensitisation of porous, wettable substrates (e.g. paper, fabric), resulting in locally adsorbed layers of water molecules in the contact regions.
- Reaction(s) with lipids that may occur across the double bonds of unsaturated free fatty acids and other similar compounds.

The strong dependence of the SO_2 reaction on the relative humidity in the chamber during treatment tends to support the theory that the main reaction occurring is the water-phase fixation mechanism, although the observation that marks can still be developed on wetted surfaces indicates that reactions with lipids also occur.

The development of fingermarks by the radioactive SO_2 process and subsequent autoradiography is illustrated schematically in Figure 7.31.

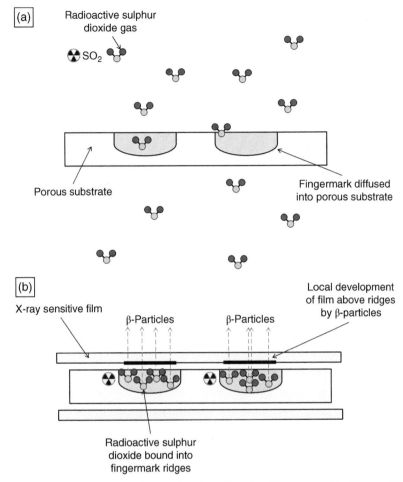

Figure 7.31   Schematic diagram illustrating the radioactive SO_2 process: (a) SO_2 gas diffusing through porous substrate and (b) autoradiography of sample with radioactive sulphur bound into fingermark ridges.

7.6.3   The radioactive sulphur dioxide process

Early equipment for the processing of items with radioactive sulphur dioxide utilised cylinders containing ^{35}S-labelled sulphur dioxide gas (Spedding et al., 1970), providing a direct feed into the processing chamber. This was found impractical because of large distances of pipework that needed to be maintained free of leaks. The method that was latterly recommended for this process was the generation of radioactive sulphur dioxide gas from the combustion of filter paper impregnated with ^{35}S-labelled thiourea, which was then used to treat items in a humidity-controlled cabinet.

The role of the thiourea in the process was to release sulphur dioxide as a combustion product. The radioactive sulphur dioxide sources were prepared by dissolving ^{35}S-labelled thiourea in water and decanting small aliquots of solution onto discs of filter paper. The concentration of the solution was adjusted to give a concentration of 1 mCi (millicurie) per 50 μL, with 5 μL being impregnated into each disc to give a disc content of 0.1 mCi of thiourea.

The 55% relative humidity level in the chamber and concentration of radioactive thiourea used in the process were chosen to give the optimum conditions identified in early experimental work (Anon, 1971) and to provide the conditions for selective adsorption of water molecules thought to contribute to reactions fixing sulphur dioxide into the fingermark.

To treat items with radioactive sulphur dioxide, the thiourea-impregnated filter paper disc was loaded into the crucible chamber of the apparatus. Items were then suspended in the main chamber, which was sealed and brought to a relative humidity of 55%. The apparatus used is illustrated in Figure 7.32.

The impregnated disc was then ignited, and the predetermined concentration of radioactive SO_2 released during combustion was allowed to fill the processing chamber. Once the processing cycle was completed, residual gas was vented into an activated carbon trap. The concentration of SO_2 was monitored throughout processing, and when it had returned to the level prior to commencing treatment, items were removed from the chamber.

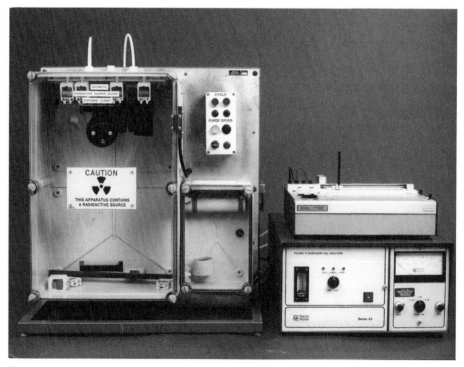

Figure 7.32 The apparatus used for radioactive sulphur dioxide processing. Reproduced courtesy of the Home Office.

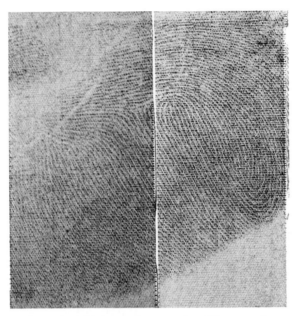

Figure 7.33 Autoradiograph of fabric sample exposed to different environments and treated with radioactive sulphur dioxide. Reproduced courtesy of the Home Office.

To reveal the fingermarks, items were sandwiched between two sheets of X-ray film and then placed in a press. Activity was monitored with a Geiger counter to calculate exposure times, typically 7–10 days. As outlined in Section 7.6.2, β-particles emitted from sulphur dioxide fixed in the fingermark ridges selectively develop the X-ray film. An autoradiograph produced from radioactive sulphur dioxide treatment of a fabric sample is shown in Figure 7.33.

The process involved constant monitoring of all items of laboratory equipment, clothing and items that came into contact with radioactive material and the disposal of contaminated articles in an approved fashion.

7.7 Other fuming techniques

7.7.1 Outline history of the process

There are several other ways in which vapour phase processes can be used to enhance fingermarks, some of which are outlined in Section 7.7.2.

In a review of techniques for development of latent marks, Micik (1974) listed three fuming techniques: iodine, hydrogen fluoride (for etching fingermarks on glass) and the burning of substances including camphor and magnesium to produce fumes that selectively deposit particles on fingermark ridges.

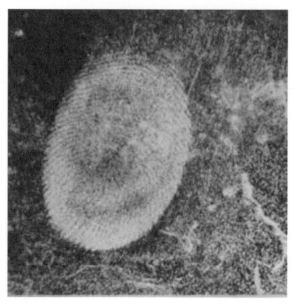

Figure 7.34 Fingermarks on a metal surface developed by anthracene fuming. Reproduced courtesy of the Home Office.

Almog and Gabay (1980) investigated the development of fingermarks on paper by the fuming of fluorescent chemicals. Good results were reported for anthranilic acid (for fresh marks), anthracene (for older marks) and antimony trichloride. In some cases the fluorescent chemical was selectively deposited on the ridges; in other cases deposition occurred on the background only.

Peacock (1982) further explored anthracene fuming both in vacuum and under ambient conditions on metal and plastic surfaces. It was found that sublimation in air gave better results than vacuum deposition, and although the process did develop fingermarks on plastics, it was not as effective as other processes already available. Results on metals were more promising, and anthracene fuming was found to be more effective than iodine fuming over a range of different metal surfaces (Figure 7.34).

Haque (1982) considered the fuming of naphthalene and camphor, followed by iodine fuming and dusting with magnetic powder. This sequential approach appeared to give good results for marks on plastic bags. Haque also explored the development of marks on polymers using the fumes of halogenated hydrocarbons such as dichloromethane and chloroform to selectively attack the surface. The technique worked well on polystyrene but was ineffective on vinyl and thermoset plastics and did not work at all on polyethylene.

Fuming has also been reported in combination with other processes for the revelation of fingermarks. Meylan et al. (1990) described the fuming of ammonium hydrogen carbonate after exposure of a paper surface to a corona discharge.

This combined treatment produced fluorescent fingermarks that could be excited by ultraviolet light. This technique was further investigated by Davies et al. (2000), who carried out an analysis of the fluorescent products and suggested that lipid derivatives were responsible for the fluorescence observed.

In addition to the hydrofluoric acid fuming process mentioned by Micik, other acid fuming techniques have been considered. Bentsen et al. (1996) tri-alled nitric acid fuming for development of fingermarks on brass cartridge cases by selective etching, and Broniek and Knaap (2002) proposed hydrochloric acid fuming as a technique for revealing fingermarks on thermal receipts, in this case by the formation of a dark green reaction product on the fingermark ridges. The highly corrosive nature of these substances meant that such techniques have not been widely adopted for operational use because of the precautions required for their use.

A novel process that has been recently reported by Kelly et al. (2008) is the use of disulphur dinitride, allowed to sublime under a static vacuum. This has been reported to be capable of developing fingermarks on a wide range of surfaces including paper, fabric, cling film and metals, possibly by formation of the blue-black SN_x polymer (Figure 7.35).

Williams et al. (2011) have reported sublimation of copper phthalocyanine using a vacuum desiccator and a resistive heater to heat the substance to 400°C. The process was found to develop marks with deep blue ridge patterns on light-coloured porous surfaces but was less successful on plastic bags and ceramic tiles.

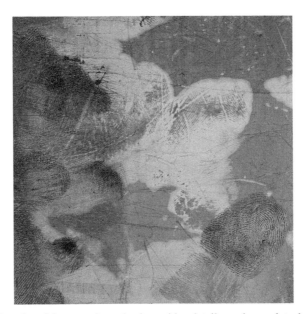

Figure 7.35 A series of fingermarks and palmar ridge detail on a brass plate developed using disulphur dinitride.

7.7.2 Theory

Because many different types of substance have been used in vapour phase processes for the development of fingermarks, there is no single mechanism that applies
to all chemicals. A range of mechanisms may operate, and some of these are outlined in Table 7.1, together with some of the processes that they are applicable to.

Table 7.1   Overview of vapour phase process and the mechanisms by which fingermarks are
revealed.

Mechanism	Processes
Absorption of coloured vapours into fingermark residues	Occurs for iodine (and other halogens such as bromine) and also copper phthalocyanine
Chemical reaction between fumes and fingermark residues to form a coloured or fluorescent reaction product	An example of this is the black product formed by osmium tetroxide fumes or the green product of hydrochloric acid fuming
Catalysis of a polymerisation reaction by fingermark residues, promoting the growth of a solid polymer phase from the gaseous monomer	Occurs during the cyanoacrylate fuming process and also possibly the recently reported disulphur dinitride process (Figure 7.36)
Selective deposition of coloured or fluorescent particulates on fingermark ridges (or background)	Observed for fuming of anthracene, antimony trichloride, camphor and naphthalene
Selective etching/attack of fingermark ridges (or background) by fumes of acid or other chemicals	Seen for hydrogen fluoride on glass, nitric acid on brass and chloroform on polystyrene

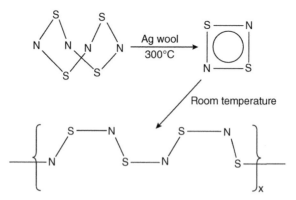

Figure 7.36   Proposed mechanism for the formation of SN_x polymer from S_2N_2. Image
reproduced courtesy of Loughborough University.

References

Albinson R A, 'The Development of Latent Fingerprints on Fabric', Draft Home Office SRDB Report No. 72/84 (Unpublished).

Almog J, Gabay A, 'Chemical Reagents for the Development of Latent Fingerprints. III: Visualisation of Latent Fingerprints by Fluorescent Reagents in Vapor Phase', J. Forensic Sci., vol 25(2), (1980), p 408–410.

Almog J, Gabay A, 'A Modified Super Glue Technique – The Use of Polycyanoacrylate for Fingerprint Development', J. Forensic Sci., vol 31(1), (1986), p 250–253.

Almog J, Sasson Y, Anati A, 'Chemical Reagents for the Development of Latent Fingerprints II: Controlled Addition of Water Vapor to Iodine Fumes – A Solution to the Ageing Problem', J. Forensic Sci., vol 24(2), (1979), p 431–436.

Anon 'Report of an Informal Symposium on Fingerprints Held at AWRE Aldermaston on 2 December 1970', Home Office PSDB Report 2.71, March 1971.

Bandey H (ed.), 'Fingermark Visualisation Manual', Home Office, 2014.

Bentolila A, Totre J, Zozulia I, Levin-Elad M, Domb A J, 'Fluorescent Cyanoacrylate Monomers and Polymers for Fingermark Development', Macromolecules, vol 46, (2013), p 4822–4828.

Bentsen R K, Brown J K, Dinsmore A, Harvey K K, Kee T G, 'Post Firing Visualisation of Fingerprints on Spent Cartridge Cases', Sci. Justice, vol 36(1), (1996), p 3–8.

Besonen J A, 'Heat Acceleration of the Super Glue Fuming Method for Development of Latent Fingerprints', Identif. News, February 1983, p 3–4.

Broniek B, Knaap W, 'Latent Fingerprint Development on Thermal Paper Using Muriatic (Hydrochloric) Acid', J. Forensic Identif., vol 54(4), (2002), p 427–432.

Casault P, Gilbert N, Daoust B, 'Comparison of Various Alkyl Cyanoacrylates for Fingerprint Development', Can. Soc. Forensic Sci. J., vol 50(1), (2016), p 1–22.

Chu P W L, 'Assessment of the Reactions between Lipophilic Reagents for Fingerprint Development and Typical Fatty Constituents Found in Latent Fingerprints', MSc project Report submitted to the Chemistry Department of Loughborough University, September 2011.

Davies L M, Jones N E, Brennan J S, Bramble S K, 'A New Visibly-Excited Fluorescent Component in Latent Fingerprint Residue Induced by Gaseous Electrical Discharge', J. Forensic Sci., vol 45(6), (2000), p 1294–1298.

Downham R P, Sears V G, Mehmet S, 'Pseudo-Operational Investigation into the Development of Latent Fingerprints on Flexible Plastic Packaging Films', J. Forensic Identif., vol 62(6), (2012), p 661–682.

Farrugia K J, Deacon P, Fraser J, 'Evaluation of Lumicyano™ Cyanoacrylate Fuming Process for the Development of Latent Fingermarks on Plastic Carrier Bags by Means of a Pseudo Operational Comparative Trial', Sci. Justice, vol 54(2), (2014), p 126–132.

Fraser J, Sturrock K R, Deacon P, Bleay S, Bremner D H, 'Visualisation of Fingermarks and Grab Impressions on Fabrics. Part 1: Gold/Zinc Vacuum Metal Deposition', Forensic Sci. Int., vol 208(1–3), (2011), p 74–78.

Godsell J W, 'Successful Application of the Radio-Active Sulphur Dioxide Method to Development of Latent Fingermarks on Genuine and Forged Bank Notes in Operational Cases', Home Office PSDB Technical Note 1/72, 1972.

Godsell J W, Vincent P G, 'Comparative Study of Radio-Active Sulphur Dioxide, Ninhydrin and Silver Nitrate from the Point of View of Their Efficiency for Developing Latent Fingerprints on Paper', Home Office PSDB Technical Memorandum 1/73, 1973.

Grant R L, Lyth H F, Hockey J A, 'Detecting Fingerprints on Paper', Nature, vol 200, (1963a), p 1348.

Grant R L, Lyth H F, Hockey J A, 'A New Method of Detecting Fingerprints on Paper', J. Forensic Sci. Soc., vol 4(2), (1963b), p 85–86.

Groeneveld G, Kuijer S, de Puit M, 'Preparation of Cyanoacrylate Derivatives and Comparison of Dual Action Cyanoacrylate Formulations', Sci. Justice, vol 54(1), (2014), p 42–48.

Guraratne A, Knaggs C, Stansbury D, 'Vacuum Metal Deposition: Comparing Conventional Gold/Zinc to Aluminium VMD', Identification Canada, vol. 30(2), (2007), p 40–62.

Haines S A, 'Latent Fingerprint Development – A New Technique', Canadian Police News Magazine, (1982), p 22–23.

Hambley D S, 'The Physics of Vacuum Evaporation Development of Latent Fingerprints', PhD Thesis, The Royal Holloway College, University of London, 1972.

Haque F, 'Organic Vapours for Developing Latent Fingerprints on Non-porous Surfaces', Fingerprint Report No. 7, Chemistry Department, University of Ottawa, March 1982.

Hebrand J, Donche A, Jaret Y, Loyan S, 'Revelation of Fingerprints with Cyanoacrylate Vapours Traditional Treatment/Vacuum Treatment', Proceedings of the International Symposium on Fingerprint Detection and Identification, Ne'urim, Israel, 26–30 June 1995, p 67–78.

Jones N, Stoilovic M, Lennard C, Roux C, 'Vacuum Metal Deposition: Factors Affecting Normal and Reverse Development of Latent Fingerprints on Polyethylene Substrates', Forensic Sci. Int., vol 115, (2001a), p 73–88.

Jones N, Stoilovic M, Lennard C, Roux C, 'Vacuum Metal Deposition: Developing Latent Fingerprints on Polyethylene Substrates after the Deposition of Excess Gold', Forensic Sci. Int., vol 123, (2001b), p 5–12.

Jones N, Mansour D, Stoilovic M, Lennard C, Roux C, 'The Influence of Polymer Type, Print Donor and Age on the Quality of Fingerprints Developed on Plastic Substrates Using Vacuum Metal Deposition', Forensic Sci. Int., vol 124, (2001c), p 167–177.

Kelly P F, King R S P, Mortimer R J, 'Fingerprint and Inkjet Trace Imaging Using Disulfur Dinitride', Chem. Commun., (2008), p 6111–6113.

Kendall F G, Rehn B W, 'Rapid Method of Super Glue Fuming Application for the Development of Latent Fingerprints', J. Forensic Sci., vol 28(3), (1983), p 777–780.

Kent T (ed.), 'Manual of Fingerprint Development Techniques', 1st ed., Home Office, 1986, ISBN 0-86252-230-7.

Kent T, Thomas G L, Reynoldson T E, East H W, 'A Vacuum Coating Technique for the Development of Latent Fingerprints on Polythene', J. Forensic Sci. Soc., vol 16(2), (1976), p 93–101.

Khuu A, Chadwick S, Spindler X, Lam R, Moret S, Roux C, 'Evaluation of One-Step Luminescent Cyanoacrylate Fuming', Forensic Sci. Int., vol 263, (2016), p 126–131.

Knighting S, Fraser J, Sturrock K, Deacon P, Bleay S, Bremner D H, 'Visualisation of Fingermarks and Grab Impressions on Dark Fabrics Using Silver Vacuum Metal Deposition', Sci. Justice, vol 53(3), (2013), p 309–314.

Larsen J K, 'The Starch Powder-Steam Method of Fixing Iodine Fumed Latent Prints', Identification, July 1962, p 3–5.

Lewis L A, Smithwick R W III, Devault G L, Bolinger B, Lewis S A Sr, 'Processes Involved in the Development of Latent Fingerprints Using the Cyanoacrylate Fuming Method', J. Forensic Sci., vol 46(2), (2001), p 241–246.

Mankidy P J, Rajagopalan R, Foley H C, 'Influence of Initiators on the Growth of Poly(ethyl 2-cyanoacrylate) Nanofibers', Polymer, vol 49, (2008), p 2235–2242.

Martindale W E II, 'Cyanoacrylate Fuming as a Method for Rapid Development of Latent Finger-prints Utilizing Anhydrous Sodium Carbonate as a Dry Catalyst', Identif. News, November 1983, p 13.

Mashiko K, Ishizaki M, 'Latent Fingerprint Processing: Iodine-7,8-Benzoflavone Method', Identif. News, vol 27(11), (1977), p 3–5.

McLaren C, Lennard C, Stoilovic M, 'Methylamine Pretreatment of Dry Latent Fingermarks on Polyethylene for Enhanced Detection by Cyanoacrylate Fuming', J. Forensic Identif., vol 60(2), (2010), p 199–222.

McLaughlin A R, 'Chemicals and Their Application for Developing Latent Prints', Identification, July 1961, p 3–7.

Menzel E R, Burt J A, Sinor T W, Tubach-Ley W B, Jordan K J, 'Laser Detection of Latent Finger-prints: Treatment with Glue Containing Ester', J. Forensic Sci., vol 28(2), (1983), p 307–317.

Meylan N, Lennard C, Margot P, 'Use of a Gaseous Electrical Discharge to Induce Luminescence in Latent Fingerprints', Forensic Sci. Int., vol 45, (1990), p 73–83.

Micik W, 'Latent Print Techniques', Identification, October 1974, p 3–9.

Mitchell C A, 'The Detection of Fingerprints on Documents', Analyst, vol 45, (1920), p 122–129.

Morris J R, 'An Examination of the Chemical Literature on Fingerprint Technology for the Period 1890 to August 1974', SSCD Memo 359, AWRE, October 1974.

Olenik J H, 'Super Glue, A Modified Technique for the Development of Latent Fingerprints', J. Forensic Sci., vol 29(3), (1984), p 881–884.

Olsen R D, 'The Oils of Latent Fingerprints', Fingerprint Identif. Mag., vol 56(7), (1975), p 3–12.

Olsen R D Sr, 'A Practical Fluorescent Dye Staining Technique for Cyanoacrylate-Developed Latent Prints', Identif. News, April 1984, p 5, 11–12.

Paine M, Bandey H L, Bleay S M, Willson H, 'The Effect of Relative Humidity on the Effective-ness of the Cyanoacrylate Fuming Process for Fingermark Development and on the Micro-structure of the Developed Marks', Forensic Sci. Int., vol 212(1), (2011), 130–142.

Peacock P M, 'The Development of Latent Fingerprints by the Evaporation of Anthracene', Poly-technic of the South Bank Report, February 1982.

Philipson D, Bleay S, 'Alternative Metal Processes for Vacuum Metal Deposition', J. Forensic Identif., vol 57(2), (2007), p 252–273.

Prete C, Galmiche L, Quenum-Possy-Berry F-G, Allain C, Thiburce N, Colard T, 'Lumicy-ano™: A New Fluorescent Cyanoacrylate for a One-Step Luminescent Latent Fingermark Development', Forensic Sci. Int., vol 233(1), (2013), p 104–112.

Quinche N, Margot P, 'Coulier, Paul-Jean (1824–1890): A Precursor in the History of Fingermark Detection and Their Potential Use for Identifying Their Source (1863)', J. Forensic Identif., vol 60(2), (2010), p 129–134.

Sears V G, 'I$_2$ Experiments and Notes 1987', Unpublished PSDB project file, 1987.

Smith B E, 'The Role of the Fingerprint Branch at New Scotland Yard Working in Support of the Police Officers Investigating the Provisional IRA Bombing Campaign in England 1973–1976', Proceedings of EC Working Group II, Sub-Group on Forensic Science and Related Matters, Fingerprint Symposium Held at London, 4–5 March 1981, p 69–80.

Spedding D J, 'Detection of Latent Fingerprints with $^{35}SO_2$', Nature, vol 229, (1971), p 123–124.

Spedding D J, Rowlands R P, Heard M J, 'A Method for the Detection of Fingerprints on Paper Using Sulphur-35 Sulphur Dioxide', AERE Harwell Memorandum M 2293, 28 February 1970.

Stroud P T, 'Some Comments on Finger Print Development by Vacuum Deposition', AWRE report Nuclear Research Note 5/71 (1971).

Stroud P T, 'Further Comments on Finger Print Development by Vacuum Deposition', AWRE report Nuclear Research Note 10/72 (1972).

Tahtouh M, Despland P, Shimmon R, Kalman J R, Reedy B J, 'The Application of Infrared Chemical Imaging to the Detection and Enhancement of Latent Fingerprints: Method Optimisation and Further Findings', J. Forensic Sci., vol 52(5), (2007), p 1089–1096.

Theys P, Lepareux A, Chevet G, Ceccaldi P F, 'New Technique for Bringing Out Latent Fingerprints on Paper: Vacuum Metallisation', Int. Crim. Police Rev. Part, vol 217, (1968), p 106–108.

Thiburce N, Becue A, Champod C, Crispino F, 'Design of a Control Slide for Cyanoacrylate Polymerisation: Application to the CA-Bluestar Sequence', J. Forensic Identif., vol 61(3), (2011), p 232–249.

Trowell F, 'A Method for Fixing Latent Fingerprints Developed with Iodine', J. Forensic Sci. Soc., vol 15, (1975), p 189–195.

Wargacki S P, Lewis L A, Dadmun M D, 'Understanding the Chemistry of the Development of Latent Fingerprints by Superglue Fuming', J. Forensic Sci., vol 52(5), (2007), p 1057–1062.

Wargacki S P, Lewis L A, Dadmun M D, 'Enhancing the Quality of Aged Latent Fingerprints Developed by Superglue Fuming: Loss and Replenishment of Initiator', J. Forensic Sci., vol 53(5), (2008), p 1138–1144.

Watkin J E, Wilkinson D A, Misner A H, Yamashita A B, 'Cyanoacrylate Fuming of Latent Prints – Vacuum versus Heat/Humidity', Identification Canada, July/August/September 1994, p 15–19.

Weaver D E, 'A One-Step Fluorescent Cyanoacrylate Fingerprint Development Technology', J. Forensic Identif., vol 43(5), (1993), p 481–492.

Wells A C, 'An Autoradiographic Technique for Revealing Fingerprints on Intractable Surfaces Using Radioactive Sulphur Dioxide', AERE Harwell Report R7635, September 1975.

Williams G, ap Llwyd Dafydd H, Watts A, McMurray N, 'Latent Fingermark Visualisation Using Reduced-Pressure Sublimation of Copper Phthalocyanine', Forensic Sci. Int., vol 204(1–3), (2011), p e28–e31.

Wood L W, 'The Discovery of Super Glue Fuming', Fingerprint Whorld, vol 16(64), (1991), p 117–118.

Yu I-H, Jou S, Chen C-M, Wang K-C, Pang L-J, 'Development of Latent Fingerprint by ZnO Deposition', Forensic Sci. Int., vol 207(1), (2011), p 14–18.

Further reading

Bandey H, Kent T, 'Superglue Treatment of Crime Scenes – A Trial of the Effectiveness of the Mason Vactron SUPERfume Process', PSDB Publication No. 30/03, 2003.

Fallano J F, 'Alternatives to "Alternate Light Sources": How to Achieve a Greater Print Yield with Cyanoacrylate Fuming', J. Forensic Identif., vol 42(2), (1992), p 91–95.

Froude J H Jr, 'The Super Glue Fuming Wand: A Preliminary Evaluation', J Forensic Identif., vol 46(1), (1996), p 19–31.

Fung T C, Grimwood K, Shimmon R, Spindler X, Maynard P, Lennard C, Roux C, 'Investigation of Hydrogen Cyanide Generation from the Cyanoacrylate Fuming Process Used for Latent Fingermark Detection', Forensic Sci. Int., vol 212(1–3), (2011), p 143–149.

Gellar B, Springer E, Almog J, 'Field Devices for Cyanoacrylate Fuming: A Comparative Analysis', J. Forensic Identif., vol 48(4), (1998), p 442–450.

Goode G C, Morris J R, Wells J M, 'The Application of Radioactive Bromine Isotopes for the Visualisation of Latent Fingerprints', J. Radioanal Chem., vol 48, (1979), p 17–28.

Grady D P, 'Cyanoacrylate Fuming: Accelerating by Heat within a Vacuum', J. Forensic Identif., vol 49(4), (1999), p 377–387.

Harvey K K, Dinsmore A, Brown J K, Burns D T, 'Detection of Latent Fingerprints by Vacuum Cyanoacrylate Fuming – An Improved System', Fingerprint Whorld, vol 26(99), (2000), p 29–31.

Kendall F G, 'Super Glue Fuming for the Development of Latent Fingerprints', Identif. News, vol 27(5), (1982), p 3–5.

Kent T, Winfield P, 'Superglue Fingerprint Development – Atmospheric Pressure and High Humidity, or Vacuum Deposition', Proceedings of the International Symposium on Fingerprint Detection and Identification, Ne'urim, Israel, 26–30 June 1995, p 55–66.

Mazella W D, Lennard C J, 'An Additional Study of Cyanoacrylate Stains', J. Forensic Identif., vol 45(1), (1995), p 5–18.

McCarthy M M, 'Evaluation of Ardrox as a Luminescent Stain for Cyanoacrylate Processed Latent Impressions', J. Forensic Identif., vol 40(2), (1990), p 75–80.

Mock J P, 'Super Glue Fuming Techniques – A Comparison Between Methods of Acceleration', Identif. News, November 1984, p 7, 10–11.

Stoilovic M, Kobus H J, Warrener R N, 'Luminescent Enhancement of Fingerprints Developed with Super Glue: A Case Example', Fingerprint Whorld, July 1983, p 17–18.

Tissier P, Didierjean J-C, Prud'homme C, Pichard J, Crispino F, 'A "Cyanoacrylate Case" for Developing Fingerprints in Cars', Sci. Justice, vol 39(3), (1999), p 163–166.

Vaughn J M, 'Laser Fingerprint Development: Simplified Vapour Dye Staining', Identif. News, January 1985, p 3–12.

Velthuis S, de Puit M, 'Studies Toward the Development of a Positive Control Test for the Cyanoacrylate Fuming Technique Using Artificial Sweat', J. Forensic Identif., vol 61(1), (2011), p 16–29.

Wilkinson D A, Misner A H, 'A Comparison of Thenoyl Europium Chelate with Ardrox and Rhodamine 6G for the Fluorescent Detection of Cyanoacrylate Prints', J. Forensic Identif., vol 44(4), (1994), p 387–406.

8

Solid phase selective deposition techniques

Stephen M. Bleay

Home Office Centre for Applied Science and Technology, Sandridge, UK

Key points

- The principal solid phase deposition process is powdering, which is the most widely used process for fingermark development.

- Selective adhesion of solid particles to fingermarks does not involve a chemical reaction with fingermark constituents, and hence these processes are relatively low impact.

8.1 Introduction

There are several development techniques that function by the selective deposition of solid material onto fingermark ridges or the background. This deposition may originate from a solid, liquid or vapour phase, but in all cases the essential factor is that the deposition rate on the fingermark ridges differs sufficiently from that on the background, enabling the fingermark to be readily distinguished. This chapter is specifically concerned with processes where the material deposited is already in the solid phase when it is applied to the surface. Such processes will generally have less detrimental impact on the surface and on subsequent fingermark enhancement than those processes that involve exposure to a liquid, and therefore processes of this type tend to be used towards the beginning of processing sequences.

The first of these processes is powdering, which has been used since the late 19th century (Faulds, 1912) and relies on the selective adhesion of solid particulates to

---

Fingerprint Development Techniques: Theory and Application, First Edition.
Stephen M. Bleay, Ruth S. Croxton and Marcel de Puit.

the fingermark ridges. There has been little change to the basic process since then, although many types of powder have been produced and different methods of applying them to the surface have been considered, including magnetic applicators (MacDonell, 1962), electrostatic powdering (Roy, 1976) and aerosol spray cans.

The principal advance in the 21st century relating to the powdering process has been the introduction of functionalised nanoparticles as powdering media. Powders with a wide range of functionalities are available. Some have been specifically tagged with antibodies so that they chemically bind to specific constituents of natural sweat, metabolised substances excreted in sweat or specific contaminants such as human blood (Frascione et al., 2012). Other types of functionalised nanoparticle adhere to fingermarks by conventional adhesion mechanisms but have additional functionality in that they can act as enhancers for subsequent analytical techniques (e.g. MALDI or SALDI) used to obtain chemical information from the mark (Rowell et al., 2009).

The other process described in this section is electrostatic document analysis (ESDA). This process was developed in the mid-1970s, initially for development of fingermarks on fabrics (Foster and Morantz, 1977). It was found to be relatively ineffective in this role but subsequently found to give better results for developing electrostatic images of fingermarks on paper and better still in detecting indented writing on documents (Foster and Morantz, 1979). The technique was ultimately introduced for document examination rather than fingermark enhancement and has become used worldwide for this purpose. The disadvantage of the process for fingermark enhancement is that effectiveness tends to fall rapidly as the age of the mark increases and it is ineffective on items that have been wetted. However, it is non-destructive in that there is no direct contact between the item and the developer powder, and it is still capable of developing marks that are not subsequently developed by any chemical process.

8.2   Current operational use

Powders remain the most commonly used tool worldwide, being simple, effective, cheap and versatile. Powders can be used on non-porous and semi-porous surfaces both at crime scenes and in a laboratory, and marks are developed rapidly. Powders should not be used on sticky or heavily contaminated surfaces because the particles will adhere across the entire surface and the fingermark may not be readily discriminated.

The fundamental process has changed little since first being proposed in the 19th century, with some of the earliest brush and powder combinations still being in use today. Initial powder formulations tended to be granular in form and black, white or grey in colour to give contrast with a range of different surfaces. Although granular powders are still used, metal flake powders (in particular aluminium) are now the most widely used type of powder in the United Kingdom, primarily because of their compatibility with the subsequent lifting process. Lifting of marks enables rapid collection of large numbers of marks from a crime scene without the time constraints of imaging in situ but may result in a deterioration in quality. The other type of powders that has found increasing application is magnetic powders, available in both granular and flake forms, both of which tend to give better results on textured surfaces than granular or metal flake powders. Fluorescent powders are also available, in both granular and magnetic forms. Although not widely used in the United Kingdom, they do find more widespread application in other countries around the world.

Marks developed by powders probably account for the largest number of fingermark identifications worldwide; in the United Kingdom alone approximately 50% of the ~50 000 fingerprint identifications per annum arise from marks developed using this process. It is therefore evident that even the small percentage improvements that can be achieved by selection of the optimum powder and brush combination for a particular surface have the potential to provide significant operational benefits.

Different types of nanoparticle are becoming commercially available, although many of the reported types are still in research or developmental stage. If operational benefits can be demonstrated in their use, they may increasingly displace some of the existing powder types and find a market niche.

The ESDA process is not generally used as a primary fingermark enhancement technique because it is less sensitive than other techniques for developing fingermarks on porous surfaces and is ineffective on marks more than 24 h old. However, it may reveal fingermarks when used as part of an integrated strategy for retrieval of forensic evidence, ESDA being mostly non-destructive to fingerprint evidence unless pre-humidification is used. In this respect, ESDA could be more widely applied for its original purpose of fingermark enhancement.

8.3   Powders

8.3.1   Outline history of the process

Late 1800s: Faulds (1912) stated that Forgeot was already conducting experiments into methods for enhancing fingermarks by powdering.

1905: Faulds described formulations for different colours of powder and the different types of animal hair brush required for optimum results.

1920: Mitchell described a wide range of different coloured powders that had been considered for fingermark enhancement, including mercury–chalk (hydrargyrum-cum-creta), graphite, lamp black, ferric oxide, magnesium carbonate, aniline dye stuffs, lycopodium powder–Sudan Red mixture, red lead oxide, lead carbonate, lead iodide and lead acetate.

1934: Brose reported the first use of fluorescent and phosphorescent powders (anthracene and zinc sulphide) to overcome interfering background patterns, using long-wave ultraviolet radiation to promote luminescence and phosphorescence, respectively.

1962: MacDonell introduced the 'Magna Brush' for the application of magnetic granular powders, consisting of a retractable bar magnet within a non-magnetic cover material. A 'brush' of magnetic powder was formed around the tip of the applicator that could then be used to powder the surface.

Early 1970s: Aluminium flake powder in combination with lifting introduced as the principal powdering process by the Metropolitan Police (Lambourne, 1984).

1976: Roy reported research into electrostatic powdering and outlined equipment and types of powder that could be used for enhancement of marks using a contactless, electrostatic powdering method. This was not ultimately pursued further.

1991: James et al. developed a magnetic flake powder ('Magneta Flake') designed to combine advantageous features of both metal flake and magnetic granular powders (James et al., 1991a, 1991b, 1991c).

2004–2007: Bandey and co-workers reported results of comprehensive, comparative studies between metal flake, granular, magnetic flake and magnetic granular powders on a range of different surface types (Bandey, 2004; Bandey and Gibson, 2006; Bandey and Hardy, 2006; Bandey, 2007).

8.3.2 Theory

All types of powder used for fingermark enhancement utilise adhesion mechanisms that occur between the particulate material in the powder and the material in the fingermark ridges. For the process to be effective, the affinity of the powder to the fingermark must be greater than that of the powder to the surface, so that selective deposition occurs.

There are many mechanisms that may play a role in the selective adhesion of particles to fingermark deposits, and more than one of these mechanisms may operate for any given powder type. The factors that may influence adhesion include, but are not exclusively restricted to, the following:

• Particle shape

• Surface chemistry of the powder particle

• Electrostatic charge on the particle (and surface)

• Adhesion to grease

• Wetting of particles by liquids

Particle shape can affect the way in which particles adhere to the surface in several ways. Whereas granular powders tend to be spherical in shape, or have low aspect ratios, flake powders are flat and have high aspect ratios. This means that when the different particle types are applied to the surface, the flat shape of flake powders gives them a higher surface area of contact with the fingermark deposits. The shape will also affect the way in which particles move across the surface, which is particularly relevant when powders are being applied using a fibre brush. The low aspect ratio granular powders can roll across the surface, whereas flake powders are more likely to slide. This mode of movement may make particular mechanisms of adhesion more or less likely.

Modifying the surface chemistry can influence the mode of adhesion of a powder particle to the fingermark. Zimon (1969) describes how particle adhesion to a solid surface in air occurs partly due to molecular forces. By changing the surface chemistry of the powder particle, and therefore the type of molecules present at the surface, the interaction between that particle and the medium it adheres to will be changed. Surface coatings have been shown to influence the effectiveness of metal flake powders (both magnetic and non-magnetic) during fingermark development. James et al. (1991a, 1991b) demonstrated that the presence of stearic acid coatings was necessary for fingermark enhancement using magnetic flake powders and that optimum results were obtained for a coating thickness of 70 nm. Most aluminium flake powders also have stearic acid coatings. In these cases lipophilic interactions may be occurring between the stearic acid coating and closely related fatty acids present in the fingermark.

Zimon (1969) states that if particles are highly charged, the value of the attractive Coulomb forces to the surface may exceed that of other contributions to adhesion. Fingermarks may possess some residual electrical charge soon after deposition, and if charged particles are used for powdering, they may become attracted to the mark (Figure 8.1).

Although Roy (1976) investigated ways of utilising this effect for enhancing fingermark development using charged powders such as calcium tungstate, it is not the major mechanism used in any of the types of powder currently used at crime scenes. The contact of the brush on the surface during powdering tends to remove residual

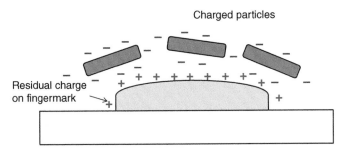

Figure 8.1 Schematic diagram showing electrostatic attraction between charged particles and the residual charge on a fingermark.

static charge from the fingermark, and therefore it is considered that this mechanism does not generally play a role.

The presence of viscous, greasy constituents in a fingermark can contribute to the mechanisms by which powders adhere to it. For small, low aspect ratio particles that can roll across the surface, the presence of a high viscosity medium may cause the particle to slow and ultimately be trapped within the fingermark (Figure 8.2).

For cases where the fingermark contains lower viscosity liquids such as water, other adhesive mechanisms may operate. Firstly, the liquid may be able to wet the surface of the powder particle, thus giving a greater contact area for weak attractive interactions. The second mechanism that may operate is the capillary force of the liquid caused by surface tension. In atmospheres of relative humidity in excess of 70% the increase observed in the adhesion of microscopic particles is due to capillary forces, illustrated schematically in Figure 8.3.

Wertheim (1997) suggests 'huffing' (blowing warm or hot air or breathing over the mark) as a means of improving the effectiveness of powders on marks that may have dried out. It is thought that this practice rehumidifies the mark and makes this mechanism of adhesion more likely.

The powdering process is not necessarily complete once the initial layer of particles has adhered to the fingermark. It may be necessary for additional layers of particles to adhere for the fingermark to become sufficiently visible, and in this situation the process of auto-adhesion (the interaction between individual powder particles) becomes important, more so for flake powders than for granular powders, because flake powder particles have large surface areas over which they can interact.

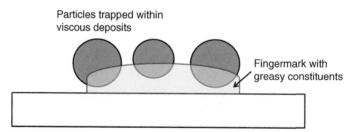

Figure 8.2   Schematic diagram showing trapping of low aspect ratio particles within the viscous constituents of a fingermark.

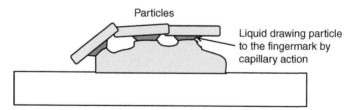

Figure 8.3   Schematic diagram showing wetting and drawing of high aspect ratio particles to a fingermark by low viscosity liquid constituents.

For aluminium flake powders, it is known that marks can be built up by successive passes of the brush, indicating that strong auto-adhesive bonds do exist between aluminium powder particles. For magnetic flake powders, marks are usually developed using a single sweep of the applicator, with further passes thought to 'fill in' or reduce the quality of the fingermark. This indicates that auto-adhesive forces between magnetic flake particles are weaker and the magnetised particles may even repel each other.

8.3.3 The powders process

The types of powder currently in widespread use can be grouped into several main classes, these being as follows:

- Metal flake powder (e.g. aluminium and bronze)
- Granular powder (black and white)
- Magnetic granular powders
- Magnetic flake powder
- Fluorescent powders

The abovementioned categories represent a general classification, and many individual powder blends are available in the world market, some of which could be described by more than one category. There is no one powder that will consistently develop marks of optimal quality on all types of surface, and powders (and their method of application) should be selected on the basis of the type of surface that is present.

The types of powder that are in routine use in the United Kingdom are metal flake, granular, magnetic granular and magnetic flake powders. The uses of different types of powders in the process are described in greater detail in the succeeding text.

8.3.3.1 *Metal flake powder*

The particulates most commonly used as metal flake powders are aluminium and brass (also commonly described as 'bronze' or 'gold' due to their colour). Both types of powder contain metal flakes with smooth surfaces and jagged edges. The diameter of the particles falls within the range 1–12 μm and the thickness is approximately 0.5 μm (Figure 8.4). The flakes are coated with stearic acid during the milling process to prevent clumping.

Metal flake powders are most effective on smooth, non-porous surfaces, with aluminium being particularly effective on glass. Aluminium will develop marks of good contrast on most surfaces, but where developed marks will not be readily seen

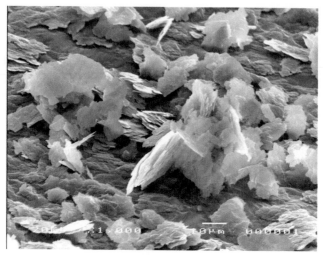

Figure 8.4   Scanning electron micrographs of a representative aluminium powder. Reproduced courtesy of the Home Office.

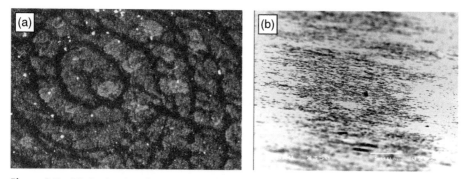

Figure 8.5   Marks developed using aluminium flake powder, (a) optical micrograph of a mark on a dark surface and (b) scanning electron micrograph of a powdered ridge. Reproduced courtesy of the Home Office.

(e.g. on silver-painted surfaces), brass flake powder can be used instead. Images of marks enhanced using aluminium flake powder are illustrated in Figure 8.5.

The most effective application method for use with metal flake powder is the Zephyr-style glass fibre brush (Figure 8.6).

In comparative tests (Bandey, 2004), this type of brush gave the optimum combination of ridge detail, contrast and minimal brush damage to the developed mark. This is because the glass fibre brush retained the powder well and released it gradually, making it well suited to the progressive build-up of the aluminium particulates on the mark that is required for this type of powder.

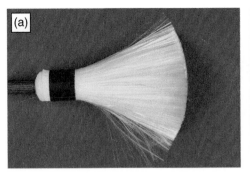
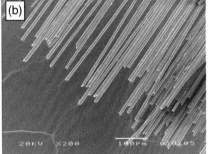

Figure 8.6 Pictures of Zephyr-style glass fibre brushes: (a) visual image and (b) scanning electron micrograph. Reproduced courtesy of the Home Office.

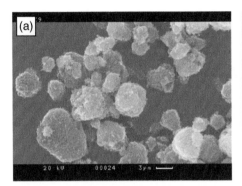
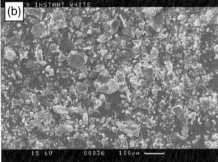

Figure 8.7 Scanning electron micrographs of typical (a) black and (b) white granular powder. Reproduced courtesy of the Home Office.

8.3.3.2 Granular powders

Most black granular powders are carbon based, produced by pyrolysis of organic compounds (e.g. lamp black). The example shown in Figure 8.7a consists of amorphous, elemental carbon with a particle size in the range 5–10 μm and an irregular (but smooth) shape.

White powders are more varied in composition and may contain more than one particle type. Figure 8.7b shows an example that consists of large flakes of magnesium silicate (20–100 μm in size) that may act as a carrier for the smaller granules of titanium dioxide (mostly <1 μm). Other white powders such as chalk (calcium carbonate) may also be encountered.

Granular powders are generally considered as less sensitive than other types of powder, and their small, low aspect ratio particles may become readily trapped by surface features. Black granular powder is suggested for use on some smooth surfaces and can be considered as an alternative to brass flake powder on silver-coloured surfaces. White granular powder can be used on dark-coloured surfaces,

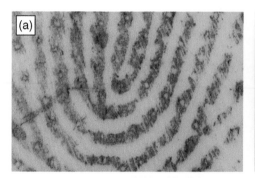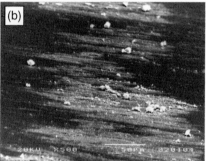

Figure 8.8 Marks developed using granular powders: (a) optical micrograph of a black granular powder mark on a light surface and (b) scanning electron micrograph of a powdered ridge. Reproduced courtesy of the Home Office.

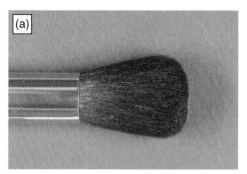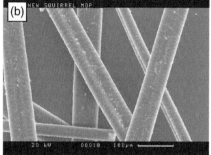

Figure 8.9 Pictures of animal (squirrel) hair mop style brushes, visual image and scanning electron micrograph. Reproduced courtesy of the Home Office.

but other types of light powder (aluminium flake, magnetic flake) may give better results. However, granular powders are likely to adhere to the mark by different mechanisms to flake powders, and there may be benefit in using the two types in sequence. Examples of marks developed using granular powders are illustrated in Figure 8.8.

Squirrel hair, mop-style brushes (Figure 8.9) are the most widely used brush for use with granular powders. Animal hair brushes do not retain powder particularly well, and the brush may have to be regularly recharged when powdering large areas.

8.3.3.3 *Magnetic granular powders*

A range of different magnetic granular powders are available in colours ranging from black to white to give contrast with the surface. Black magnetic powders are most commonly used and these consist of large magnetic carrier particles of elemental iron (20–200 μm) and smaller non-magnetic particles of iron oxide

(Fe_3O_4) with a particle size in the range 3–12 µm (Figure 8.10). The larger particles act as a carrier medium for the smaller particles, which selectively adhere to the fingermark ridges.

Magnetic granular powder is generally most effective on textured surfaces and u-PVC (Bandey and Hardy, 2006). The best results have been observed with dark-coloured powders (black and 'jet black') with lighter powder types (e.g. grey, silver) found to be lower in sensitivity. White magnetic powder, although less effective than grey and silver magnetic granular powders, may still have applications for enhancing marks on dark, textured surfaces when contrast is an issue. Examples of marks developed using magnetic granular powders are illustrated in Figure 8.11.

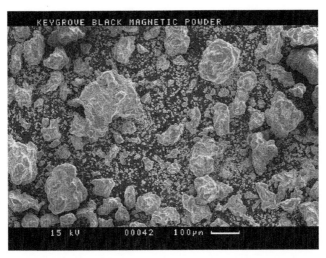

Figure 8.10 Scanning electron micrograph of a representative magnetic granular powder. Reproduced courtesy of the Home Office.

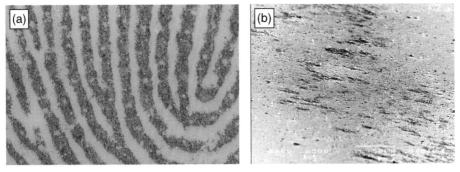

Figure 8.11 Marks developed using magnetic granular powders: (a) optical micrograph of a mark on a dark surface and (b) scanning electron micrograph of a powdered ridge. Reproduced courtesy of the Home Office.

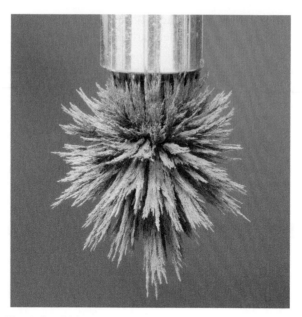

Figure 8.12   A 'brush' formed on a magnetic wand by a black magnetic powder.

Magnetic granular powders are applied using magnetic wand applicators, where a small magnet at the tip of the wand picks up a 'brush' of powder when dipped into the powder container (Figure 8.12).

This powder 'brush' is then applied to the surface, thus avoiding any direct contact between the applicator and the surface and minimising the possibility of damage to the mark (James et al., 1991c). Although such powders are relatively easy to apply to horizontal surfaces, application to vertical surfaces is less straightforward and powder may drop off. Ease of application to a particular surface should be taken into consideration when selecting the powder to use.

8.3.3.4   *Magnetic flake powders*

The first of these types of powder was Magneta Flake, developed in the early 1990s (James et al., 1991a, 1991b, 1991c) and produced by milling spherical carbonyl iron with 3–5% stearic acid in an appropriate solvent to produce a smooth edged flake with particle sizes in the range 10–60 μm (Figure 8.13). Other types of magnetic flake powder are now available.

Magneta Flake powder is slightly less sensitive than black magnetic powder on textured surfaces, but may provide a more contrasting development technique on dark textured surfaces. It can also be used on most smooth surfaces although application can be difficult and inconsistent. Examples of marks developed using magnetic granular powders are illustrated in Figure 8.14.

Magnetic flake powders are generally applied to the surface with a magnetic wand applicator, as for magnetic granular powders.

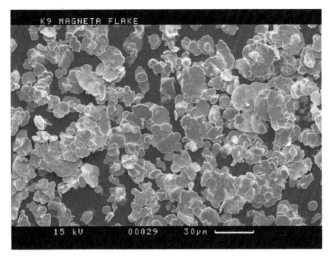

Figure 8.13 Scanning electron micrograph of a representative magnetic flake powder. Reproduced courtesy of the Home Office.

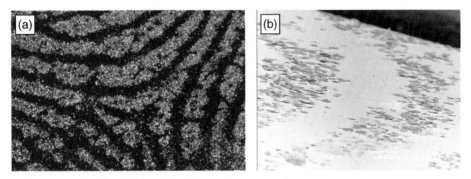

Figure 8.14 Marks developed using magnetic flake powders: (a) optical micrograph of a mark on a dark surface and (b) scanning electron micrograph of a powdered ridge. Reproduced courtesy of the Home Office.

8.3.3.5 *Fluorescent powders*

Fluorescent powders are available in a range of different colours including red, orange, green and yellow. Most powders currently available use large organic particles such as cornstarch to as carriers for the fine fluorescent dye particles (Figure 8.15).

Fluorescent powders may have applications on highly coloured and/or textured surfaces where it may be difficult to visualise marks developed by other powders and can be applied with a range of different types of brush. Another potential application of these powders is to enhance marks developed using cyanoacrylate fuming that cannot be treated with fluorescent dye solutions.

Recent developments of fluorescent powders include powders with anti-Stokes properties (Ma et al., 2011; Drabarek et al., 2012) and powders with fluorescence in

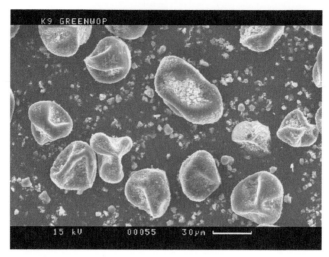

Figure 8.15 Scanning electron micrograph of a representative fluorescent powder. Reproduced courtesy of the Home Office.

the infrared region of the spectrum (King et al., 2015; Errington et al., 2016). Both these types of powder are produced to improve visualisation of fingermarks on patterned, coloured surfaces, by significantly reducing the likelihood of developed marks being obscured by background fluorescence.

8.3.3.6 *Powdering and lifting*

An important decision once marks have been powdered is to consider whether any marks that have been developed should be imaged in situ or whether they should be lifted from the surface. Each of these processes has advantages and disadvantages associated with it, and the type of powder that has been used to develop the mark will also influence the decision of which route to take.

Lifting involves using an adhesive lifting medium to remove traces of the developed mark from the surface. The process is described separately in greater detail in Chapter 15. The advantages of lifting are that a large number of marks can be collected quickly from the crime scene, it overcomes issues associated with trying to image marks on highly shaped, textured or coloured surfaces, and the lift can be kept as a first-generation permanent record of the mark.

The disadvantages of lifting are that by lifting the mark from the surface, potentially important contextual information about the environment the mark was found in may be removed and that the quality of the lifted mark may be degraded from that originally developed on the surface. This is because some of the powder will remain on the developed mark, whilst the remainder adheres to the lifting medium, and therefore the lifted mark will only imperfectly replicate the detail originally developed. For many marks this will not be a major issue, but for others it may degrade the quality of a potentially identifiable mark to one that is considered insufficient for comparison.

Lifting is a process most compatible with flake powders because the developed marks consist of layers of flat particles that can readily separate from each other due to weak interlayer bonding. It is less appropriate to granular and magnetic granular powders, which have particles strongly attached to the fingermark residue, resulting in less carryover of powder particles to the lifting medium. This may result in a greater degradation in quality of the lifted mark for these powder types.

8.4 ESDA

8.4.1 Outline history of the process

Mid 1970s: Foster and Morantz at the London College of Printing developed equipment for electrostatically charging and imaging fingermarks on fabrics under contract to the UK Home Office. Issues associated with rapid charge decay were overcome by covering the surface with a thin layer of polyester and producing the charge image on the thin polymer film (Foster and Morantz, 1977).

1979: During further tests into electrostatic fingermark enhancement on paper, it was observed (Foster and Morantz, 1979; Young, 1979) that the process is particularly effective for enhancing indentations in paper surfaces and it is subsequently commercialised for this purpose.

An example of fingermarks detected on paper using ESDA is shown in Figure 8.16.

8.4.2 Theory

The precise mechanism of why electrostatic images of fingermarks are formed during the ESDA process has not been conclusively established.

It is known that the application of a corona charge spraying device (known as a corotron) across the surface of a thin polyester film in intimate contact with the surface sets up electrostatic fringing fields that are locally concentrated at features on the item such as indentations or fingermarks. These charge patterns are subsequently revealed by the application of a cascade powder (a mixture of carrier beads (fine glass spheres) and toner particles (carbon black)) that results in preferential deposition of the toner particles in regions where the charge patterns are present (Figure 8.17).

Foster and Morantz (1979) originally proposed that the formation of the fringing fields could be explained by a simple capacitance theory. In this theory, the fingermarks produce a local increase in dielectric constant in the paper substrate because of the

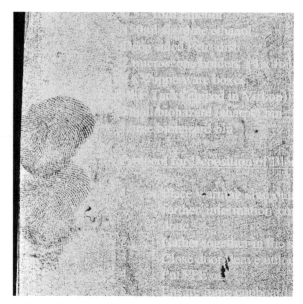

Figure 8.16 Fingermarks developed by ESDA on a paper document.

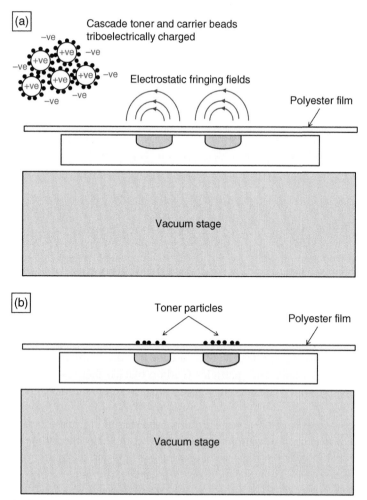

(a) Cascade toner and carrier beads triboelectrically charged

−ve +ve −ve
−ve +ve +ve −ve
+ve +ve +ve −ve
−ve −ve

Electrostatic fringing fields

Polyester film

Vacuum stage

(b) Toner particles

Polyester film

Vacuum stage

Figure 8.17 Schematic diagrams showing toner development of electrostatic images, (a) development of electrostatic fringing fields on the polymer film and (b) selective adherence of toner particles to regions where fields are present.

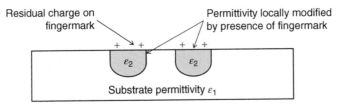

Figure 8.18 Schematic diagram illustrating local modification of the dielectric constant (permittivity) of the paper substrate by the fingermark.

presence of water and other high permittivity constituents and the filling of air gaps in the paper by the fingermark (Figure 8.18).

However, capacitance variations cannot be the only mechanism that can operate because it is noted that very deep indented writing impressions (which would give also give large local changes in capacitance) sometimes do not develop with ESDA.

Kent (1986) later proposed that the development of indented writing could be explained by damage and abrasion of surface fibres caused by lateral movement between sheets of paper during the writing process, resulting in areas that charge in a different way from the rest of the surface. However, it is unlikely that sufficient surface damage would be caused by contact from a finger for this to be the dominant mechanism for fingermark enhancement.

Another theory proposed to explain the improved performance of ESDA, which was often observed after pre-humidification of the article was termed 'surface variation theory' (Wanxiang and Xiaoling, 1987), which considered that after humidification the paper no longer behaved as a dielectric but had sufficient moisture content to be effectively considered as a conductor.

Surface variation theory considered that the variation of electrostatic potential on the polymer film was influenced by the level of intimate contact formed between the polymer film and the paper. This in turn would be affected by variations in the surface features of the paper such as porosity and texture (which may also be modified by the presence of the fingermark). This could explain why deep indentations, where the film may not physically contact the paper, do not always produce results using ESDA. As fingermarks are progressively absorbed into the porous surface, their effect on the surface will also progressively reduce, and this may explain the reduction in effectiveness for ESDA observed on marks over 24 h old.

8.4.3 The ESDA process

The ESDA process utilises specialist equipment designed purposefully and available from several manufacturers. Its use is restricted to thin, porous items that can fit on the vacuum stage (typically documents).

The item to be treated is first drawn down onto a vacuum stage. A thin (~3.5 µm) polyester film is laid over the top of the item so that the film is drawn down to form intimate contact with the surface, ensuring that the film is free from creases that may otherwise physically trap toner beads instead of allowing them to be electrically attracted to the fringing fields.

With the film in place, charge is applied to a charge-spraying device known as a corotron or corona wand (a thin wire held at high voltage within a shielded metal enclosure). The corona wand is then passed over the surface of the film in a series of sweeps, without actually making contact with the surface itself and without following too regular a pattern. The charged surface is then left to stand for a short period to allow the fringing fields that form the charge pattern to develop.

The vacuum stage is then tilted and the cascade toner shaken across the surface. The angle of tilt is such that the glass carrier beads easily roll across the surface, but the carbon black toner particles carried by them may be retained by the electrostatic charge pattern developed on the surface. Application of the toner is continued until it is considered that optimum development of fingermarks has occurred.

The developed marks are very fragile and should be either imaged in situ, preserved by laminating the polyester film with a clear adhesive acetate sheet or lifted.

8.5 Nanoparticle powders

8.5.1 Outline history of the process

Because of the wide range of nanoparticle technologies being considered for fingermark enhancement, it is difficult to provide a definitive timeline for the history of the process, but research into these techniques has increased significantly since the early 2000s. A comprehensive review of nanoparticle technologies used for fingermark detection has been conducted elsewhere (Becue and Cantu, in Ramotowski, 2013).

This section exclusively considers nanoparticles that are used as dusting powders. It is separated from the section Powders because the theory associated with fingermark enhancement using certain types of functionalised nanoparticle differs significantly from that of conventional powders.

8.5.2 Theory

There are two principal ways in which functionalised nanoparticles have been used as a solid deposition process for fingermark enhancement. Functionalised nanoparticles may also be used as aqueous suspensions, but this is potentially more damaging to the substrate and considered outside the scope of this chapter.

In the first approach, the nanoparticle is functionalised using antibodies so that it specifically binds to one or more constituents present within the fingermark. Additional functional species may also be incorporated so that the tagged nanoparticle may also have, for example, fluorescent properties, making it easier to detect.

Nanoparticles tagged with a range of different antibodies have been produced for the purposes of fingermark enhancement, applied either in solid form or from an aqueous medium. These include the following:

- Drug metabolites (Leggett et al., 2007)
- Proteins in blood plasma (Reinholz, 2008)
- Skin proteins (Drapel et al., 2008)
- Body fluids (Frascione et al., 2012)
- Amino acids (Spindler et al., 2011; Wood et al., 2013)

The nanoparticles used as the basis of the functionalised system also vary, with gold, iron oxide, titanium dioxide and silica all being reported.

Antibodies will not bind directly to the nanoparticles, so the nanoparticle must first be treated so that linking molecules can be attached to its surface and the antibodies attached to the linking molecule in a subsequent treatment. A schematic representation of a generic antibody tagged nanoparticle is illustrated in Figure 8.19.

When these functionalised nanoparticles are applied to the surface and fingermark, under appropriate conditions the antibodies specifically bind to the fingermark constituents that they have been designed to interact with (Figure 8.20) and do not bind to other regions of the fingermark or surface.

For the second type of nanoparticle powder that may be encountered, the functionalised nanoparticle binds to the fingermark by similar mechanisms to those outlined for the abovementioned conventional powders. The additional functionality incorporated into the nanoparticle during manufacture can include fluorescent or magnetic properties. The use of nanoparticles has been claimed to give enhanced definition of third-level detail (such as pores) within the fingermark compared with that observed in equivalent marks developed using conventional powders. However,

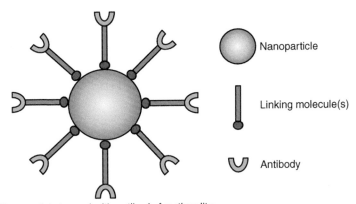

Nanoparticle tagged with antibody functionality

Figure 8.19 Schematic diagram of a generic functionalised nanoparticle.

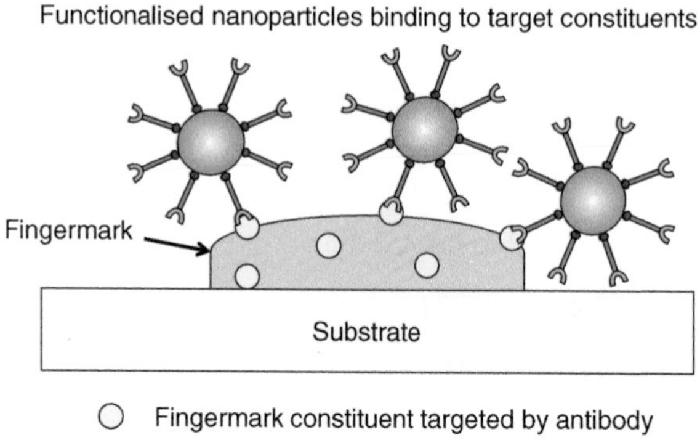

Functionalised nanoparticles binding to target constituents

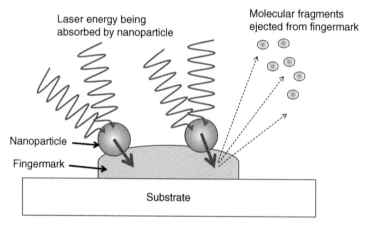

Figure 8.20   Schematic diagram of constituent-specific binding of functionalised nanoparticles.

Figure 8.21   Schematic diagram showing how nanoparticles act as matrix enhancers for processes producing ionisation of the fingermark.

developing the mark is not the sole function of the powder, and it can also be used as a 'matrix enhancer' for subsequent analytical techniques such as SALDI and MALDI (Chapter 15), where the particle strongly absorbs the incident laser energy and concentrates it into the fingermark (Figure 8.21). This increases the subsequent ionisation yield from the fingermark and assists with subsequent compositional mapping and analysis of the mark (Rowell et al., 2009).

8.5.3   The nanoparticle powders process

Nanoparticle powders can be applied to the surface by similar methods proposed for conventional powders, namely brushes, magnetic applicators, electrostatic application and aerosol spraying. The exact method of application will depend on the specific type of nanoparticle being used.

It may be necessary to have a means of removing excess nanoparticles from the surface for the mark to be seen. This may be by washing with water, but in the case of the systems reported by Frascione et al. (2012), a magnetic nanoparticle is used, and the excess particles removed using a magnet.

References

Bandey H L, 'The Powders Process, Study 1: Evaluation of Fingerprint Brushes for Use with Aluminium Powder', PSDB Fingerprint Development and Imaging Newsletter, Special Edition, Publication No. 54/04, (2004).

Bandey H L, 'Fingerprint Powders Guidelines', HOSDB Publication No. 09/07, (2007).

Bandey H L, Gibson A P, 'The Powders Process, Study 2: Evaluation of Fingerprint Powders on Smooth Surfaces', HOSDB Fingerprint Development and Imaging Newsletter, Special Edition, Publication No. 08/06, (2006).

Bandey H L, Hardy T, 'The Powders Process, Study 3: Evaluation of Fingerprint Powders on Textured Surfaces and U-PVC', HOSDB Fingerprint and Footwear Forensics Newsletter, Special Edition, Publication No. 67/06, (2006).

Brose H L, 'Finger-Print Detection', Analyst, vol 59, (1934), p 25–27.

Drabarek B, Siejca A, Moszczyński J, Konior B, 'Applying Anti-Stokes Phosphors in Development of Fingerprints on Surfaces Characterized by Strong Luminescence', J. Forensic Identif., vol 62(1), (2012), p 28–35.

Drapel V, Becue A, Champod C, Margot P, 'Identification of Promising Antigenic Components in Latent Fingermark Residues', Forensic Sci. Int., vol 184(1–3), 2008, p 47–53.

Errington B, Lawson G, Lewis S W, Smith G D, 'Micronised Egptian Blue pigment: A Novel Near-Infrared Luminescent Fingerprint Dusting Powder', Dyes Pigm., vol 132, (2016), p 310–315.

Faulds H, 'Guide to Fingerprint Identification', Wood, Mitchell and Co., Hanley, (1905).

Faulds H, 'Dactylography, or the Study of Fingerprints', Milner, Halifax, (1912).

Foster D J, Morantz D J, 'The Detection of Fingerprints on Fabrics by the Development of Electrostatic Images', Final Report on PSDB contract, London College of Printing, (1977).

Foster D J, Morantz D J, 'An Electrostatic Imaging Technique for the Detection of Indented Impressions in Documents', Forensic Sci. Int., vol 13, (1979), p 51–54.

Frascione N, Thorogate R, Daniel B, Jickells S, 'Detection and Identification of Body Fluid Stains Using Antibody-Nanoparticle Conjugates', Analyst, vol 137, (2012), p 508–512.

James J D, Pounds C A, Wilshire B, 'Flake Metal Powders for Revealing Latent Fingerprints', J. Forensic Sci., vol 36(5), (1991a), p 1368–1375.

James J D, Pounds C A, Wilshire B, 'Production and Characterisation of Flake Metal Powders for Fingerprint Detection', Powder Metall., vol 34(1), (1991b), p 39–43.

James J D, Pounds C A, Wilshire B, 'Obliteration of Latent Fingerprints', J. Forensic Sci., vol 36(5), (1991c), p 1376–1386.

Kent T, 'The Electrostatic Development of Fingerprints and Indented Writing – A Review', unpublished HO SRDB paper, (1986).

King R S P, Hallett P M, Foster D, 'Seeing into the Infrared: A Novel IR Fluorescent Fingerprint Powder', Forensic Sci. Int., vol 249, (2015), p e21–e26.

Lambourne G, 'The Fingerprint Story', Harrap, London, (1984).

Leggett R, Lee-Smith E E, Jickells S M, Russell D A, 'Intelligent Fingerprinting: Simultaneous Identification of Drug Metabolites and Individuals by Using Antibody-Functionalized Nanoparticles', Angew. Chem. Int. Ed., vol 46(22), (2007), p 4100–4103.

Ma R, Bullock E, Maynard P, Reedy B, Shimmon R, Lennard C, Roux C, McDonagh A, 'Fingermark Detection on Non-Porous and Semi-Porous Surfaces Using NaYF4:Er,Yb Up-converter Particles', Forensic Sci. Int., vol 207(1–3), (2011), p 145–149.

MacDonell H L, 'Recent Developments in Processing Latent Finger Prints', Identif. News, August 1962, p 3–18.

Mitchell C A, 'The Detection of Fingerprints on Documents', Analyst, vol 45, (1920), p 122–129.

Ramotowski R (ed.), 'Lee and Gaensslen's Advances in Fingerprint Technology', 3rd Edition, CRC Press, Boca Raton, 2013.

Reinholz A D, 'Albumin Development Method to Visualize Friction Ridge Detail on Porous Surfaces', J. Forensic Identif., vol 58(5), (2008), p 524–539.

Rowell F, Hudson K, Seviour J, 'Detection of Drugs and their Metabolites in Dusted Latent Fingermarks by Mass Spectrometry', Analyst, vol 134(4), (2009), p 701–707.

Roy P, 'Electrostatic Powder Development of Fingerprints at Scenes of Crime', HO PSDB Research Note 13/76, (1976).

Spindler X, Hofstetter O, McDonagh A M, Roux C P, Lennard C J, 'Enhancement of Latent Fingermarks on Non-Porous Surfaces Using Anti-L-Amino Acid Antibodies Conjugated to Gold Nanoparticles', Chem. Commun., vol 47(19), (2011), p 5602–5604.

Wanxiang L, Xiaoling C, 'Electrostatic Imaging Technique: A Study of Its Principle and the Effect of Experimental Condition on Imaging', presented at IAFS Vancouver, 2–7 August 1987.

Wertheim P A, 'Magnetic Powder', Minutiae, The Lightning Powder Co. Newsletter, 43 (July–August 1997).

Wood M, Maynard P J, Spindler X, Roux C P, Lennard C J, 'Selective Targeting of Fingermarks Using Immunogenic Techniques', Aust. J. Forensic Sci., vol 45(2), (2013), p 211–226.

Young P A, 'Equipment for the Detection of Indented Impressions', HO PSDB Tech. Memo. No. 8/79, (1979).

Zimon A D, 'Adhesion of Dust and Powder', Plenum Press, New York, (1969).

9

Amino acid reagents

Stephen M. Bleay

Home Office Centre for Applied Science and Technology, Sandridge, UK

Key points

- Amino acid reagents are generally the most effective processes for development of marks on porous surfaces.

- Although many different amino acid reagents have been considered, only three (ninhydrin, DFO and 1,2-indandione) are in widespread use.

- Because amino acids are water soluble, amino acid reagents are not effective on surfaces that have been wetted.

9.1 Introduction

The most important class of reagents for the enhancement of fingermarks on porous surfaces are those that react with the amino acid constituents of fingermarks to yield a coloured and/or fluorescent product. The amino acid reagents described in this chapter fall into two categories: those that theoretically give the same reaction product regardless of the amino acid involved in the reaction and those that give reaction products that retain some characteristic groups associated with the original amino acid involved in the reaction. These are summarised in Table 9.1. In some cases the reaction may not proceed to completion, and intermediate compounds may be present in the developed fingermark.

The first and probably still the most operationally significant of all amino acid reagents is ninhydrin. First proposed for this purpose in the early 1950s (Oden and von Hofsten, 1954), ninhydrin gives a visible purple reaction product 'Ruhemann's purple' with amino acids, and most marks develop within minutes under optimal

---

Fingerprint Development Techniques: Theory and Application, First Edition.
Stephen M. Bleay, Ruth S. Croxton and Marcel de Puit.
© 2018 John Wiley & Sons Ltd. Published 2018 by John Wiley & Sons Ltd.

Table 9.1 Amino acid reagents categorised by the type of reaction product formed with amino acids.

Reagents giving reaction products independent of amino acid	Reagents giving reaction products characteristic of amino acid
Ninhydrin	Fluorescamine
1,8-Diazafluoren-9-one (DFO)	o-Phthalaldehyde
1,2-Indandione	Genipin
Ninhydrin analogues	NBD chloride
Alloxan	Dansyl chloride
Lawsone	Dimethylaminocinnemaldehyde
Isatin	Dimethylaminobenzaldehyde

conditions of temperature and humidity. Although other related chemicals such as alloxan were evaluated as fingermark enhancement reagents soon afterwards (Morris, 1974), none of these were found to be as effective as ninhydrin. The synthesis of the fluorescent amino acid reagents fluorescamine (Udenfriend et al., 1972) and o-phthalaldehyde (Benson and Hare, 1975) in the late 1960s/early 1970s led to investigations of their use for fingermark enhancement. Although potentially more sensitive than ninhydrin, neither of these reagents ultimately found widespread use because the long-wave ultraviolet radiation used to excite fluorescence in the fingermark also caused strong fluorescence of the optical brighteners used in many modern paper types, making the fingermark difficult to distinguish. However, the concept that reagents producing fluorescent reaction products could be more effective than those producing coloured products prompted further research.

The use of metal salts to change the colour of the ninhydrin reaction product was first proposed in the late 1970s (Morris, 1978), but it was later found that some of these metal complexes were also fluorescent (Herod and Menzel, 1982). Metal toning became used as a post-treatment for ninhydrin, increasing the overall number of marks detected, but two processing steps were still required to produce fluorescent marks. The first operationally significant reagent to produce fluorescent marks in a single processing step was 1,8-diazafluoren-9-one (DFO), first introduced in 1990 (Grigg et al., 1990). DFO developed significantly more marks than ninhydrin and could also be used before it in a processing sequence. It subsequently found widespread use, but research continued into analogues of ninhydrin and DFO in the hope that one of these could give further improvements in performance. The most significant compound arising from this research was 1,2-indandione (Hauze et al., 1998), and much research has subsequently been carried out to compare its performance with that of DFO. The discovery that metal salts could be introduced into the 1,2-indandione formulation to enhance both the intensity of fluorescence and the consistency of the results obtained in environments where ambient humidity can be variable (Stoilovic et al., 2007) has resulted in a significant increase in the operational use of 1,2-indandione.

Other recent research into amino acid reagents has focused on the identification of 'dual action' reagents, those that are capable of developing marks that are both

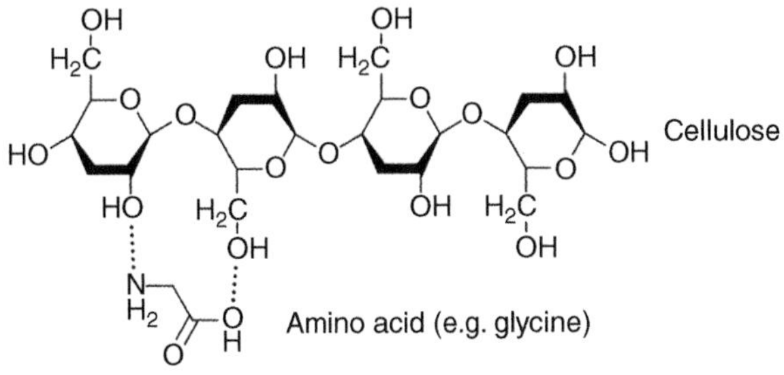

Figure 9.1 Chemical bonding schematic showing how amino acids can form hydrogen bonds with sites along a cellulose fibre.

strongly coloured and fluorescent in a single-stage process. These have included ninhydrin analogues such as 5-methylthioninhydrin and 5-methoxyninhydrin with zinc salts incorporated into the formulation (Almog et al., 2008) and also natural products such as genipin (Almog et al., 2004; Levinton-Shamuilov et al., 2005). However, none of these reagents have yet shown sufficient advantages in performance to have led to widespread operational use.

One of the attractions of the amino acid reagents for the development of finger-marks on paper substrates is that amino acids can form hydrogen bonds with the cellulose present in paper (Figure 9.1). This means that amino acids do not readily migrate from the original area of contact with the finger and ridge detail in older fingermarks can remain crisp unless they have been exposed to high humidity. The interactions between amino acids, cellulose and different amino acid reagents have been studied in detail by Spindler et al. (2011, 2015), showing the importance of both the cellulose and the amino acid reagent used in the quality of the developed mark and the different ways in which the reaction products interact with the cellulose in the paper. During the reaction with 1,2-indandione, cellulose is proposed to have a catalytic role in the early stages of the reaction with amino acids and also binds water molecules that are required for the reaction to proceed. It also plays a role in the stabilisation of the fluorescent reaction product, and it was subsequently shown that the nature of this interaction varies according to the amino acid reagent used and the location of the sites on the reaction product available for hydrogen bonding.

However, despite these interactions with cellulose, it should be noted that none of the amino acid reagents are suitable for use on surfaces that have been wetted or exposed to high humidity. This is because the amino acids are water soluble and are either washed away or diffused when exposed to these conditions.

9.2 Current operational use

The three amino acid reagents that are in widespread operational use worldwide are ninhydrin, DFO and 1,2-indandione.

Ninhydrin remains one of the most effective, versatile and widely used reagents for porous surfaces, and many formulations have been proposed. The purple reaction product means that enhanced marks can be easily visualised without the need for any specialist light sources. It is most widely applied as a single process for rapid treatment for large numbers of paper items but may also develop additional marks when used after DFO (and 1,2-indandione) in sequential treatments. It may also be used on painted and wallpapered walls at crime scenes, although when used in this way it is not possible to apply the optimised development conditions of elevated temperature and humidity. When applied at crime scenes, marks are generally allowed to develop at room temperature and the scene re-examined 10–14 days later.

Until the 2000s, DFO was recognised as the single most effective amino acid reagent and was routinely used where sequential treatments were being carried out on porous exhibits in laboratories. The need to use fluorescence examination to view most of the enhanced marks has meant that ninhydrin tends to be favoured in cases where only a single treatment is being carried out. DFO is less versatile than ninhydrin because the higher temperatures and processing times required for the marks to develop preclude its use at crime scenes.

1,2-Indandione has displaced DFO in several countries as the preferred amino acid reagent when optimum sensitivity in fingermark enhancement is required. On many porous surfaces, especially brown paper and cardboard, 1,2-indandione now appears to be consistently more effective than DFO. In common with DFO, fluorescence examination is required to visualise developed marks, and it is therefore unlikely to displace ninhydrin for use in large-scale processing of articles.

1,2-Indandione has greater potential than DFO for use at crime scenes because its reaction with amino acids can proceed at lower temperatures than that of DFO. It is currently not widely used in this role, and some reformulation may be required prior to more widespread use.

Ninhydrin, DFO and 1,2-indandione are capable of enhancing marks in blood in addition to latent marks, via reactions with amine groups in the proteins present.

More detailed descriptions of ninhydrin, DFO and 1,2-indandione are given in the following sections, together with less detailed summaries of many of the other amino acid reagents that have also been considered for use in fingermark enhancement.

9.3 Ninhydrin

9.3.1 Outline history of the process

1910: Ninhydrin was first synthesised by Ruhemann (1910a, 1910b).

1911–1913: Abderhalden and Schmidt observed reactions between ninhydrin, proteins and certain body fluids including sweat (Abderhalden and Schmidt, 1911, 1913).

1948: Dent characterised reaction products formed between ninhydrin and a wide range of amine-containing substances, including those found in body fluids.

1954: Oden and von Hofsten proposed ninhydrin in acetone solvent as a method for enhancing fingermarks.

1969: Crown proposed a revised formulation based on petroleum ether solvent to reduce issues associated with ink running during processing of documents.

1974: Morris and Goode published a non-flammable ninhydrin formulation using a chlorofluorocarbon (CFC) solvent.

1975: Linde first suggested the use of elevated temperature and relative humidity to increase the effectiveness of ninhydrin.

1978: Morris reported the use of toning using metal salts to change the colour of the ninhydrin reaction product.

1982: Herod and Menzel observed that some complexes formed by metal toning are also fluorescent.

1997: Hewlett et al. developed non-flammable, non-ozone-depleting ninhydrin formulations based on hydrofluoroether (HFE) and hydrofluorocarbon (HFC) carrier solvents (Hewlett and Sears, 1997; Hewlett et al., 1997).

2007: Almog et al. showed that zinc salts can be incorporated into ninhydrin formulations to give similar results to post-treatment by zinc toning.

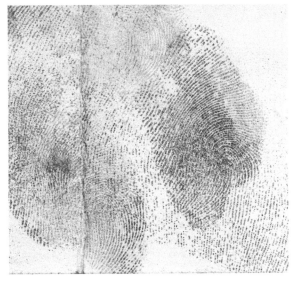

Figure 9.2 Fingermarks on white copier paper developed using ninhydrin.

9.3.2 Theory

Because ninhydrin is a widely used reagent and has many applications outside fin-germark enhancement, there have been many studies into its reaction mechanisms with amino acids and the resultant formation of the Ruhemann's purple reaction product. Some of the most comprehensive studies into the reactions include those by McCaldin (1960), Friedman and Sigel (1966), Friedman and Williams (1974), Yuferov (1971) and Joullie et al. (1991).

The reaction mechanism outlined in Figure 9.3 is typical of the generally accepted reaction pathway between ninhydrin and amino acids. In this reaction ninhydrin reacts with the amine group of the amino acid to form Ruhemann's purple, assuming the reaction proceeds to completion. Some of the studies referenced earlier have investigated the ninhydrin reaction mechanisms that occur with individual amino acids and explored the effect of varying the effect of varying conditions (e.g. pH) on the outcome. In some studies attempts have been made to identify all the intermediate compounds that are formed during the reaction.

In the context of fingermark enhancement, it is observed that the colour of developed fingermarks is very rarely the characteristic colour of Ruhemann's purple and in practice can vary from almost red to deep purple. This arises for several reasons. The colour of the reaction products that are formed between ninhydrin and the

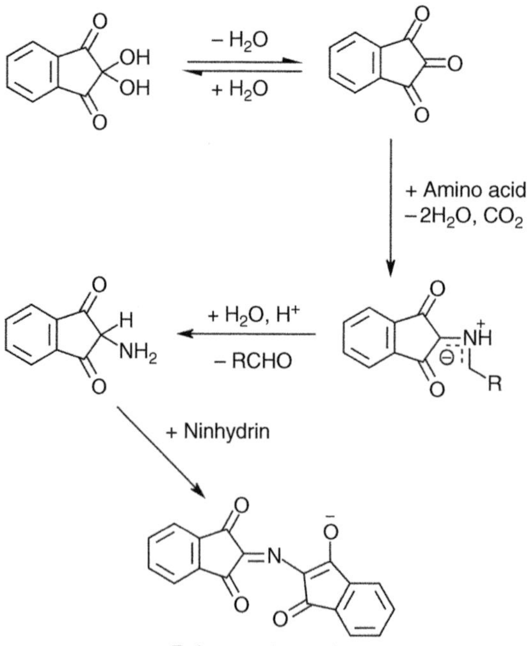

Figure 9.3   Generally accepted reaction pathway between ninhydrin and amino acids to form Ruhemann's purple.

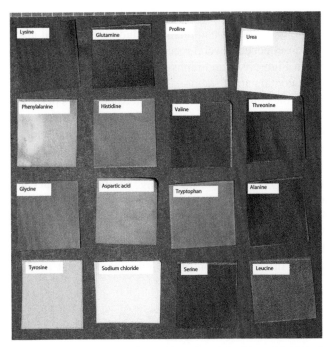

Figure 9.4 Coloured reaction products formed between ninhydrin and 0.1 M solutions of amino acids and other eccrine constituents deposited onto filter paper. Reproduced courtesy of the Home Office.

different amino acids is not uniformly purple (Figure 9.4), possibly because the reaction shown in Figure 9.3 may not proceed to completion for all the constituents in the mark. The reaction conditions will also influence reaction kinetics, and there are coloured intermediate imine and aldimine compounds in the full ninhydrin reaction scheme where the reaction may stop if the acidity is not high enough. A pH of <5 is required for the reaction to proceed past the intermediate product, but it is also possible for the reaction to proceed to the colourless hydrindantin product instead of to Ruhemann's purple when acidity is lower than pH 2. The actual colour of the intermediate imine compound is dependent on the -R groups attached to the active species, which will in turn influence the colour of the mark developed.

Fingermarks do not only contain amino acids, and other compounds may be present that can react with ninhydrin. A wide range of coloured reaction products are known to form in reactions between ninhydrin and different amine-containing substances. A comprehensive study was conducted by Dent (1948), who investigated 60 different compounds and recorded the colour of their reaction products with ninhydrin. For some of these substances, the reaction with ninhydrin cannot proceed to the Ruhemann's purple product because they do not have the structure required to react beyond the coloured intermediate compounds. It has also been shown in other studies (Cashman et al., 1979; Dutt and Poh, 1980) that ninhydrin can be used to detect phenethylamines and other basic drugs. Some of these substances or their metabolites may be present in fingermarks, either through handling or ingestion, and other contaminants including blood will also give positive reactions. As a consequence, several reaction mechanisms may operate in addition to that outlined in Figure 9.4, and ninhydrin may develop some additional fingermarks that do not contain amino acids.

The structure of the complex formed between Ruhemann's purple and metal salts has also been investigated, and the generic structure is shown in Figure 9.5.

Most of these complexes are coloured in nature, but some of them (most notably those formed with zinc and cadmium) are also fluorescent. Studies by Lennard et al. (1987) established that there were two different coloured zinc/Ruhemann's purple complexes that could be formed during toning: an orange product and another that appeared magenta/pink. The fluorescence of these complexes differed, with the magenta/pink product being more fluorescent than the orange one. These differences were attributed to the amount of water bound into the complex, and it was considered that humidification during toning is an important factor in providing sufficient water to drive formation of the more fluorescent product. Figure 9.6

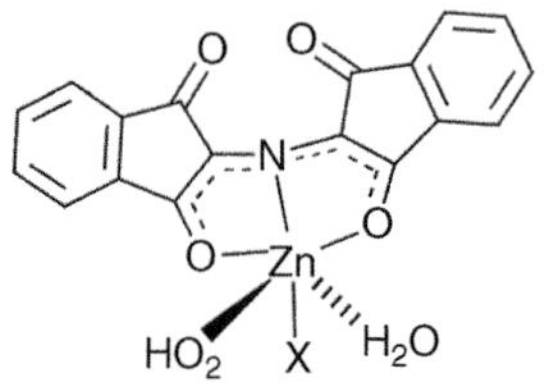

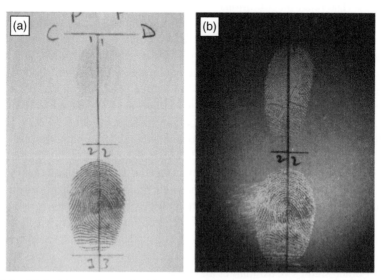

Figure 9.5 Complex formed between zinc salt and Ruhemann's purple, in some cases giving rise to colour changes and fluorescence.

Figure 9.6 Ninhydrin marks toned with zinc chloride solution, (a) viewed under room lighting and (b) viewed using fluorescence examination. Reproduced courtesy of the Home Office.

illustrates the visible appearance of marks treated with zinc chloride toning solution and the same marks when viewed using fluorescence examination. In this case it is the orange reaction product that has been formed.

9.3.3 The ninhydrin process

The following ninhydrin formulation is that recommended by the UK Home Office (Bandey, 2014). It involves the initial preparation of a concentrated solution, which can be diluted to give a working solution for use when required. This is because the working solution only has a limited stability in air before precipitation of ninhydrin occurs; this may be partly attributed to the evaporation of the HFE7100 (methoxy-nonafluorobutane) in air, which lowers the temperature of the solution, thus promoting precipitation.

Concentrated solution

Ninhydrin	25 g
Absolute ethanol	225 mL
Ethyl acetate	10 mL
Glacial acetic acid	25 mL

Working solution

Concentrated solution	52 mL
HFE7100	1 L

The roles of the constituents in the formulation are as follows:

Ninhydrin	The principal active component and reveals fingermarks by means of the (primarily) purple product formed in its reactions with amino acids and proteins. It has limited solubility in the main carrier solvent and is present in as high a concentration as possible without making the working solution rapidly unstable.
Ethanol	Required to ensure solubility of ninhydrin in the carrier solvent. Absolute ethanol is used so that the water required in the reaction is solely provided by the humidity oven and thus carefully controlled.
Ethyl acetate	Added as a co-solvent to inhibit the esterification reaction by shifting its equilibrium towards formation of ethanol and acetic acid. This prevents production of water droplets during processing, which may otherwise cause diffusion of fingermark ridges.
Acetic acid, water	Required to catalyse the reaction of the intermediate indantrione molecule with amino acids, the water being supplied in a controlled manner by the humidity oven. The acetic acid content is kept as low as possible to minimise any ink diffusion on documents being treated, but there is also a balance to be achieved in having sufficient acid present to ensure the reaction proceeds to the formation of Ruhemann's purple. This is of particular relevance for alkaline paper types such as magazine pages, which have high filler contents and may remove the hydrogen ions provided by the acetic acid.

| HFE7100 | The main carrier solvent for ninhydrin. HFE7100 meets the criteria of being non-toxic and non-flammable and causing minimal damage to documentary evidence. It is, however, expensive and a specially designed shallow dipping tray can be used to minimise usage of solution. |

To carry out processing using ninhydrin, articles are drawn through a shallow tray of working solution so that all areas of the article are wetted, or working solution is applied to the surface using a brush. Treated articles are then allowed to dry before being processed in a humidity-controlled oven, with most marks having developed after 5 min.

The processing conditions used in the humidity oven are 80°C and 65% relative humidity (RH). These conditions are selected because heating accelerates the reaction and the development of fingermarks, but temperatures in excess of 100°C may cause unwanted background reactions and possibly cause damage to the paper. The optimum level of RH during processing has been determined as approximately 65% at 80°C. At lower levels of humidity, not all marks will develop, and at higher humidity levels, unwanted reactions may occur with the background, potentially obscuring marks.

Developed fingermarks can be photographed immediately, but further marks can continue to develop for up to 2 weeks (although development has been observed to continue for 13 weeks in some cases) during which articles should ideally be kept in the dark. The time marks take to develop is dependent on the surface and may be related to pH because more acidic papers such as cheques generally develop more marks.

If toning is to be carried out after development of marks, the use of a zinc chloride-based toning solution is recommended, an example formulation being given as follows.

Toning solution

Zinc chloride	6 g
Absolute ethanol	50 mL
Propan-2-ol	10 mL
Acetic acid	10 mL
HFE7100	200 mL

This solution is then sprayed lightly over the marks to be treated and the article then retreated in the humidity oven at 80°C and 65% RH. Humidity is required to accelerate complex formation with the metal salt, the reaction occurring in less than 5 min at 65% RH. Zinc chloride is preferred over cadmium salts for fluorescent toning because of the toxicity of cadmium and its salts.

As discussed earlier, the marks developed by ninhydrin can vary in colour from reddish purple to deep purple, being influenced by the composition of the mark and the substrate it is deposited on.

After toning with zinc salts, the marks become either pink or orange in colour and are fluorescent. The excitation maximum occurs at approximately 500 nm and the

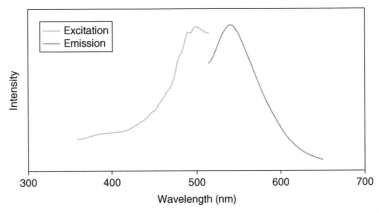

Figure 9.7   Measured excitation and emission spectra for ninhydrin toned with zinc chloride.

emission maximum at approximately 540 nm (Figure 9.7). Fluorescence examination is generally conducted using light sources with emission in the blue-green region of the spectrum, using an orange viewing filter (such as Schott glass OG550) to view the yellow-orange fluorescence.

9.4   1,8-Diazafluoren-9-one

9.4.1   Outline history of the process

1950: Druey first synthesised DFO as part of a study into phenanthroline quinones and diazafluorenes (Druey and Schmidt, 1950).

1989: DFO was synthesised at Queen's University Belfast under contract from the Home Office Central Research Establishment for use as a fingermark enhancement reagent, and trials were subsequently conducted at laboratories worldwide.

1990: Pounds et al. published the first journal paper detailing the use of DFO for fingermark enhancement.

1991: Masters et al. reported the sequential use of DFO before ninhydrin to increase fingermark recovery.

1993: Hardwick et al. reported refinements to the DFO formulation and illustrate the effect of temperature on development rate.

1998: First publication of non-ozone-depleting formulations based on hydrofluoroethers (HFE) (Didierjean et al., 1998; Rajtar, 2000; Sears and Hewlett, 2003).

2001: Conn et al. investigated toning of DFO with metal salts but found it of limited benefit.

Figure 9.8 shows an example of a mark developed on paper using DFO.

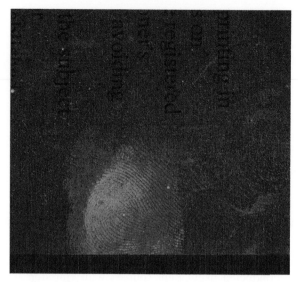

Figure 9.8 Mark developed on paper using DFO.

9.4.2 Theory

The reaction product formed between DFO and amino acids is a pale red/pink in colour but is also fluorescent. Studies into the reaction mechanism for formation of this product have been conducted by Grigg et al. (1990) and Wilkinson (2000). Initial work by Grigg focused on isolating the red reaction product formed between DFO and various α-amino acids and analysing its structure, which was found to be closely related to the protonated Ruhemann's purple structure developed with nin-hydrin. Wilkinson later performed X-ray crystallography on the reaction product and confirmed that its structure consisted of two DFO molecules linked by a bridg-ing nitrogen atom. In the crystalline product analysed, hydrogen-bonded bridges were observed between molecules of the reaction product, with water molecules forming the linkages.

In addition to studies of the reaction product, Wilkinson investigated the reaction with a single amino acid (L-alanine) and used a range of analytical techniques including NMR and GC-MS to identify intermediate products formed during the reaction.

Wilkinson proposed that the DFO reaction with amino acids is similar to that of ninhydrin, although it is assisted by the initial formation of a hemiketal from reac-tion between the DFO molecule and the methanol in the solvent mixture. The result-ant hemiketal has a higher reactivity with amino acids than the original DFO molecule. The nitrogen atom of the amino acid is then able to attack the hemiketal at the electron-deficient carbon in the polarised carbonyl, with resultant loss of water. This produces an aromatic imine retaining the alkyl fragment of the amino acid, which then undergoes decarboxylation to form another intermediate product.

Hydrolysis then occurs at the nitrogen–carbon double bond to produce an aromatic amine and acetaldehyde with the aromatic amine finally reacting with another DFO molecule to form the red fluorescent reaction product.

The reaction mechanisms proposed from these studies are illustrated in Figures 9.9 and 9.10.

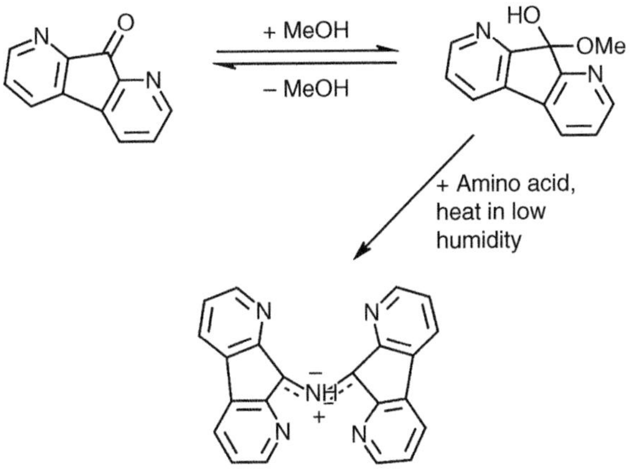

Figure 9.9   Proposed mechanism for formation of hemiketal.

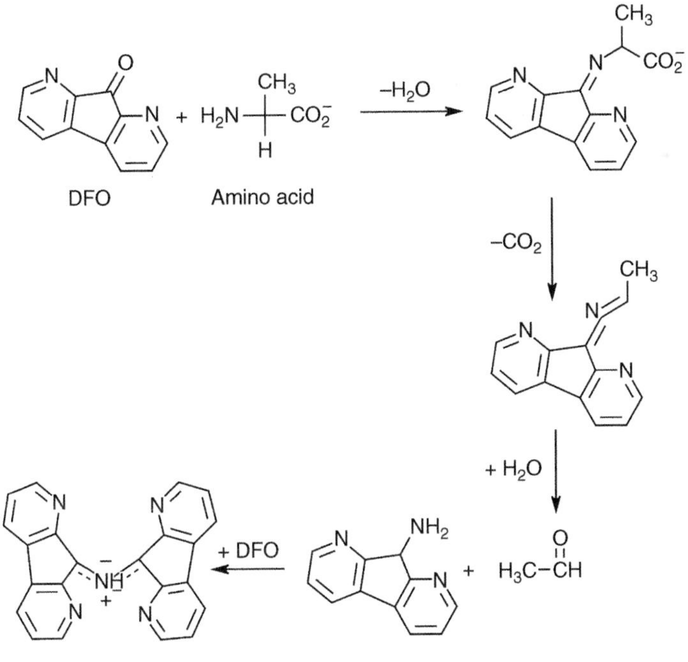

Figure 9.10   Proposed reaction path of DFO with amino acids (Wilkinson, 2000).

The reaction products that are formed between different amino acids and DFO are generally pale red/pink in colour, with some exceptions (e.g. proline, which gives a blue product). The principal mode of viewing DFO is fluorescence examination, and all of the reaction products produce an orange fluorescence when illuminated using green light (Figure 9.11).

The reaction between DFO and amino acids is not thought to proceed to completion for all amino acids and has been shown by Figuera et al. (2015) not to consume all of the amino acids that are present in the fingermark. This is consistent with both experimental and operational observations that ninhydrin will develop additional marks when used sequentially after DFO, because amino acids (and some amine-containing contaminants) may remain available to react.

9.4.3 The DFO process

The DFO process detailed here is that recommended by the UK Home Office (Bandey, 2014). The process uses a single working solution, produced from:

DFO	0.25 g
Methanol	30 mL
Acetic acid	20 mL
HFE71DE (HFE7100 premixed with *trans*-1,2-dichloroethylene)	275 mL
HFE7100	725 mL

The roles of the constituents in the formulation are as follows.

DFO	The role of DFO is to react with amino acids present in fingermarks to give the fluorescent reaction product. In this particular formulation, the primary purpose of DFO is to produce a fluorescent product, and therefore the presence of any coloured reaction product is of secondary importance. The formulation uses 0.25 g of DFO per litre, found to give the maximum intensity of fluorescence. Any increase in DFO content will make the coloured product more intense (although still far less visible than the purple of ninhydrin) but does not enhance fluorescence. Quantities of >0.2 g DFO per litre are essential for the reaction to occur, and quantities of >0.75 g cannot be dissolved.
Methanol	An essential component of the DFO formulation, allowing DFO to form hemiketals that in turn have greater reactivity with amino acids. Longer-chain alcohols are not as effective in this role. The formulation uses as little methanol as possible due to its toxic nature.
Acetic acid	Added to acidify the solution. If acidification is not carried out, virtually no fingermarks are developed. Propanoic acid can be used in place of acetic acid but has no performance benefit, whereas formic acid rapidly esterifies with the methanol component of the formulation, producing water as an unwanted by-product. This is undesirable as the presence of water causes phase separation of the solution, reducing the amount of DFO in the non-polar phase available for fingermark development.

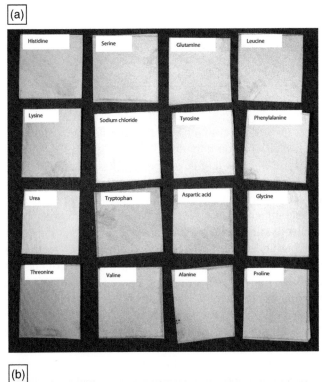

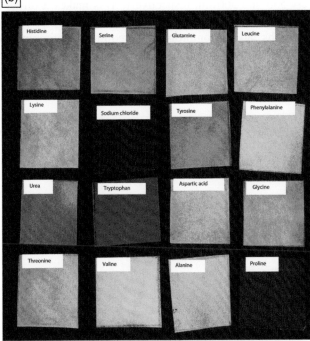

Figure 9.11 Reaction products formed between DFO and 0.1 M solutions of amino acids and other eccrine constituents deposited onto filter paper, (a) viewed under white light and (b) by fluorescence examination. Reproduced courtesy of the Home Office.

HFE7100,	Used as the principal carrier solvent for DFO. The addition of *trans*-1,2-
HFE71DE	dichloroethylene as a co-solvent (i.e. in the HFE71DE component of
	the formulation) appears to be important for the development of greater
	quantities of brighter fluorescent fingermarks although the reasons for this
	are not firmly established.

To carry out processing using DFO, articles are drawn through a shallow tray of working solution, or working solution is applied to the surface using a brush. Once dry, articles are heated in a non-humidified oven at 100°C for 20 min, followed by examination in white light (where developed marks may be detected due to their pale pink colour) and subsequent fluorescence examination.

Although the DFO reaction will proceed quicker at higher temperatures, process-ing at 100°C is recommended to give a combination of a reasonably short develop-ment time combined with a reduced risk of any damage that may occur to articles (e.g. paper charring and melting of plastic windows in envelopes). A processing time of 10 min was originally recommended, but this was extended to 20 min fol-lowing studies using a luminance meter that showed that for a significant majority of articles, optimum fluorescence was only obtained after this period.

Marks developed using DFO are generally only faintly visible and of a pale pink/red colour. They are best viewed using fluorescence examination, the excitation and emission spectra being shown in Figure 9.12.

It can be seen that the excitation and emission maxima are very close together, at approximately 555 and 560 nm, respectively. This makes it difficult to identify combinations of light source and filter that fully utilise either the peak excitation or emission wavelengths, and a compromise is required. Optimum fluorescence is obtained when using illumination in the green region of the spectrum (e.g. a 532 nm laser), and the resultant orange fluorescence should be viewed through an orange filter such as Schott glass OG570.

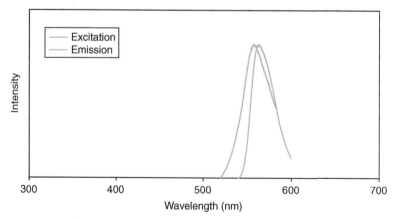

Figure 9.12   Excitation and emission spectra of DFO.

The broad emission spectrum of DFO means that for surfaces where appreciable background fluorescence occurs when illuminated with green light, better results may be obtained using yellow illumination sources (such as a 577 nm laser) in conjunction with red filters (e.g. Schott glass RG610). DFO will still fluoresce under these conditions whereas the background fluorescence may be considerably reduced. This is particularly relevant for many types of brown and coloured paper.

9.5   1,2-Indandione

9.5.1   Outline history of the process

1997: Joullie and co-workers at the University of Pennsylvania synthesised and assessed a range of amino acid reagents and identified 1,2-indandione as having potential for fingermark enhancement (Ramotowski et al., 1997; Hauze et al., 1998).

1999: Almog et al. reported the first operational trials of 1,2-indandione.

2003: Gardner and Hewlett observed that post-treatment using zinc salts can be used to enhance fluorescence of marks developed using 1,2-indandione.

2007: Stoilovic et al. reported incorporation of zinc salts into the 1,2-indandione formulation to increase its stability and effectiveness.

The appearance of developed marks under white light and fluorescence examination is shown in Figure 9.13.

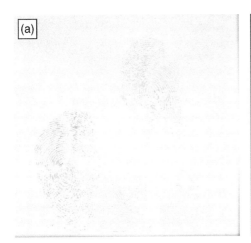
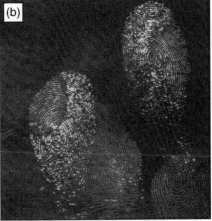

Figure 9.13   Marks developed using 1,2-indandione on paper, viewed (a) under white light and (b) using fluorescence examination. Reproduced courtesy of the Home Office.

9.5.2 Theory

1,2-Indandione is closely structurally and chemically related to ninhydrin, and it has been proposed that its reaction with amino acids is also very similar. A proposed reaction path is illustrated in Figure 9.14. The Ruhemann's purple analogue that is formed as the reaction product is becoming more commonly known as Joullie's pink, after the researcher that first reported the synthesis of the molecule (Joullie et al., 1991).

Marks developed using formulations that have a high content of 1,2-indandione may exhibit a pink colouration, but in common with DFO the developed marks are best observed using fluorescence examination.

It was considered until recently that the presence of methanol was not necessary for the 1,2-indandione reaction to proceed and could instead inhibit it. This is because indandione is known to form stable hemiketals with methanol that may prevent the subsequent reaction with amino acids taking place. Whilst this may be true of the original 1,2-indandione formulations, more recently it has been proposed that zinc salts are added to the formulation to improve stability of the solutions and fluorescence of the developed marks. Studies have shown that when methanol is added to these more complex formulations (Nicolasora, 2014), it can have further beneficial effects on fluorescence, so there may be more complex interactions occurring than that outlined in Figure 9.14.

The addition of zinc salts to the formulation produces reaction products that have consistent excitation and emission spectra across a wide range of amino acids. 1,2-Indandione formulations without zinc salt additions exhibited significant variability in the fluorescence of the products formed with different amino acids (Spindler

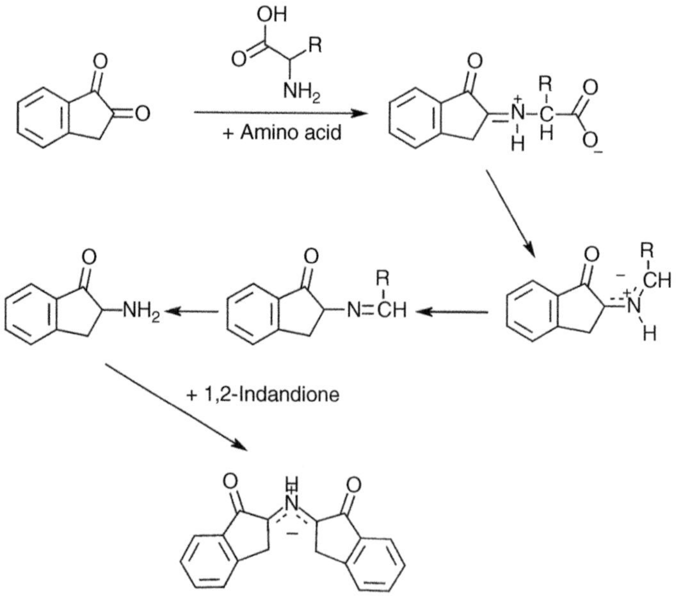

Figure 9.14   Proposed reaction pathway for 1,2-indandione with amino acids.

et al., 2009), and it was proposed that the role of Zn^{2+} present is to act as a Lewis acid catalyst in driving the formation of the fluorescent reaction product. Spindler et al. (2011) conducted further extensive studies of the role of zinc chloride and published a reaction mechanism showing its contribution to formation of the Joullie's pink reaction product.

The appearance of filter papers impregnated with a range of amino acids and other eccrine constituents after processing with 1,2-indandione is illustrated in Figure 9.15.

9.5.3 The 1,2-indandione process

The process described as follows is that used in the most recent trials conducted in the United Kingdom (Bandey, 2017), and other effective formulations have also been published (Bicknell and Ramotowski, 2008; Serrano and Sturelle, 2010) or have already been implemented operationally. The process uses a single working solution, produced from:

1,2-Indandione	0.25 g
Ethyl acetate	45 mL
Methanol	45 mL
Acetic acid	10 mL
$ZnCl_2$ stock solution	1 mL
HFE7100	1 L

where the zinc chloride stock solution consists of:

Zinc chloride	0.1 g
Ethyl acetate	4 mL
Acetic acid	1 mL

The roles of the constituents in the formulation are as follows:

1,2-Indandione	The role of 1,2-indandione is to react with amino acids present in finger-print residues to give a fluorescent reaction product. 0.25 g 1,2-indandione per litre of solution gives the optimum fluorescence level in the developed mark. Higher concentrations can give a more intense pink colour, but in common with the DFO formulation, fluorescence is regarded as the most important characteristic.
Ethyl acetate	90 mL of ethyl acetate per litre of solution is added as a co-solvent.
Acetic acid	10 mL of acetic acid per litre of solution gives the optimum fluorescence of fingerprints without increasing undesirable background fluorescence to a level where it begins to obscure marks.

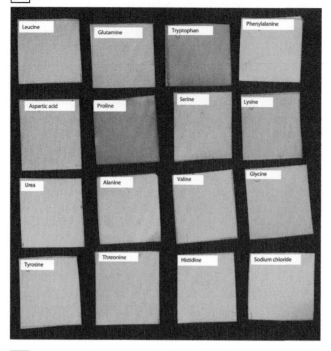

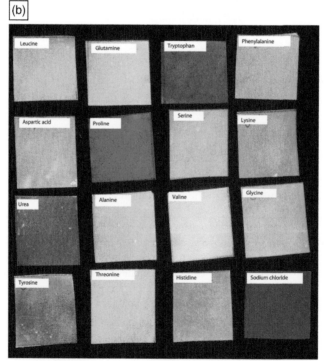

Figure 9.15 Reaction products formed between 1,2-indandione and 0.1 M solutions of amino acids and other eccrine constituents deposited onto filter paper, (a) viewed under white light and (b) by fluorescence examination. Reproduced courtesy of the Home Office.

Methanol	Increases the solubility of 1,2-indandione in the working solution and probably interacts with zinc chloride in driving the reaction towards higher yield of the fluorescent product. Content minimised to reduce the risk of causing diffusion of marks.
HFE7100	Used as the principal carrier solvent for 1,2-indandione and selected as a proven non-flammable, non-toxic solvent for fingerprint formulations.
ZnCl₂ stock solution	Acts as a Lewis acid catalyst, stabilising intermediate products and promoting formation of the fluorescent reaction product.

To carry out processing using this 1,2-indandione formulation, the same conditions for DFO are used. Articles are drawn through a shallow tray of working solution, or working solution is applied to the surface using a brush.

Once dry, articles are heated in a non-humidified oven at 100°C for 10 min, followed by examination in white light (where developed marks may be detected due to their pale pink colour) and subsequent fluorescence examination.

Other researchers have proposed alternative processing conditions, Bicknell and Ramotowski (2008) suggesting the use of a humidified oven using the same conditions for ninhydrin where the humidity level of the paper is below a critical level and other operational users (Stoilovic et al., 2007) recommending a shorter processing time of 10 s at 165°C in a hot press. The use of higher processing temperatures may cause damage to some lighter paper types, and this should be taken into account when selecting processing conditions. In addition, the physical contact involved during processing in a hot press may contribute to high background development (Nicolasora, 2014; Dyer, 2015), and therefore heating in an oven is preferred for the formulation given earlier.

'Dry' formulations of 1,2-indandione have been produced for the development of fingermarks on documents to avoid any risk of ink running. One dry formulation consists of:

1,2-Indandione	0.25 g
Ethyl acetate	9 mL
Acetic acid	2 mL
HFE7100	89 mL

Sheets of copy paper are dipped into this solution and allowed to dry, and the article to be treated is then placed between two of these pre-impregnated pages and pressed at ~150°C for approximately 15 s.

An alternative 'dry' formulation has been proposed for use on thermal papers (Patton et al., 2010).

The formulation of 1,2-indandione mentioned has been produced with the intention of maximising the number of marks seen by fluorescence examination rather than increasing the intensity of the visible pink product. The excitation and emission spectra for 1,2-indandione are shown in Figure 9.16.

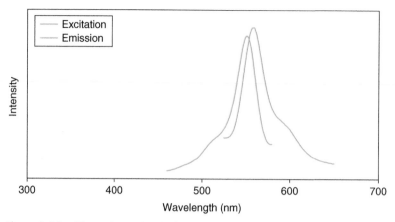

Figure 9.16   Absorption and emission spectra measured for 1,2-indandione-zinc.

Similarly to DFO, the excitation and emission maxima are very close together, approximately 555 and 560 nm, respectively. The optimum viewing conditions for fluorescence are also similar, using green light for illumination and viewing through an orange filter such as the Schott glass OG570. The colour of fluorescence obtained from 1,2-indandione is yellow-orange, in comparison with the orange product from DFO.

9.6   Ninhydrin analogues

9.6.1   Outline history of the process

1982: Almog et al. reported the first comprehensive studies of ninhydrin analogues for specific application as fingermark enhancement reagents, identifying benzo[f] ninhydrin as having particular potential for operational use.

1985: Menzel and Almog reported that toning of benzo[f]ninhydrin with metal salts produces highly fluorescent complexes.

1986: Lennard et al. reported the synthesis and assessment of a further range of ninhydrin analogues, including 5-methoxyninhydrin.

1987: Almog published further studies of ninhydrin analogues, related compounds and their reactions with amino acids.

1992: Almog et al. reported the synthesis and evaluation of a range of thioninhydrins, including 5-methylthioninhydrin.

2000: A joint Israeli/UK study evaluated benzo[f]ninhydrin against ninhydrin and found no operational benefit for the ninhydrin analogue.

2008: Almog et al. proposed 'dual action' reagents based on 5-methoxyninhydrin and 5-methylthioninhydrin with additions of zinc salts to their formulations.

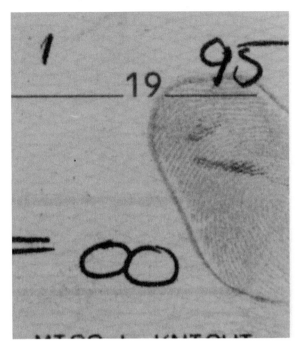

Figure 9.17 A fingermark developed on a cheque using benzo[f]ninhydrin. Reproduced courtesy of the Home Office.

5-MTN is the only one of the ninhydrin analogues currently manufactured for forensic use. Some others are commercially available for other applications (e.g. 5-methoxyninhydrin), but their price makes their purchase prohibitive and there appears to be no significant operational benefit in their use. Figure 9.17 shows a mark developed using benzo[f]ninhydrin, a ninhydrin analogue that has been previously considered for operational use.

9.6.2 Theory

It is thought that all ninhydrin analogues essentially react with amino acids in a similar way to ninhydrin itself, and the reaction product is also a linked double molecule characteristic of the parent compound. For those analogues that are capable of forming complexes with metal salts, it is thought that the structure of these complexes is also analogous to that observed for ninhydrin.

The chemical structures of ninhydrin and the analogues that have been mostly widely researched for applications in fingermark enhancement are illustrated in Figure 9.18.

The principal colours of the reaction products formed with amino acids differ from the dark purple observed for ninhydrin and can vary significantly in colour,

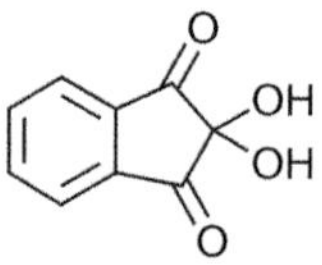

Ninhydrin

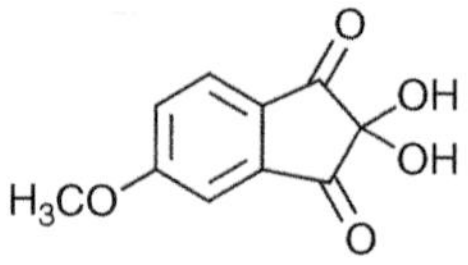

5-Methoxyninhydrin

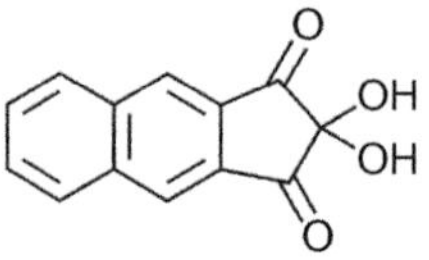

Benzo[f]ninhydrin

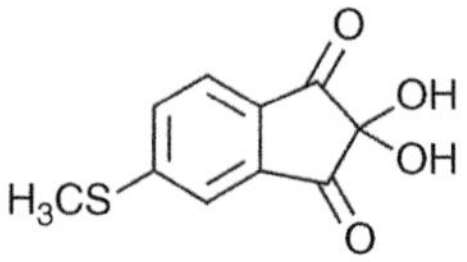

5-Methylthioninhydrin

Figure 9.18 Structures of some of the principal ninhydrin analogues.

from dark green observed for benzo[f]ninhydrin, deep red/pink for 5-methoxyninhydrin and pink/purple for 5-methylthioninhydrin. Some examples of reaction products obtained from different amino acids are illustrated in Figure 9.19.

9.6.3 Ninhydrin analogue processes

There is no single recognised formulation involving ninhydrin analogues in operational use. The formulations that have been used for some of the published comparisons between ninhydrin analogues, ninhydrin and DFO are summarised as follows.

Benzo[f]ninhydrin working solution (Almog et al., 2000)

Benzo[f]ninhydrin	6 g
Methanol	60 mL
Acetic acid	30 mL
Methyl acetate	60 mL
1,1,2-Trichloro-1,2,2-trifluoroethane (CFC113)	850 mL

5-Methylthioninhydrin-zinc concentrated solution (Porpiglia et al., 2012):

5-Methylthioninhydrin	2.5 g
Absolute ethanol	225 mL
Ethyl acetate	10 mL
Acetic acid	25 mL

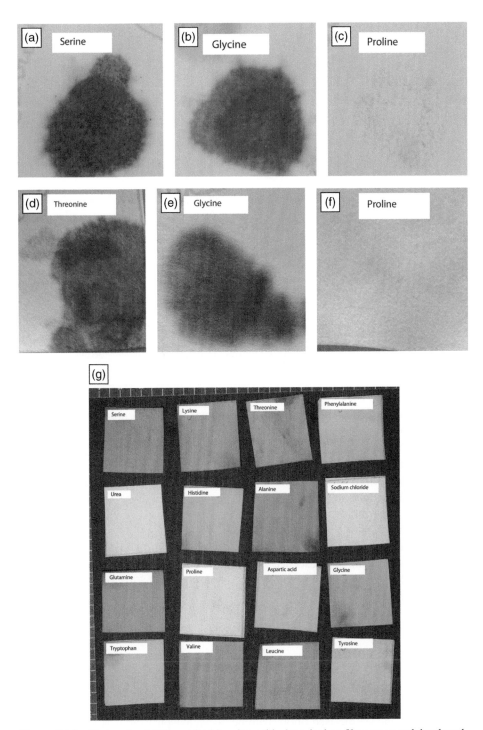

Figure 9.19 Test spots of different 0.1 M amino acids deposited on filter paper and developed using ninhydrin analogues: (a–c) benzo[f]ninhydrin, dark green principal reaction product; (d–f) 5-methoxyninhydrin, red/purple principal reaction product; and (g) 5-methylthioninhydrin, pale purple reaction product, all viewed using white light. Analogous results for proline also shown. Reproduced courtesy of Loughborough University and the Home Office.

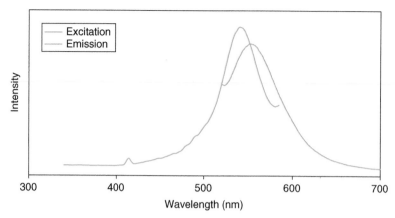

Figure 9.20 Measured excitation and emission spectra for 5-methylthioninhydrin-zinc.

5-Methylthioninhydrin-zinc working solution (Porpiglia et al., 2012):

Concentrated solution	52 mL
ZnCl$_2$ stock solution (2 g of ZnCl$_2$ in 50 mL absolute ethanol)	36 mL
HFE7100	1 L

Most formulations based on ninhydrin analogues have been processed using the same conditions as the parent compound, that is, by dipping the article or brushing solution onto the surface, allowing it to dry and then using a humidity-controlled cabinet and elevated temperature to develop the marks.

Marks developed using all these ninhydrin analogues can be converted to fluorescent products by the addition of zinc salts to the formulation. The fluorescence spectra obtained from 5-methylthioninhydrin with additions of zinc salts is illustrated in Figure 9.20.

The excitation maximum is approximately 540 nm and the emission maximum approximately 555 nm. Fluorescence examination generally uses green light as illumination and an orange viewing filter (e.g. Schott glass OG 570), similarly to DFO and 1,2-indandione.

9.7   Fluorescamine

9.7.1   Outline history of the process

1972: Udenfriend synthesised fluorescamine (4-phenylspiro[furan-2(3H), 1′-phtha-lan]-3,3′-dione) as a fluorescent reagent for automated assay of amino acids (Udenfriend, 1972; Udenfriend et al., 1972).

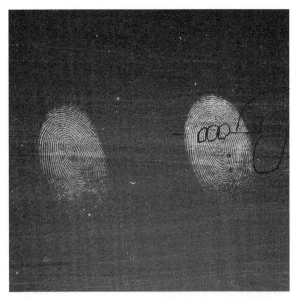

Figure 9.21   Marks developed using fluorescamine on a matt emulsion painted wall. Reproduced courtesy of the Home Office.

1976: Ohki first proposed fluorescamine for as a reagent for fingermark enhancement.

1979: Lee and Attard conducted comparative studies between fluorescamine, ninhydrin and *o*-phthalaldehyde for fingermark enhancement and find fluorescamine to have some advantages over ninhydrin.

Fluorescamine was not widely adopted for fingermark enhancement, and there are several reasons for this. The principal solvent used in the formulation is acetone, which is highly flammable and causes ink on documents to run. The fluorescamine solution is also unstable in contact with water and is more difficult to store than ninhydrin. The long-wave ultraviolet radiation required to visualise the developed fingermarks also excites optical brighteners used in most modern papers, making developed marks more difficult to see against the fluorescing background. On surfaces such as matt-painted walls, background fluorescence is less of an issue and marks may be more clearly seen (Figure 9.21).

9.7.2   Theory

Fluorescamine reacts with the amine groups of amino acids and peptides present in fingermarks to produce a fluorescent product, and the reaction that occurs is summarised in Figure 9.22.

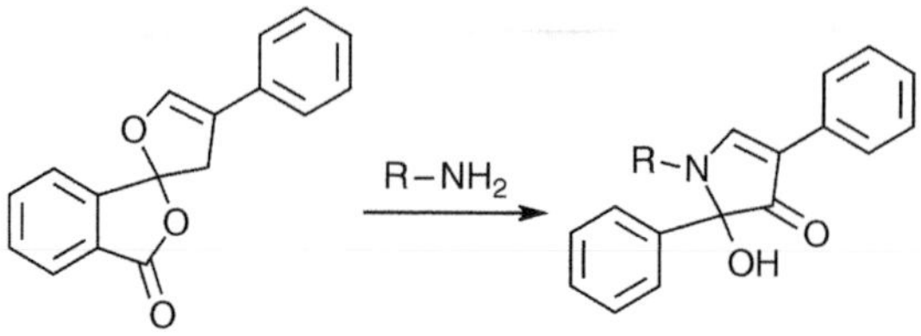

Figure 9.22   Reaction of fluorescamine with amines to form fluorescent products.

The fluorescent product formed by this reaction is visualised by fluorescence examination using an excitation wavelength of approximately 390 nm (long-wave ultraviolet) that produces a visible (pale blue) emission in the region 475–495 nm. The fluorescence of the reaction product is consistent across a range of different amino acids (Figure 9.23).

9.7.3   The fluorescamine process

The following formulation is that proposed by Ohki (1976) and utilises a working solution that is ideally made just before use:

Fluorescamine	15 mg
Triethylamine	0.1 mL
Acetone	100 mL

In this formulation, acetone is the principal solvent, and the small addition of triethylamine acts as an organic base, replacing the aqueous bases proposed in earlier formulations that were found to diffuse ridge detail. Fluorescamine is the active constituent and reacts with the amine groups of amino acids and peptides present in fingermarks to form a fluorescent reaction product.

These constituents were mixed together and then sprayed using an atomiser onto the surface being treated or applied using a brush. The reaction occurs at room temperature without the need for humidification, and fluorescent marks develop within a few minutes after application.

However, the reagent also had some disadvantages in that the working solution did not have long term stability and could be hydrolysed by water to a non-fluorescent product.

Marks enhanced using fluorescamine are not visible by eye and can only be observed using fluorescence examination. Excitation uses a UV-A radiation source outputting at approximately 365 nm, with the resultant fluorescence maximum occurring at approximately 445 nm (Figure 9.24). Fluorescence is best viewed through a pale yellow viewing filter such as the Schott glass GG395.

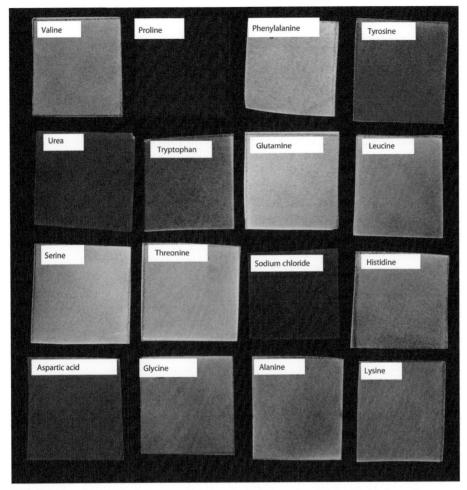

Figure 9.23   Reaction products formed between fluorescamine and 0.1 M solutions of amino acids and other eccrine constituents deposited onto filter paper, viewed by fluorescence examination. Reproduced courtesy of the Home Office.

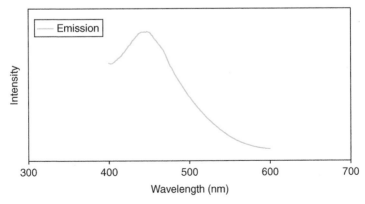

Figure 9.24   Measured emission spectra for fluorescamine.

9.8 *o*-Phthalaldehyde

9.8.1 Outline history of the process

1975: Benson and Hare proposed the use of *o*-phthalaldehyde for fingermark enhancement.

1978: Mayer et al. and Ohki independently proposed revised formulations for *o*-phthalaldehyde, offering potential advantages over fluorescamine formulations of reduced cost and increased stability in the presence of water.

1979: Lee and Attard conducted comparative studies between *o*-phthalaldehyde, fluorescamine and ninhydrin for fingermark enhancement.

1990: Fischer reported a simpler and less hazardous two-stage formulation involving immersion in *o*-phthalaldehyde solution and then spraying with dilute nitric acid, which produces a product with different fluorescence characteristics.

The reagent has not subsequently been widely used for fingermark detection for similar reasons to those given for fluorescamine. Of the three reagents (*o*-phthalaldehyde, fluorescamine and ninhydrin) assessed in the early 1970s, ninhydrin was found to be the easiest to use, with the visible marks produced being easier to image. *o*-Phthalaldehyde solution can be unstable in contact with air and is best stored under an inert gas, which makes it less practical than ninhydrin for routine use.

9.8.2 Theory

o-Phthalaldehyde undergoes a chemical reaction with any primary amines that may be present in fingermark deposits to form fluorescent reaction products. These reaction products have an optimum excitation wavelength of approximately 340 nm and an emission of approximately 455 nm.

Research has indicated that the fluorescent reaction products are 1-alkylthio-2-alkyl-substituted isoindoles (Simons and Johnson, 1976; Lee and Drescher, 1978; Svedas et al., 1980). An example of one of the reactions proposed for *o*-phthalaldehyde with amino acids in the presence of a sulphur-containing compound such as 2-mercaptoethanol is given in Figure 9.25.

9.8.3 The *o*-phthalaldehyde process

The formulation proposed by Lee and Attard (1979) was made up as a two-part formulation with an aqueous base, where:

Solution A	
Boric acid	2.5 g
Distilled water	95 mL

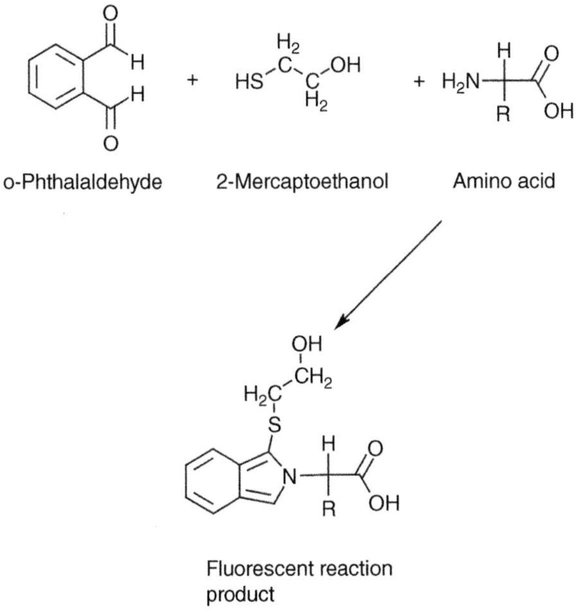

Figure 9.25 Proposed reaction between *o*-phthalaldehyde, 2-mercaptoethanol and α-amino acids.

pH adjusted to 10.40 with additions of 6 M potassium hydroxide

| Brij 35 detergent | 0.3 mL |
| 2-Mercaptoethanol | 0.2 mL |

Solution B

| *o*-Phthalaldehyde | 0.5 g |
| Methanol | 1 mL |

The solutions were mixed together and then sprayed.
Ohki (1978) proposed an alternative, 1-part solution with an organic base

o-Phthalaldehyde	40 mg
95% ethanol	1 mL
Chloroform	50 mL
Triethylamine	0.5 mL
2-Mercaptoethanol	0.1 mL

Again, the solution was sprayed onto the surface being treated.

In the aqueous formulation, potassium hydroxide provides the basic environment required for the reaction to proceed, whilst in the one-part solution triethylamine acts an organic base.

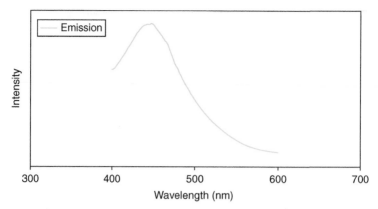

Figure 9.26   Measured emission spectra for *o*-phthalaldehyde.

The 2-mercaptoethanol constituent of both formulations is essential for the reaction to proceed and forms part of the fluorescent reaction product. Other sulphur-containing substances including ethanethiol and sodium sulphite have been used in this role in similar formulations used for amino acid assays.

o-Phthalaldehyde is the active constituent that reacts with amino acids, and methanol or a combination of ethanol and chloroform is used as solvent for it.

Marks enhanced using *o*-phthalaldehyde are mostly not visible by eye, although may occasionally be distinguished as pale grey ridge detail. They can be observed using fluorescence examination with an UV-A radiation source outputting at approximately 365 nm, with the resultant fluorescence maximum occurring at approximately 440 nm (Figure 9.26). Fluorescence is best viewed through a pale yellow viewing filter such as the Schott glass GG395.

The two-part system later proposed by Fischer did not use 2-mercaptoethanol and involved preparation of a solution consisting of 0.25 g *o*-phthalaldehyde in 100 mL acetone. The exhibits were dipped in this solution for 15 s and then sprayed with a second solution of 1% nitric acid in acetone, marks finally being developed by application of a steam iron. Unlike the previous formulations, heat was required to develop marks and fluorescence was produced by illumination with blue light rather than ultraviolet radiation, suggesting that the reaction products formed by this route were different. A solution of 5 mL of denatured ethanol mixed with 95 mL of CFC113 could be used in place of acetone to give non-flammable formulations.

9.9   Genipin

9.9.1   Outline history of the process

2004: Almog et al. first proposed genipin as an amino acid reagent for fingermark enhancement, producing dark blue visible marks with a red fluorescence.

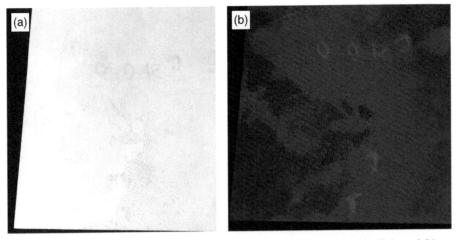

Figure 9.27 Marks on paper developed using genipin, viewed (a) under white light and (b) under fluorescence examination. Reproduced courtesy of the Home Office.

2005: Levinton-Shamuilov et al. reported further results on genipin and present an improved formulation.

2007: Almog et al. compared genipin with other 'dual action' reagents, 5-methoxyninhydrin-zinc and 5-methylthioninhydrin-zinc.

Genipin is not routinely used on operational work because it is not as effective as ninhydrin in developing visible coloured marks and not as effective as DFO or 1,2-indandione in developing fluorescent marks. However, it has been observed that on certain paper types (e.g. red paper used in Chinese gift envelopes), genipin may give better results than ninhydrin, DFO and 1,2-indandione. Consequently there may be niche applications for this type of reagent, particularly where the higher excitation and emission wavelengths required to visualise the fluorescent product reduce any background fluorescence from the paper and/or any inks that may be present. An example of a mark developed using genipin is shown in Figure 9.27.

9.9.2 Theory

Studies into the reactions between genipin and amino acids (Levinton-Shamuilov et al., 2005) have established that slightly different reactions will occur between genipin and the different amino acids present in the fingermark. Some of the blue reaction products produced have been identified, and the proposed reaction is shown in Figure 9.28.

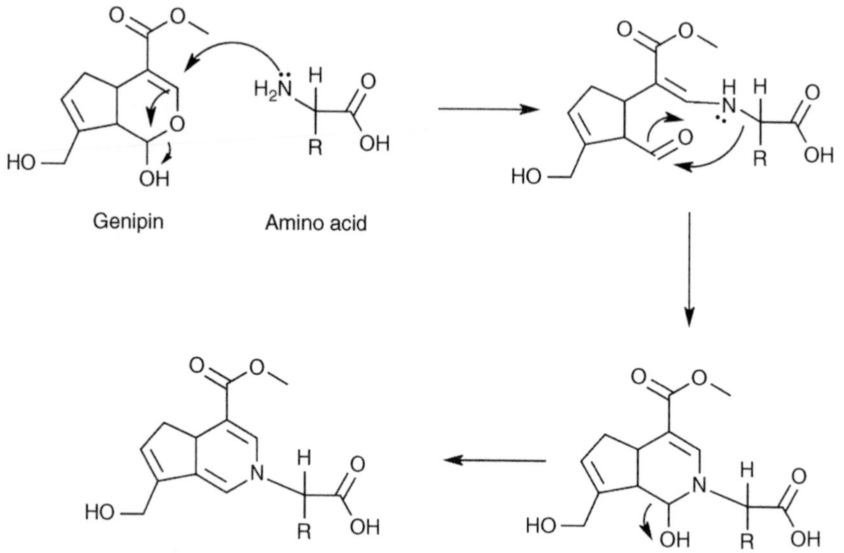

Figure 9.28 Proposed reaction mechanism for genipin with amino acids.

In common with many other amino acid reagents, not all reactions with amino acids proceed at the same rate or result in products with similar visible or fluorescent characteristics. This is illustrated for genipin in Figure 9.29.

9.9.3 The genipin process

The optimised formulation published by Levinton-Shamuilov et al. (2005) consists of a working solution:

Genipin	1.7 g
Absolute ethanol	57 mL
Ethyl acetate	86 mL
HFE7100	587 mL

The constituents and their roles in the formulation are the same as reported for ninhydrin, with the exception that acetic acid is not used in the genipin formulation.

For development of marks using genipin, the exhibit is dipped in the genipin solution, allowed to dry and then processed in a humidified over under the same conditions as ninhydrin (80°C, 65% RH) for 10 min.

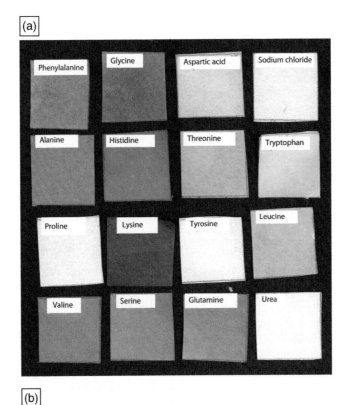

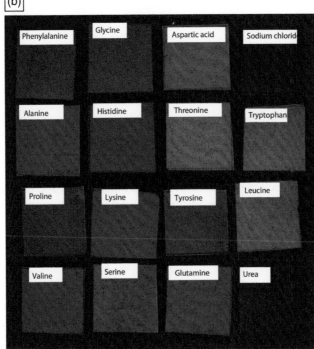

Figure 9.29 Reaction products formed between genipin and 0.1 M solutions of amino acids and other eccrine constituents deposited onto filter paper, viewed (a) under white light and (b) by fluorescence examination. Reproduced courtesy of the Home Office.

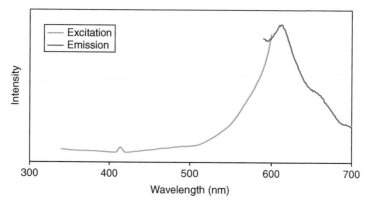

Figure 9.30 Measured excitation and emission spectra for genipin.

Marks developed using genipin are blue in colour, although the intensity of colour in the developed marks may vary. Weakly coloured marks may be better viewed using fluorescence examination, the measured fluorescence spectra being illustrated in Figure 9.30.

There is no clearly defined excitation maximum, and many wavelengths of light, ranging from green and green-yellow to yellow, can be used to excite fluorescence. The resultant red fluorescence occurs with a peak emission at approximately 610 nm and is viewed through a red filter such as the Schott glass RG610.

9.10　Lawsone

9.10.1　Outline history of the process

2008: Jelly et al. first reported fingermark enhancement using lawsone (2-hydroxy-1,4-naphthoquinone), a component of henna.

Lawsone has not yet found any significant operational applications. The visible colour of the developed marks is weak, and the longer times and higher processing temperatures required for fingermark development make it less attractive than several other amino acid reagents.

9.10.2　Theory

Lawsone is another compound that reacts with amino acids to give a reaction product consisting of two linked molecules, resembling Ruhemann's purple in general

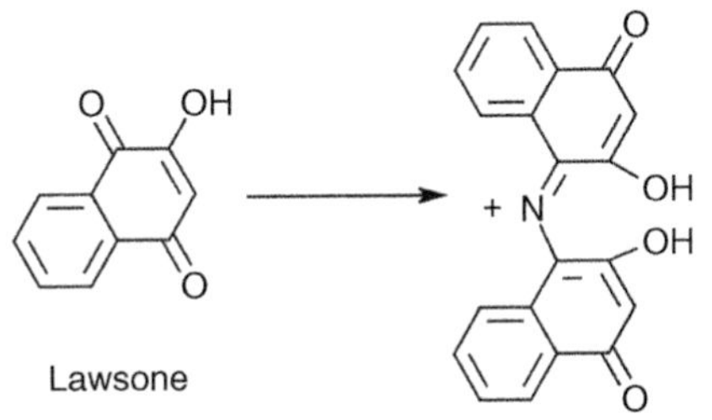

Figure 9.31 Structure of lawsone and the proposed reaction product with amino acids.

structural form (Figure 9.31). The reaction product formed with fingermarks is pale brown but is more readily visualised by fluorescence examination rather than as a visible mark (Figure 9.32).

9.10.3 The lawsone process

The formulation proposed by Jelly et al. (2008) consists of a single working solution:

Lawsone	0.1 g
Ethyl acetate	100 mL
HFE7100	400 mL

In this formulation the ethyl acetate is the principal solvent for lawsone, the active constituent that reacts with amino acids. HFE7100 is used as a non-flammable carrier solvent.

The development process for lawsone involves dipping the exhibit, allowing it to dry and then heating to 150°C for 1 h in a dry oven. The reaction with amino acids that forms fluorescent reaction products is less favourable than those for DFO, 1,2-indandione and ninhydrin, and higher temperatures and longer reaction times are necessary for it to proceed to completion.

Marks developed using lawsone may sometimes be seen as faint brown ridges but in most cases can only be detected by fluorescence examination. Lawsone does not appear to exhibit specific excitation and emission maxima (Figure 9.33), with both occurring over a broad range. Fluorescence can be viewed using illumination in the green, green-yellow or yellow regions of the spectrum, viewing the emission through an orange or red filter such as a Schott glass OG590 or RG610.

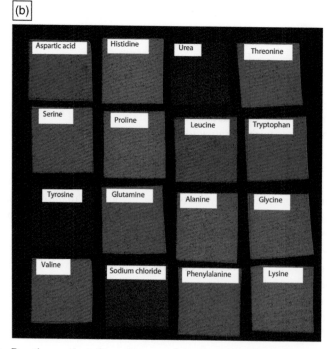

Figure 9.32 Reaction products formed between lawsone and 0.1 M solutions of amino acids and other eccrine constituents deposited onto filter paper, viewed (a) under white light and (b) by fluorescence examination. Reproduced courtesy of the Home Office.

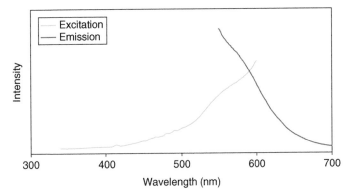

Figure 9.33 Measured excitation and emission spectra for lawsone.

9.11 Alloxan

9.11.1 Outline history of the process

1911: Ruhemann conducted a series of experiments that demonstrated that alloxan and ninhydrin must be closely related compounds because of the similar nature of their reactions.

1950s: Alloxan formulations for fingermark development were consequently reported in Japan in the late 1950s (Motosada, 1957).

1987: Almog included alloxan in a comparison with a range of ninhydrin analogues and finds it inferior in every respect.

Alloxan has not been used as a fingermark reagent for many years because it has been found to be significantly less sensitive than the currently available processes that react with amino acids.

9.11.2 Theory

Alloxan is closely related to ninhydrin in terms of chemical structure, and its reaction with amino acids is also directly analogous to that with ninhydrin, with a Ruhemann's purple analogue being formed as a result. The reaction product is orange-yellow in colour, and the structures of alloxan and the reaction product are shown in Figure 9.34.

9.11.3 The alloxan process

No operational alloxan formulations have been reported. The alloxan formulation used in the comparisons conducted by Almog (1987) was a 1–2% solution of alloxan in absolute ethanol, with a 1% addition of acetic acid.

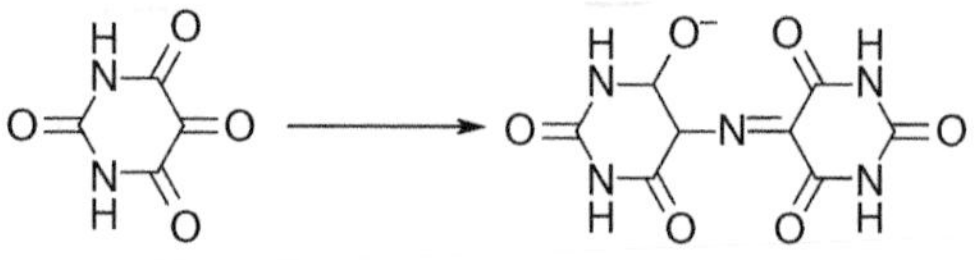

Alloxan   Ruhemann's purple
                                       analogue

Figure 9.34 Structures of alloxan and the corresponding Ruhemann's purple analogue.

9.12   4-Chloro-7-nitrobenzofuran chloride

9.12.1   Outline history of the process

Late 1960s: 4-Chloro-7-nitrobenzofuran (NBD) chloride was first synthesised.

1973: Fager et al. reported the use of NBD chloride for amino acid detection in thin-layer chromatography.

1979: Salares et al. suggested that NBD chloride with illumination from a 488 nm laser is a more sensitive reagent for fingermark detection than ninhydrin.

1983: Warrener et al. suggested a filtered arc lamp as an alternative means of exciting fluorescence in marks developed using NBD chloride.

1984: Stoilovic et al. conducted a comprehensive comparison with ninhydrin and find NBD chloride to be more sensitive.

1987: Creer and Brennan reported the operational benefits of using NBD chloride in processing sequences.

NBD chloride ceased to be regularly used when DFO was first introduced into operational use. It is not as effective in developing fingermarks as DFO or 1,2-indandione, and there are concerns about it being a suspected mutagenic compound. It was not as specific for amino acids as reagents such as DFO and ninhydrin and was sometimes observed to react with additives in papers and inks to give high levels of background fluorescence.

9.12.2   Theory

NBD chloride is a non-fluorescent compound that reacts with amino acids to produce a fluorescent reaction product that retains the –R group of the individual amino acid, as shown in Figure 9.35.

Examples of the visible and fluorescent appearance of the reaction between NBD chloride and amino acids can be seen in Figure 9.36.

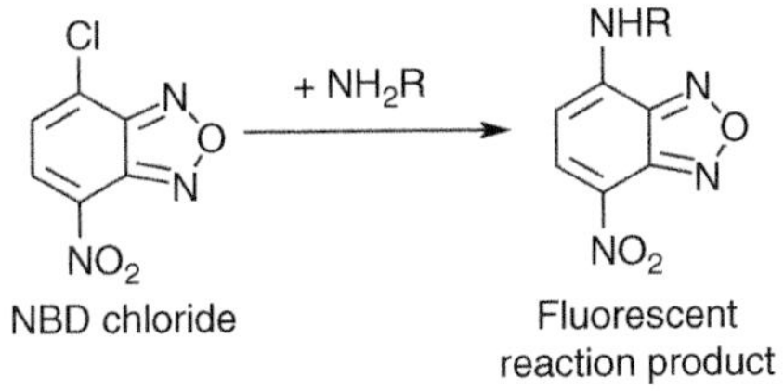

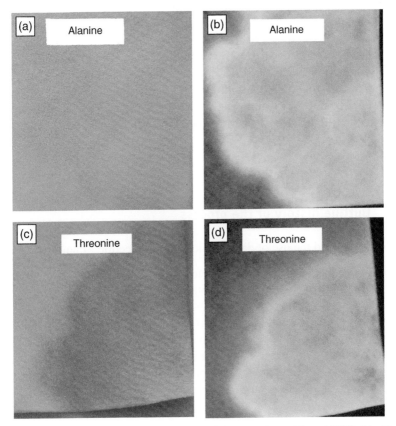

Figure 9.35 Fluorescent product formed by reaction between NBD chloride and amino acids.

Figure 9.36 Reaction products formed between different amino acids and NBD chloride, (a) alanine reaction product, white light, (b) alanine reaction product, fluorescence, (c) threonine reaction product, white light, (d) threonine reaction product, fluorescence. Reproduced courtesy of Loughborough University.

9.12.3   The NBD chloride process

A published formulation for NBD chloride (Salares et al., 1979) consisted of

NBD chloride	20 mg
Absolute ethanol	2 mL
CFC113	20 mL

Ethanol (alternatively acetonitrile) is used as the principal solvent for NBD chloride, and CFC113 was used as a non-flammable carrier solvent.

The resultant solution was sprayed, or used as a dip bath, and then the treated article allowed to dry and then heated for 10 min in the range 90–110°C.

The marks developed using NBD chloride are faint brown and are better visualised using fluorescence examination. Excitation can be achieved over a broad wavelength range, from long-wave ultraviolet to green, and the emission maximum occurs at approximately 540 nm. Fluorescence is best viewed through a yellow-orange viewing filter such as the Schott glass OG550.

9.13   Dansyl chloride

9.13.1   Outline history of the process

1970: Seiler outlined the use of dansyl chloride for detection of amino acids.

1985: Burt and Menzel reported a comparison with ninhydrin and suggested that dansyl chloride may be more sensitive in some circumstances.

The process is not in regular operational use, and no extensive comparative studies have been carried out with other amino acid reagents to establish its effectiveness. Dansyl chloride is corrosive and potentially explosive under certain conditions and is therefore not recommended for regular use for health and safety reasons.

9.13.2   Theory

The dansylation reaction of amino acids is described in detail elsewhere (Seiler, 1970). The reaction product formed by the reaction of dansyl chloride with fingermark residues is similar to that of NBD chloride, with the chlorine atom being replaced by the -NHR group characteristic of the amino acid (Figure 9.37). The reaction product has been shown to absorb at 360 nm (long-wave ultraviolet) with an emission maximum at around 475 nm.

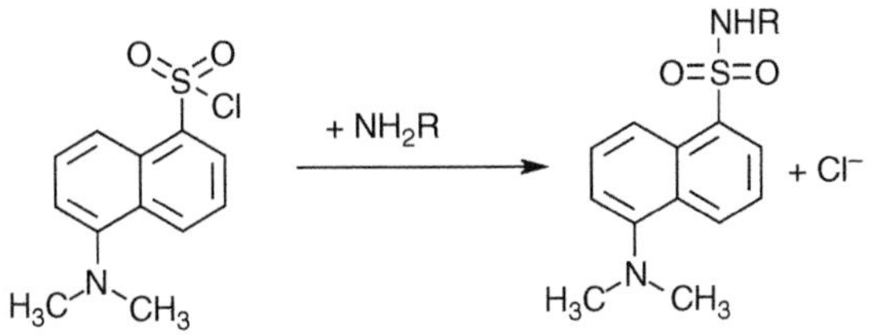

Dansyl chloride

Figure 9.37 Reaction between dansyl chloride and amino acids.

9.13.3 The dansyl chloride process

There are no optimised, published formulations for dansyl chloride. The formulations that have been published are simple, consisting only of dansyl chloride and its principal solvent:

Dansyl chloride	0.2 g
Acetone	100 mL

The pH of this formulation is adjusted to pH 10 using additions of 8 M potassium hydroxide and then applied by spraying.

The marks enhanced using dansyl chloride are not visible and require fluorescence examination to be visualised. Marks are excited using long-wave ultraviolet radiation and emission occurs in the blue-green region with a maximum at 475 nm. Viewing the fluorescence requires a pale yellow filter such as the Schott glass GG455.

9.14 Dimethylaminocinnemaldehyde and dimethylaminobenzaldehyde

9.14.1 Outline history of the process

1973: Dimethylaminocinnemaldehyde (DMAC) was first proposed as a fingermark development reagent by Morris et al. (1973) using a solution dipping process to target urea, giving a magenta reaction product (see Chapter 10).

1995: Brennan et al. reported the use of DMAC fuming to develop marks on a range of substrates, with the marks developed being fluorescent in nature.

1995: Ramotowski outlined the use of DMAC as a contact transfer process for enhancing marks on paper.

2013: Fritz et al. proposed dimethylaminobenzaldehyde (DMAB) for fingermark development.

The DMAC contact transfer process does find operational use in some niche applications, primarily in the development of fingermarks on thermal papers where it may be important to retain the printed text and it is not possible to apply heat to the article. The marks developed are fluorescent (Figure 9.38). DMAB has only recently been re-evaluated, but does not appear to be as effective as other amino acid reagents available for fingermark enhancement.

9.14.2 Theory

DMAB and DMAC are closely related compounds and are expected to react similarly with amino acids. Their structures are illustrated in Figure 9.39.

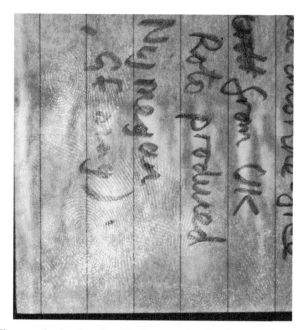

Figure 9.38 Fingermarks developed on lined notepaper using the contact transfer DMAC process.

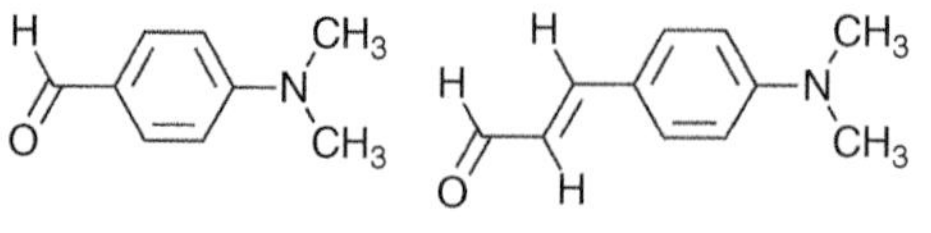

Figure 9.39 The structures of DMAB and DMAC.

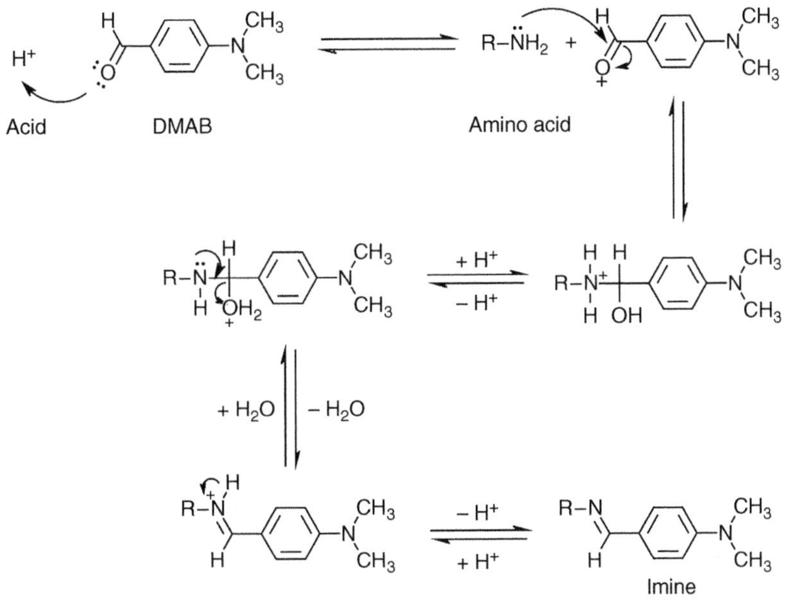

Figure 9.40   Reaction mechanism between DMAB and amino acids.

The reactions that occur between DMAC and DMAB with amino acids when used as fuming or contact reagents are different from the reaction that occurs between DMAC and urea to give a magenta-coloured product (see Chapter 10).

Fritz et al. (2015a, 2015b) have recently studied the reactions of DMAC and DMAB as amino acid reagents and have suggested that DMAC and DMAB react with primary amines to form imines, as illustrated in Figure 9.40.

The reaction products formed between DMAC and amino acids are fluorescent (Figure 9.41). A detailed analysis by Fritz et al. (2015a, 2015b) indicated small shifts in the maximum emission for the reaction product formed with different amino acids, and it is possible that a range of reaction products are in fact formed. Note that in contrast with other amino acid reagents, the reaction between DMAC and proline appears to produce the most intensely fluorescent product.

9.14.3   The DMAB and DMAC processes

The DMAC contact transfer process first proposed by Ramotowski (1995) utilises impregnated sheets of paper that are produced by dipping in a solution comprising 0.25 g of DMAC dissolved in 100 mL of ethanol. The sheets are then allowed to dry.

The article to be treated is sandwiched between two sheets of impregnated paper, placed in a press and left overnight, generating DMAC vapours that interact

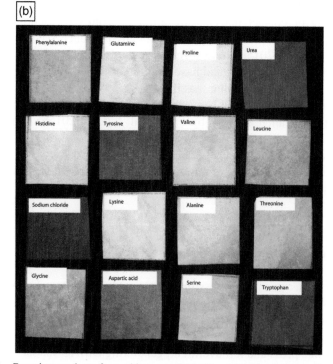

Figure 9.41   Reaction products formed between DMAC and 0.1 M solutions of amino acids and other eccrine constituents deposited onto filter paper, viewed (a) under white light and (b) by fluorescence examination. Reproduced courtesy of the Home Office.

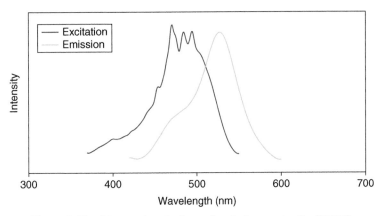

Figure 9.42   Measured excitation and emission spectra for DMAC.

with amino acids to produce the fluorescent product. Alternatively, a heated press can be used to accelerate the reaction, which takes approximately 30 s at 100°C. Heating at higher temperatures can result in excessive background fluorescence.

Marks enhanced using DMAC can occasionally be seen as darker yellow ridges against the lighter yellow colouration of the background but generally require fluorescence examination to be seen. Excitation occurs over a broad range with a maximum at approximately 480 nm, and the emission spectrum has a maximum at approximately 525 nm (Figure 9.42).

Fluorescence examination utilises illumination in the blue, blue-green or green regions of the spectrum, with fluorescence viewed through a yellow-orange filter such as the Schott glass OG530 or OG550.

The DMAB formulation used by Fritz et al. (2013) consists of:

Concentrated solution

DMAB	1 g
Ethyl acetate	22 mL
Acetic acid	3 mL

Working solution

Concentrated solution	10 mL
HFE7100	90 mL

Articles are dipped in the working solution, allowed to dry the heated in a dry oven at 150°C for 20 min or in a hot press at approximately 160°C for 20 s.

References

Abderhalden E, Schmidt H, 'On the Use of Triketohydrinenehydrate for Tracing Proteins and Their Stages of Decomposition', Z Physiol Chem (Ger), vol 72, (1911), p 37–43.

Abderhalden E, Schmidt H, 'Some Observations and Tests on Triketohydrinenehydrate', Z Physiol Chem (Ger), vol 85, (1913), p 143.

Almog J, 'Reagents for Chemical Development of Latent Fingerprints: Vicinal Triketones – Their Reaction with Amino Acids and with Latent Fingerprints on Paper', J Forensic Sci, vol 32(6), (1987), p 1565–1573.

Almog J, Hirshfield A, Klug J T, 'Reagents for the Chemical Development of Latent Fingerprints: Synthesis and Properties of Some Ninhydrin Analogues', J Forensic Sci, vol 27(4), (1982), p 912–917.

Almog J, Hirshfield A, Frank A, Grant H, Harel Z, Ittah Y, '5-Methylthio Ninhydrin and Related Compounds: A Novel Class of Fluorogenic Fingerprint Reagents', J Forensic Sci, vol 37(3), (1992), p 688–694.

Almog J, Springer E, Wisener S, Frank A, Khodzhaev O, Lidor R, et al, 'Latent Fingerprint Visualisation by 1,2-Indanedione and Related Compounds: Preliminary Results', J Forensic Sci, vol 44(1), (1999), p 114–118.

Almog J, Sears V G, Springer E, Hewlett D F, Walker S, Wisener S, Lidor R, Bahar E, 'Reagents for the Chemical Development of Latent Fingerprints: Scope and Limitations of Benzo[f]ninhydrin in Comparison to Ninhydrin', J Forensic Sci, vol 45(3), (2000), p 538–544.

Almog J, Cohen Y, Azoury M, Hahn T-R, 'Genipin – A Novel Fingerprint Reagent with Colorimetric and Fluorogenic Activity', J Forensic Sci, vol 49(2), (2004), p 255–257.

Almog J, Levinton-Shamuilov G, Cohen Y, Azoury M, 'Fingerprint Reagents with Dual Action: Color and Fluorescence', J Forensic Sci, vol 52(2), (2007), p 330–334.

Almog J, Klein A, Davidi I, Cohen Y, Azoury M, Levin-Elad M, 'Dual Fingerprint Reagents with Enhanced Sensitivity: 5-Methoxy- and 5-Methylthioninhydrin', J Forensic Sci, vol 53(2), (2008), p 364–367.

Bandey H L (ed.), 'Fingermark Visualisation Manual', Home Office, London, 2014.

Bandey H L, 'Fingermark Visualisation Newsletter', Home Office, London, March 2017 (accessed via https://www.gov.uk/government/collections/centre-for-applied-science-and-technology-information#fingermark-documents (accessed 24 October 2017).

Benson J R, Hare P E, 'o-Phthalaldehyde: Fluorogenic Detection of Primary Amines in the Picomole Range: Comparison with Fluorescamine and Ninhydrin', Proc Natl Acad Sci U S A, vol 72(2), (1975), p 619–622.

Bicknell D E, Ramotowski R S, 'Use of an Optimised 1,2-Indanedione Process for the Development of Latent Prints', J Forensic Sci, vol 53(5), (2008), p 1108–1116.

Brennan J, Bramble S, Crabtree S, Wright G, 'Fuming of Latent Fingerprints Using Dimethylaminocinnemaldehyde', J Forensic Identif, vol 45, (1995), p 373–380.

Burt J A, Menzel E R, 'Laser Detection of Latent Fingerprints: Difficult Surfaces', J Forensic Sci, vol 13(2), (1985), p 364–370.

Cashman P J, Beede J D, Thornton J I, 'Ninhydrin: A Color Test for the Differentiation of Phenethylamines of Abuse', J Forensic Sci Soc, vol 19, (1979), p 137–141.

Conn C, Ramsey G, Roux C, Lennard C, 'The Effect of Metal Salt Treatment on the Photoluminescence of DFO-Treated Fingerprints', Forensic Sci Int, vol 116, (2001), p 117–123.

Creer K E, Brennan J S, 'The Work of the Serious Crime Unit', Proceedings of the International Forensic Symposium on Latent Prints, 7–10 July 1987, FBI Academy, Quantico, VA, p 91–99.

Crown D A, 'The Development of Latent Fingerprints with Ninhydrin', J Crim Law Criminol Police Sci, vol 60(2), (1969), p 258–264.

Dent C E, 'A Study of the Behaviour of Some Sixty Amino-Acids and Other Ninhydrin-Reacting Substances on Phenol-'Collidine' Filter-Paper Chromatograms, with Notes as to the Occurrence of Some of Them in Biological Fluids', Biochem J, vol 43, (1948), p 169–180.

Didierjean C, Debart M-H, Crispino F, 'New Formulation of DFO in HFE7100', Fingerprint Whorld, vol 24(94), (1998), p 163–167.

Druey J, Schmidt P, 'Phenanthroline Quinones and Diazafluorenes', Helv Chim Acta, vol 33 (1950), p 1080–1087.

Dutt M C, Poh T T, 'Use of Ninhydrin as a Spray Reagent for the Detection of Some Basic Drugs on Thin Layer Chromatograms', J Chromatogr, vol 195, (1980), p 133–138.

Dyer R-M, 'Determination of the Optimal Conditions for Using 1,2-Indandione as a Fingermark Development Technique', Home Office CAST student placement report, July 2015.

Fager R S, Kutina C B, Abrahamson E W, 'The Use of NBD Chloride (4-Chloro-7-nitrobenzo-2-oxa-1,3-diazole) in Detecting Amino Acids and as an N-Terminal Reagent', Anal Biochem, vol 53, (1973), p 290–294.

Figuera M M, Xu X, de Puit M, 'Performance of 1,2-Indanedione and the Need for Sequential Treatment of Fingerprints', Sci Justice, vol 55(5), (2015), p 343–346.

Fischer J F, 'A Modified o-Phthalaldehyde Technique Utilizing Blue-Green Light Excitation for Developing Luminescent Latent Prints', J Forensic Identif, vol 40(6), (1990), p 327–333.

Friedman M, Sigel C W, 'A Kinetic Study of the Ninhydrin Reaction', Biochemistry, vol 5(2), (1966), p 478–485.

Friedman M, Williams L D, 'Stoichiometry of Formation of Ruhemann's Purple in the Ninhydrin Reaction', Bioorganic Chem, vol 3, (1974), p 267–280.

Fritz P, Van Bronswijk W, Lewis S W, 'p-Dimethylaminobenzaldehyde: Preliminary Investigations into a Novel Reagent for the Detection of Latent Fingermarks on Paper Surfaces', Anal Methods, vol 5(13), (2013), p 3207–3215.

Fritz P, Van Bronswijk W, Lewis S W, 'A New p-Dimethylaminocinnamaldehyde Reagent Formulation for the Photoluminescence Detection of Latent Fingermarks on Paper', Forensic Sci Int, vol 257, (2015a), p 20–28.

Fritz P, Van Bronswijk W, Dorakumbura B, Hackshaw B, Lewis S W, 'Evaluation of a Solvent-Free p-Dimethylaminobenzaldehyde Method for Fingermark Visualisation with a Low Cost Light Source Suitable for Remote Locations', J Forensic Identif, vol 65(1), (2015b), p 67–90.

Gardner S J, Hewlett D F, 'Optimisation and Initial Evaluation of 1,2-Indandione as a Reagent for Fingerprint Detection', J Forensic Sci, vol 48(6), (2003), p 1288–1292.

Grigg R, Mongkolaussavaratana T, Pounds C A, Sivagnanam S, '1,8-Diazafluorenone and Related Compounds: A New Reagent for the Detection of α-Amino Acids and Latent Fingerprints', Tetrahedron Lett, vol 31(49), (1990), p 7215–7218.

Hardwick S, Kent T, Sears V, Winfield P, 'Improvements to the Formulation of DFO and the Effects of Heat on the Reaction with Latent Fingerprints', Fingerprint Whorld, vol 19(73), (1993), p 65–69.

Hauze D B, Petrovskaia O, Taylor B, Joullie M M, Ramotowski R, Cantu A A, '1,2-Indandiones: New Reagents for Visualising the Amino Acid Components of Latent Prints', J Forensic Sci, vol 43(4), (1998), p 744–747.

Herod D W, Menzel E R, 'Laser Detection of Latent Fingerprints: Ninhydrin Followed by Zinc Chloride', J Forensic Sci, vol 27(3), (1982), p 513–518.

Hewlett D F, Sears V G, 'Replacements for CFC113 in the Ninhydrin Process: Part 1', J Forensic Identif, vol 47(3), (1997), p 287–299.

Hewlett D F, Sears V G, Suzuki S, 'Replacements for CFC113 in the Ninhydrin Process: Part 2', J Forensic Identif, vol 47(3), (1997), p 300–306.

Jelly R, Lewis S W, Lennard C, Lim K F, Almog J, 'Lawsone: A Novel Reagent for the Detection of Latent Fingermarks on Paper Surfaces', Chem Commun, vol 39(45), (2008), p 3513–3515.

Joullie M M, Thompson T R, Nemeroff N H, 'Ninhydrin and Ninhydrin Analogs: Syntheses and Applications', Tetrahedron, vol 47(42), (1991), p 8791–8830.

Lee H C, Attard A E, 'Comparison of Fluorescamine, o-Phthalaldehyde, and Ninhydrin for the Detection and Visualization of Latent Fingerprints', J Police Sci Adm, vol 7(3), (1979), p 333–335.

Lee K S, Drescher D G, 'Fluorometric Amino-Acid Analysis with o-Phthadialdehyde (OPA)', Int J Biochem, vol 9, (1978), p 457–467.

Lennard C J, Margot P A, Stoilovic M, Warrener R N, 'Synthesis of Ninhydrin Analogues and Their Application to Fingerprint Development: Preliminary Results', J Forensic Sci Soc, vol 26, (1986), p 323–328.

Lennard C J, Margot P A, Sterns M, Warrener R N, 'Photoluminescent Enhancement of Ninhydrin Developed Fingerprints by Metal Complexation: Structural Studies of Complexes Formed Between Ruhemann's Purple and Group IIb Metal Salts', J Forensic Sci, vol 32(3), (1987), p 597–605.

Levinton-Shamuilov G, Cohen Y, Azoury M, Chaikovsky A, Almog J, 'Genipin, a Novel Fingerprint Reagent with Colorimetric and Fluorogenic Activity, Part II: Optimization, Scope and Limitations', J Forensic Sci, vol 50(6), (2005), p 1367–1371.

Linde H G, 'Latent Fingerprints by a Superior Ninhydrin Method', J Forensic Sci, vol 20, (1975), p 581–584.

Masters N, Morgan R, Shipp E, 'DFO, Its Usage and Results', J Forensic Identif, vol 41(1), (1991), p 3–10.

Mayer S W, Meilleur C P, Jones P F, 'The Use of Ortho-Phthalaldehyde for Superior Fluorescent Visualization of Latent Fingerprints', J Forensic Sci Soc, vol 18, (1978), p 233–235.

McCaldin D J, 'The Chemistry of Ninhydrin', Chem Rev, (1960), p 39–51.

Menzel E R, Almog J, 'Latent Fingerprint Development by Frequency Doubled Neodymium: Yttrium Aluminium Garnet (Nd:YAG) Laser: Benzo[f]ninhydrin', J Forensic Sci, vol 30(2), (1985), p 371–382.

Morris J R, 'An Examination of the Chemical Literature on Fingerprint Technology for the Period 1890 to August 1974', AWRE SSCD Memo. 359, October 1974.

Morris J R, 'Extensions to the NFN (Ninhydrin) Reagent for the Development of Latent Fingerprints', SSCD Memo, CRP Work Item 41A, AWRE Aldermaston, February 1978.

Morris J R, Goode G C, 'NFN – An Improved Ninhydrin Reagent for Detection of Latent Fingerprints', Police Res Bull, vol 24 (1974), p 45–53.

Morris J R, Goode G C, Godsell J W, 'Some New Developments in the Chemical Development of Latent Fingerprints', Police Res Bull, vol 21, (1973), p 31.

Motosada K, 'Detection of Fingerprints by use of Alloxan', Kagaku to Susa, vol 10(5), (1957), p 23.

Nicolasora N, 'Comparison of 1,2-Indandione Formulations and Optimisation of Development Conditions', Home Office student placement report, July 2014.

Oden S, von Hofsten B, 'Detection of Fingerprints by the Ninhydrin Reaction', Nature, March 6 (1954), p 449–450.

Ohki H, 'A New Detection Method for Latent Fingerprints with Fluorescamine', Rep Natl Res Inst Police Sci (Japan), vol 29, (1976), p 46–47.

Ohki H, 'A New Detection Method for Latent Fingerprints with o-Phthalaldehyde', Rep Natl Res Inst Police Sci (Japan), vol 31(4), (1978), p 295–300.

Patton E L T, Brown D H, Lewis S W, Detection of Latent Fingermarks on Thermal Printer Paper by Dry Contact with 1,2-Indanedione, Anal Methods, vol 2, (2010), p 631–637.

Porpiglia N, Bleay S, Fitzgerald L, Barron L, 'An Assessment of the Effectiveness of 5-Methyl-thioninhydrin within Dual Action Reagents for Latent Fingerprint Development on Paper Substrates', Sci Justice, vol 52(1), (2012), p 42–48.

Pounds C A, Grigg R, Mongkolaussavaratana T, 'The Use of 1,8-Diazafluoren-9-one (DFO) for the Fluorescent Detection of Latent Fingerprints on Paper: A Preliminary Investigation', J Forensic Sci, vol 35(1), (1990), p 169–175.

Rajtar P E, '3M Novec™ Engineer Fluid HFE-7100', Fingerprint Whorld, vol 26(102), (2000), p 143–152.

Ramotowski R, 'Fluorescence Visualisation of Latent Fingerprints on Paper Using p-Dimethyl-aminocinnamaldehyde (PDMAC)', Proceedings of the International Symposium on Finger-print Detection and Identification, Ne'urim, Israel, June 1995, p 91–94.

Ramotowski R, Cantu A A, Joullie M M, Petrovskaia O, '1,2-Indanediones: A Preliminary Evaluation of a New Class of Amino Acid Visualising Reagents', Fingerprint Whorld, vol 23(90), (1997), p 131–140.

Ruhemann S, 'Cyclic Di- and Tri-ketones', J Chem Soc Trans, vol 97, (1910a), p 1438–1449.

Ruhemann S, 'Triketohydrindene Hydrate', J Chem Soc Trans, vol 97, (1910b), p 2025–2031.

Ruhemann S, 'Triketohydrindene Hydrate: Part III, Its Relation to Alloxan', J Chem Soc, vol 23, (1911), p 792–800.

Salares V, Eves C, Carey P, 'On the Detection of Fingerprints by Laser Excited Luminescence', Forensic Sci Int, vol 14, (1979), p 229–238.

Sears V G, Hewlett D F, 'DFO Formulations in Non-ozone Depleting Solvents', Identif Can, vol 26(1), (2003), p 4–12.

Seiler N, 'Use of the Dansyl Chloride in Biochemical Analysis', in Glick E J, 'Methods of Biochemical Analysis', John Wiley & Sons, Inc., New York, 1970.

Serrano E, Sturelle V, 'Modification and Evaluation of a 1,2-Indanedione-Zinc Chloride Formula Using Petroleum Ether as a Carrier Solvent', Can Soc Forensic Sci J, vol 43(3), (2010), p 108–116.

Simons S S, Johnson D F, 'The Structure of the Fluorescent Adduct Formed in the Reaction of Ortho-Phthalaldehyde and Thiols with Amines', J Am Chem Soc, vol 98, (1976), p 7098–7099.

Spindler X, Stoilovic M, Lennard C, Lennard A, 'Spectral Variations for Reaction Products Formed Between Different Amino Acids and Latent Fingermark Detection Reagents on a Range of Cellulose-Based Substrates', J Forensic Identif, vol 59(3), (2009), p 308–324.

Spindler X, Shimmon R, Roux C, Lennard C, 'The Effect of Zinc Chloride, Humidity and the Substrate on the Reaction of 1,2-Indanedione-Zinc with Amino Acids in Latent Fingermark Secretions', Forensic Sci Int, vol. 212, (2011), p 150–157.

Spindler X, Shimmon R, Roux C, Lennard C, 'Visualising Substrate-Fingermark Interactions: Solid-State NMR Spectroscopy of Amino Acid Reagent Development on Cellulose Substrates', Forensic Sci Int, vol. 250, (2015), p 8–16.

Stoilovic M, Warrener R N, Kobus H J, 'An Evaluation of the Reagent NBD Chloride for the Production of Luminescent Fingerprints on Paper: II A Comparison with Ninhydrin', Forensic Sci Int, vol 24, (1984), p 279–284.

Stoilovic M, Lennard C, Wallace-Kunkel C, Roux C, 'Evaluation of a 1,2-Indanedione Formulation Containing Zinc Chloride for Improved Fingermark Detection on Paper', J Forensic Identif, vol 57(1), (2007), p 4–18.

Svedas V J K, Galaev I J, Borisov I L, Berezin I V, 'The Interaction of Amino Acids with O-Phthaldialdehyde; A Kinetic Study and Spectrophotometric Assay of the Reaction Product', Anal Biochem, vol. 101, (1980), p 188–195.

Udenfriend S, 'Development of a New Fluorescent Reagent and Its Application to the Automated Assay of Amino Acids and Peptides at the Picomole Level', J Res Nat Bur Stand A Phys Chem, vol 76A(6), (1972), p 637–640.

Udenfriend S, Stein S, Bohlen P, Dairman W, Leimgruber W, Weigele M, 'Fluorescamine: A Reagent for Assay of Amino Acids, Peptides, Proteins, and Primary Amines in the Picomole Range', Science, vol 178, (1972), p 871–872.

Warrener R N, Kobus H J, Stoilovic M, 'An Evaluation of the Reagent NBD Chloride for the Production of Luminescent Fingerprints on Paper: I, Support for a Xenon Arc Lamp Being a Cheaper and Valuable Alternative to an Argon Ion Laser as an Excitation Source', Forensic Sci Int, vol 23, (1983), p 179–188.

Wilkinson D, 'A Study of the Reaction Mechanism of 1,8-Diazafluoren-9-one with the Amino Acid, L-Alanine', Forensic Sci Int, vol 109(2), (2000), p 87–102.

Yuferov V P, 'On the Mechanism of Ninhydrin Reactions', Usp Biol Khim (Russ), vol 12, (1971), p 62–71.

Further reading

Almog J, Hirshfield A, '5-Methoxyninhydrin: A Reagent for the Chemical Development of Latent Fingerprints That Is Compatible with the Copper-Vapor Laser', J Forensic Sci, vol 33(4), (1988), p 1027–1030.

Almog J, Zeichner A, Shifrina S, Scharf G, 'Nitro-Benzofurazanyl Ethers – A New Series of Fluorigenic Fingerprint Reagents', J Forensic Sci, vol 32(3), (1987), p 585–596.

Azoury M, Zamir A, Oz C, Wiesner S, 'The Effect of 1,2-Indanedione, a Latent Fingerprint Reagent on Subsequent DNA Profiling', J Forensic Sci, vol 47(3), (2002), p 586–588.

Bratton R M, Juhala J A, 'DFO-Dry', J Forensic Identif, vol 45(2), (1995), p 169–172.

Cantu A A, Leben D A, Joullie M M, Heffner R J, Hark R R, 'A Comparative Examination of Several Amino Acid Reagents for Visualising Amino Acid (Glycine) on Paper', J Forensic Identif, vol 43(1), (1993), p 44–67.

Chan J, Shimmon R, Spindler X, Maynard P, Lennard C, Roux C, Stuart B H, 'An Investigation of Isatin as a Potential Reagent for Latent Fingermark Detection on Porous Surfaces', J Forensic Identif, vol 60(3), (2010), p 320–336.

Corson W B, Lawson J E, Kuhn K E, 'Alternative Applications of DFO for Non-fluorescent Visualisation', J Forensic Identif, vol 41(6), (1991), p 437–445.

Everse K E, Menzel E R, 'Sensitivity Enhancement of Ninhydrin-Treated Latent Fingerprints by Enzymes and Metal Salts', J Forensic Sci, vol 31(2), (1986), p 446–454.

Flynn J, Stoilovic M, Lennard C, 'Detection and Enhancement of Latent Fingerprints on Polymer Banknotes: A Preliminary Study', J Forensic Identif, vol 49(6), (1999), p 594–613.

Fregau C J, Germain O, Fourney R M, 'Fingerprint Enhancement Revisited and the Effects of Blood Enhancement Chemicals on Subsequent Profiler Plus Fluorescent Short Tandem Repeat

DNA Analysis of Fresh and Aged Bloody Fingerprints', J Forensic Sci, vol 45(2), (2000), p 354–380.

Hewlett D F, Sears V G, 'An Operational Trial of Two Non-ozone Depleting Ninhydrin Formulations for Latent Fingerprint Detection', J Forensic Identif, vol 49(4), (1999), p 388–396.

Hewlett D F, Winfield P G R, Clifford A A, 'The Ninhydrin Process in Supercritical Carbon Dioxide', J Forensic Sci, vol 41(3), (1996), p 487–489.

Katzung W, 'New Reagents for the Chemical Development of Latent Fingerprints on Paper and Their Possible Applications', Krim Forensische Wiss, vol 57(58), (1985), p 82–89.

Kobus H J, Stoilovic M, Warrener R N, 'A Simple Luminescent Post-ninhydrin Treatment for the Improved Visualisation of Fingerprints on Documents in Cases Where Ninhydrin Alone Gives Poor Results', Forensic Sci Int, vol 22, (1983), p 161–170.

Kobus H J, Pigou P E, Jahangiri S, Taylor B, 'Evaluation of Some Oxygen, Sulfur and Selenium Substituted Ninhydrin Analogues, Nitrophenylninhydrin and Benzo[f]furoninhydrin', J Forensic Sci, vol 47(2), (2002), p 254–259.

Lee M-L, Safille A, 'Improved Solvent System for Thin-layer Chromatography of Dns-amino Acids', J Chromatogr, vol 116, (1976), p 462–464.

Lennard C, Mazella W, 'Evaluation of Freon-free Fingerprint Reagent Formulations', Proc Meet Intl Assoc Forensic Sci, vol 4, (1995), p 296–301.

Lennard C J, Margot PA, Stoilovic M, Warrener R N, 'Synthesis and Evaluation of Ninhydrin Analogues as Reagents for the Development of Latent Fingerprints on Paper Surfaces', J Forensic Sci Soc, vol 28, (1988), p 3–23.

McComisky P, 'DFO – A Simple and Quick Method for the Development of Latent Fingerprints', Fingerprint Whorld, vol 16(62), (1990), p 64–65.

McMahon P, 'Procedure to Develop Latent Prints on Thermal Paper', Ident Can, vol 19(3), (1996), p 4–5.

Menzel E R, Mitchell K E, 'Intramolecular Energy Transfer in the Europium-Ruhemann's Purple Complex: Application to Latent Fingerprint Detection', J Forensic Sci, vol 35(1), (1990), p 35–45.

Menzel E R, Bartsch R A, Hallman J L, 'Fluorescent Metal-Ruhemann's Purple Coordination Compounds: Applications to Latent Fingerprint Detection', J Forensic Sci, vol 35(1), (1990), p 25–34

Merrick S, Gardner S, Sears V, Hewlett D, 'An Operational Trial of Ozone-Friendly DFO and 1,2-Indandione Formulations for Latent Fingerprint Detection', J Forensic Identif, vol 52(5), (2002), p 595–605.

Petruncio A V, 'A Comparative Study for the Evaluation of Two Solvents for Use in Ninhydrin Processing of Latent Print Evidence', J Forensic Identif, vol 50(5), (2000), p 462–469.

Roux C, Jones N, Lennard C, Stoilovic M, 'Evaluation of 1,2-Indanedione and 5,6-Dimethoxy-1,2-Indanedione for the Detection of Latent Fingerprints on Porous Surfaces', J Forensic Sci, vol 45(4), (2002), p 761–769.

Russell S, John G, Naccarato S, 'Modification of the 1,2-Indandione/Zinc Chloride Formula for Latent Print Development', J Forensic Identif, vol 58(2), (2008), p 182–192.

Sasson Y, Almog J, 'Chemical Reagents for the Development of Latent Fingerprints 1: Scope and Limitations of the Reagent 4-Dimethylaminocinnamaldehyde', J Forensic Sci, vol 23, (1978), p 852–855.

Schiltz E, Schnackerz K D, Gracy R W, 'Comparison of Ninhydrin, Fluorescamine, and o-Phthaldialdehyde for the Detection of Amino Acids and Peptides and Their Effects on the Recovery and Composition of Peptides from Thin-Layer Fingerprints', Anal Biochem, vol 79, (1977), p 33–41

Sears V, Batham R, Bleay S, 'The Effectiveness of 1,2-Indandione-Zinc Formulations and Comparison with HFE-Based 1,8-Diazafluoren-9-one for Fingerprint Development', J Forensic Identif, vol 59(6), (2009), p 654–678.

Stimac J T, 'Thermal Paper: Latent Friction Ridge Development via 1,2-Indanedione', J Forensic Identif, vol 53(3), (2003), p 265–271.

Stoilovic M, 'Improved Methods for DFO Development of Latent Prints', Forensic Sci Int, vol 60, (1993), p 141–153.

Stoilovic M, Warrener R N, Kobus H J, 'An Evaluation of the Reagent NBD Chloride for the Production of Luminescent Fingerprints on Paper: II, A Comparison with Ninhydrin', Forensic Sci Int, vol 24, (1984), p 279–284.

Stoilovic M, Kobus H J, Margot P A J-L, Warrener R N, 'Improved Enhancement of Ninhydrin Developed Fingerprints by Cadmium Complexation Using Low Temperature Photoluminescence Techniques', J Forensic Sci, vol 31(2), (1986), p 432–445.

Tapuhi Y, Schmidt D E, Lindner W, Karger B L, 'Dansylation of Amino Acids for High-Performance Liquid Chromatography Analysis', Anal Biochem, vol 115, (1981), p 123–129.

Wallace-Kunkel C, Roux C, Lennard C, Stoilovic M, 'The Detection and Enhancement of Latent Fingermarks on Porous Surfaces – A Survey', J Forensic Identif, vol 54(6), (2004), p 687–705.

Wallace-Kunkel C, Lennard C, Stoilovic M, Roux C, 'Optimisation and Evaluation of 1,2-Indanedione for Use as a Fingerprint Reagent and Its Application to Real Samples', Forensic Sci Int, vol 168(1), (2007), p 14–26.

Watling W J, Smith KO, 'Heptane: An Alternative to the Freon/Ninhydrin Mixture', J Forensic Identif, vol 43(2), (1993), p 131–134.

Weisener S, Springer E, Sasson Y, Almog J, 'Chemical Development of Latent Fingerprints: 1,2-Indandione Has Come of Age', J Forensic Sci, vol 46(5), (2001), p 1082–1084.

Wilkinson D, McKenzie E, Leech C, Mayowski D, Bertrand S, Walker T, 'The Results from a Canadian National Field Trial Comparing Two Formulations of 1,8-Diazafluoren-9-one (DFO) with 1,2-Indandione', Identif Can, vol 26(2), (2003), p 8–18.

10

Reagents for other eccrine constituents

Stephen M. Bleay

Home Office Centre for Applied Science and Technology, Sandridge, UK

Key points

- Reagents targeting eccrine constituents other than amino acids are not currently in widespread use.

- Issues associated with migration of the constituents within the substrate mean that diffusion of ridge detail often occurs, and such reagents are ineffective on older fingermarks.

- The constituents targeted are water soluble, and such reagents are ineffective on surfaces that have been wetted.

10.1 Introduction

Amino acid reagents have become the predominant techniques for the enhancement of fingermarks on porous surfaces; the high sensitivity of such reagents means that they will generally detect the highest numbers of marks. However, as has been described in Chapter 3, amino acids are not the only constituents of eccrine sweat that can be utilised for fingermark development. The most abundant constituents that have been targeted in this way are chlorides, which can be detected by silver nitrate, and urea, which can be targeted by 4-dimethylaminocinnamaldehyde (DMAC). However, it should also be noted that there are also other equally abundant eccrine constituents, including lactates, that have not yet been utilised for fingermark enhancement on porous surfaces.

Fingerprint Development Techniques: Theory and Application, First Edition.
Stephen M. Bleay, Ruth S. Croxton and Marcel de Puit.
© 2018 John Wiley & Sons Ltd. Published 2018 by John Wiley & Sons Ltd.

Silver nitrate was one of the earliest chemical reagents used for fingermark development, being reported for this application as early as the late 19th century (Forgeot, 1891). Until the introduction of ninhydrin in the 1950s, silver nitrate was one of only two processes widely available for developing fingermarks on paper. It remained a complementary process to ninhydrin, being used in sequence with it because the two processes target different constituents. However, after the introduction of physical developer, which not only targeted different fingermark constituents but could also develop marks on wetted porous surfaces, the use of silver nitrate progressively declined.

Following studies into fingermark composition in the late 1960s that quantified the chloride content of eccrine sweat and also identified urea as a principal constituent (Cuthbertson, 1969), research was carried out into reagents that could react with the urea present in the fingermark deposits. The result of these studies was 4-dimethyl-aminocinnamaldehyde (DMAC), which was applied to the surface in solution and reacted rapidly without heating to give a magenta-coloured product (Morris et al., 1973). This was introduced into operational use in the United Kingdom in the early 1970s but soon withdrawn when it became evident that it was ineffective on marks older than a few days. This was attributed to the rapid diffusion of the small urea molecule within the porous substrate, this diffusion being accelerated by high humidity. Urea does not appear to bind to cellulose in paper in the same way as the amino acids.

More recently interest in DMAC has been revived, but the reagent is now used as a contact transfer process that targets amino acids, described in Chapter 9.

In common with the amino acid reagents, neither silver nitrate nor DMAC is suitable for use on surfaces that have been wetted. This is because sodium and potassium chloride and urea are all highly soluble in water and will diffuse or fully dissolve when exposed to moisture.

There are other constituents of eccrine sweat that are not actively targeted by existing techniques, including several organic acids such as lactic acid, uric acid and pyruvic acid. The feasibility of using the organic acid indicator 2,6-dichlorophenol-indophenol sodium salt in ethanolic solution (Tillmann's reagent) as a fingermark enhancement reagent has been explored by Vincent (1973). This was found to be a highly sensitive reagent, but it proved difficult to control the spray method of application to prevent the dark blue background colouration obscuring the pink developed fingermarks. In theory there are many other acidic species in fingermarks (carboxylic acid groups of amino acids and fatty acids) that could interact with this reagent, and there may be merit in revisiting the process because of its ability to react with eccrine and sebaceous constituents.

10.2   Current operational use

DMAC is no longer used in its original solution dipping form. Operational experience in the 1970s demonstrated that the solution dipping process was not suitable for marks more than a few days old because of the rapid diffusion of the urea constituent.

The solution dipping formulation originally proposed (Goode and Morris, 1983) is based on CFCs and would not be acceptable for use without reformulation to a less ozone-depleting solvent.

Silver nitrate is still used for fingermark enhancement, but its applications have progressively declined. It was recommended primarily as a process for the development of marks on light-coloured, raw wood (Kent, 1986). It was later considered that physical developer was equally as effective in this application and overcame the issues associated with progressive darkening of the background on exposure to light, and hence use of silver nitrate decreased. However, it may still be used on larger wood or cardboard articles where it is difficult or impractical to apply physical developer.

On paper items, silver nitrate can develop additional marks if used sequentially after ninhydrin because it targets different constituents in eccrine sweat. However, chlorides are more affected by moisture and high humidity conditions than many other constituents. The small chloride ions are readily soluble and can migrate rapidly when water is present, so silver nitrate cannot be used on items that have been wetted. For this reason, physical developer replaced silver nitrate for sequential treatment after ninhydrin because it both targets different constituents and can be used on wetted items.

10.3   4-Dimethylaminocinnamaldehyde

10.3.1   Outline history of the process

1973: DMAC was first proposed as a fingermark development reagent by Morris, Goode and Godsell, who used a solution dipping process to target urea.

1978: Sasson and Almog described the limitations of DMAC in developing marks more than a few days old, confirming the issues observed in operational trials.

1985: Katzung first observed that marks developed using DMAC have fluorescent properties in addition to a visible magenta colour.

1987: Van Enckevort re-evaluated DMAC but also encountered issues of ridge diffusion in older marks and did not recommend it for operational use.

1995: It was later observed that DMAC had potential for use as a fuming and contact transfer process, and subsequent use focuses on these applications (Brennan et al., 1995; Ramotowski, 1995).

The appearance of the magenta reaction product produced between DMAC solution and fingermarks is illustrated in Figure 10.1.

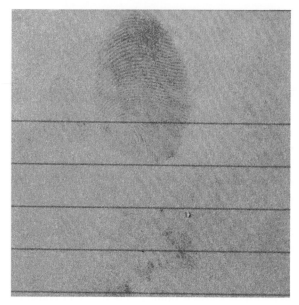

Figure 10.1   Fingermark on lined notepaper enhanced using DMAC solution.

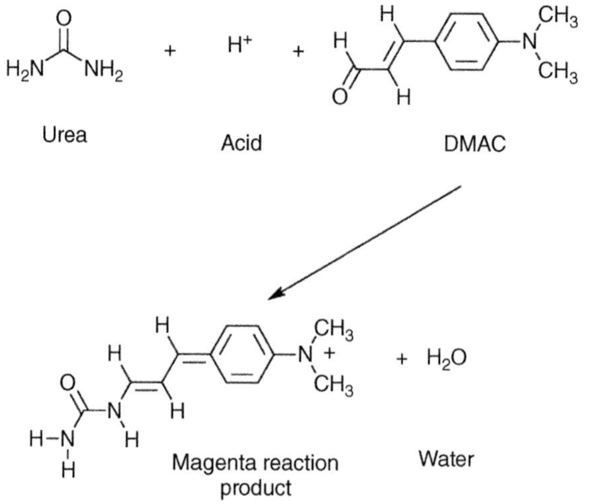

Figure 10.2   Proposed mechanism for formation of coloured product from reaction between DMAC and urea under acid conditions.

10.3.2   Theory

The magenta-coloured fingermarks that were developed by DMAC arise as a result of the formation of a coloured Schiff base through a reaction between DMAC and urea under acidic conditions (Figure 10.2).

10.3.3 The DMAC process

The formulation originally proposed by Morris et al. (1973) for solution dipping was a two-part system made up into a working solution as follows:

Solution A

DMAC	5 g
1,1,2-Trifluorotrichloroethane (CFC113)	650 mL
Absolute ethanol	350 mL

Solution B

5-Sulphosalicylic acid	20 g
1,1,2-Trifluorotrichloroethane (CFC113)	650 mL
Absolute ethanol	350 mL

Working solution

Solution A	500 mL
Solution B	500 mL

In this formulation, the ethanol acts as the principal solvent for DMAC, and the CFC113 was the carrier solvent. The 5-sulphosalicylic acid provides the acidic conditions required for the reaction to form the Schiff base.

For treatment, articles are dipped and marks develop within minutes without application of heat. Spray application is possible, but in this case the surface to be treated is first sprayed with solution A followed by a second spray of solution B.

10.4 Silver nitrate

10.4.1 Outline history of the process

1878: Aubert observed the reactions of silver nitrate with sweat and its potential to reveal traces of fingermarks on paper (Forgeot, 1891).

1969: Cuthbertson utilised silver nitrate to study the chloride composition of latent fingermarks and concluded that the optimum concentration in the formulation is 1% (Cuthbertson, 1969; Godsell, 1969).

1974: Morris and Goode proposed a modified silver nitrate process to overcome both the background darkening and the lack of control over the photochemical development step. This included converting the silver chloride to silver sulphide using thiourea, giving a more stable final product and a complexing agent,

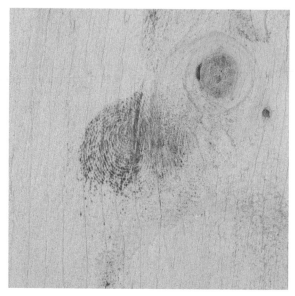

Figure 10.3   A fingermark developed on untreated wood using silver nitrate. Reproduced courtesy of the Home Office.

disodiumethylenediaminetracetic acid (Na$_2$EDTA), to form complexes with unreacted silver so that it could be washed from the surface more easily (Morris and Goode, 1974, 1976).

1998: Price and Stow proposed the use of stopping solutions based on methanol, acetic acid, glycerol and water to slow overdevelopment of the background.

An example of a mark developed on untreated wood using silver nitrate is shown in Figure 10.3.

10.4.2   Theory

The theory behind the silver nitrate process is that the silver nitrate in solution reacts with the chloride constituents of fingermarks to produce insoluble silver chloride:

$$AgNO_{3\ (aq)} + NaCl_{(aq)} \rightarrow AgCl_{(s)} + NaNO_{3\ (aq)}$$

Silver chloride is light sensitive and when exposed to light darkens rapidly as metallic silver is formed:

$$AgCl_{(s)} + h\nu \rightarrow Ag_{(s)} + \frac{1}{2}Cl_{2\ (g)}$$

The treated exhibit is therefore exposed to ultraviolet (or white) light to promote development although the optimum exposure time will vary from surface to surface and is not always easy to establish because both print and background progressively darken with time. In the case of the background, this occurs due to gradual breakdown of unreacted silver nitrate in the porous substrate, and treated articles should be stored in the dark to reduce the speed at which this occurs. Formulations designed to decrease the rate of background darkening or to wash unreacted silver from the surface have been proposed, but none have found widespread use.

10.4.3 The silver nitrate process

The formulation previously recommended for operational use by the UK Home Office was as follows:

Silver nitrate	10 g
Methanol	500 mL

In this simple formulation, methanol acts as the carrier solvent for the active silver nitrate constituent. After carrying the silver nitrate into contact with the chlorides in the mark so that reaction can occur, the methanol rapidly evaporates allowing conversion of silver chloride to silver on exposure to light. The silver nitrate concentration used in this formulation is 2%, chosen to ensure sufficient silver nitrate is present to react with all chlorides in the fingermark. Work by Cuthbertson (1969) showed that below concentrations of 1% there was insufficient reagent to react with the chloride available in the fingermark and above 10% the background colouration began to become excessive.

The article to be treated is immersed in the solution for a maximum of 5 s, or working solution is applied to the surface using a soft brush. The treated article is then allowed to dry in the dark before being exposed to light. The wavelength and power of the radiation used will influence the speed at which development occurs, with the reaction occurring most rapidly when short wavelengths are used. Short-wave ultraviolet (UVC) radiation will therefore produce more rapid development than white light of the same power. Exposure to light should continue until the mark has developed and stopped before the background starts to darken to the extent that contrast with the mark is lost.

References

Brennan J, Bramble S, Crabtree S, Wright G, 'Fuming of Latent Fingerprints Using Dimethylaminocinnamaldehyde', J Forensic Identif, vol 45, (1995), p 373–380.
Cuthbertson F, 'The Chemistry of Fingerprints', AWRE Report No. O 13/69, October 1969.
Forgeot R, 'Étude Medico-Légale des Empreintes peu Visibles ou Invisibles et Révélées par des Procédés Spéciaux', Arch d'Anthrop Crimin (French), vol 6, (1891), p 387–404.

Godsell J W, 'Chemistry of Fingerprints – A Note on the Investigation of the Chloride Content of Fingerprints and the Implications for Police and Fingerprint Technicians', HO PRDB Report No. 14/69, September 1969.

Goode G C, Morris J R, 'Latent Fingerprints: A Review of Their Origin, Composition and Methods for Detection', AWRE Report No. O 22/83, October 1983.

Katzung W, 'New Reagents for the Chemical Development of Latent Fingerprints on Paper and Their Possible Applications', Krim Forensische Wiss, vol 57, 58 (1985), p 82–89.

Kent T, 'Manual of Fingerprint Development Techniques', 1st edition, Home Office, London, 1986.

Morris J R, Goode G C, 'The Detection of Fingerprints by Chemical Techniques. Report for Period April 1972–March 1974', AWRE SSCD Memo 356, 1974.

Morris J R, Goode G C, 'Chemical Aspects of Fingerprint Technology – Report for Period April 1974–March 1976', AWRE SSCD Memo No. 396, June 1976.

Morris J R, Goode G C, Godsell J W, 'Some New Developments in the Chemical Development of Latent Fingerprints', Police Res Bull, vol 21, (1973), p 31–36.

Price D, Stow K, 'A Method for Stopping Over-development of Silver Nitrate Treated Finger and Footwear Marks', Fingerprint Whorld, vol 24(93), (1998), p 107–110.

Ramotowski R, 'Fluorescence Visualisation of Latent Fingerprints on Paper Using p-Dimethyl-aminocinnamaldehyde (PDMAC)', Proceedings of the International Symposium on Fingerprint Detection and Identification, Ne'urim, Israel, June 1995, p 91–94.

Sasson Y, Almog J, 'Chemical Reagents for the Development of Latent Fingerprints 1: Scope and Limitations of the Reagent 4-Dimethylaminocinnamaldehyde', J Forensic Sci, vol 23(4), (1978), p 852–855.

Van Enckevort H J, 'The Detection and Visualisation of Latent Fingerprints: A Review', Report No. CD 2380, Chemistry Division, Department of Scientific and Industrial Research, New Zealand, 1987.

Vincent S E, 'Finger-print Detection on Cloth', Final year Project report, Department of Chemical Physics, University of Surrey, June 1973.

Further reading

Godsell J W, Vincent P G, 'Comparative Study of Radio-Active Sulphur Dioxide, Ninhydrin and Silver Nitrate from the Point of View of Their Efficiency for Developing Latent Fingerprints on Paper', HO PSDB Tech. Memo. 1/73, 1973.

Godsell J W, Vincent P G, Lloyd D W, 'Influence of Storage of Latent Fingerprints in an Atmosphere of a Given Humidity on the Choice of the Optimum Developing Agent', HO PSDB Tech. Memo. 3/72, 1972.

Green W D, 'Modified Chemical and Physical Methods for the Detection of Latent Fingerprints', Criminologist, vol 5(16/17), (1970), p 54–62.

Kerr F M, 'A Useful Alternative to Aqueous Silver Nitrate for Fingerprinting', RCMP Gazette, vol 41(6), (1979), p 8–10.

Kirby F J, Olsen R D Sr, 'Modified Silver Nitrate Formula for Intensifying Faint Ninhydrin Prints', Forensic Photogr, vol 2(5), (1973), p 15–19.

Olsen R D Sr, 'Scott's Fingerprint Mechanics', Charles C Thomas, Springfield, 1978, ISBN 0-398-06308-7.

O'Neill M E, 'Development of Latent Finger-Prints on Paper', J Criminal Law Criminol, vol 28(3), (1937), p 432–441.

11

Lipid reagents

Stephen M. Bleay

Home Office Centre for Applied Science and Technology, Sandridge, UK

Key points

- Lipid reagents can be used to target both the sebaceous constituents of fingermarks and certain greasy contaminants that may also be present.

- They are generally less effective than other chemical processes because the constituents that they target are usually less abundant than eccrine constituents in natural marks.

- The constituents targeted by these reagents are mostly water insoluble and therefore these processes can be used on surfaces that have been wetted.

- Most lipid reagents are potentially damaging to the surfaces that they are applied to, and hence they are used towards the end of processing sequences.

11.1   Introduction

There are several fingermark enhancement processes that rely on the interactions between the reagent and the sebaceous constituents of fingermarks. In general there are few lipids and other sebaceous constituents present in naturally deposited marks, and therefore these processes tend to be less effective overall than those that target eccrine constituents. As a consequence, lipid reagents are rarely used as primary fingermark enhancement techniques unless there are strong indications that the marks may contain greasy contaminants. They can be effective when used in sequence after other techniques because they target constituents that are generally unaffected by prior application of reagents for eccrine constituents.

Fingerprint Development Techniques: Theory and Application, First Edition.
Stephen M. Bleay, Ruth S. Croxton and Marcel de Puit.
© 2018 John Wiley & Sons Ltd. Published 2018 by John Wiley & Sons Ltd.

Many of the techniques that target lipids utilise the migration of dye molecules or fluorescent species into a lipid-rich fingermark from the liquid or gas phase. The exceptions to this are ruthenium and osmium tetroxide, which undergo chemical reactions with lipids to form coloured reaction products, and europium chelate and rubeanic acid–copper acetate, which form chelates with the fatty acids present.

The first of the sebaceous reagents to be utilised was iodine fuming (described in Chapter 7), first used in the 19th century for fingermark enhancement on porous surfaces (Quinche and Margot, 2010). The reactions between osmium tetroxide and ruthenium tetroxide (RTX) and fingermarks were also observed in the early part of the 20th century (Mitchell, 1920). As synthetic dyes began to be produced on an industrial scale, they were investigated for a range of alternative applications including biological staining of tissue. It is from these applications that several of the current sebaceous reagents (Solvent Black 3, Basic Violet 3 and Oil Red O) have originated.

Sebaceous reagents have been adapted for use on the full range of surfaces encountered operationally. Solvent Black 3 is recommended for non-porous surfaces, Basic Violet 3 for adhesive surfaces and non-porous surfaces and Oil Red O for porous surfaces. Several of the techniques (iodine, Oil Red O and europium chelate) are known to work less well on older fingermarks (Figure 11.1), and it is possible that the constituents that are targeted by these techniques degrade relatively rapidly with time.

The constituents of sebaceous sweat and many greasy contaminants are water insoluble, and as a consequence, one important application of the lipid reagents is on surfaces that have been wetted.

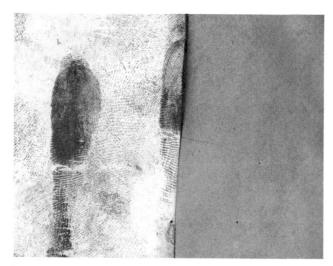

Figure 11.1   Palm and fingermarks approximately 1 year old, left-hand side treated with physical developer and right-hand side treated with Oil Red O. Reproduced courtesy of the Home Office.

11.2   Current operational use

The three lipid reagents that find most widespread operational use are Solvent Black 3, Basic Violet 3 and Oil Red O, although they are used much less frequently than other processes such as amino acid reagents and cyanoacrylate fuming.

Solvent Black 3 is recommended for use on surfaces contaminated with oils and foodstuffs (Cadd et al., 2013; Garrett and Bleay, 2013; Gaskell et al., 2013a, 2013b), but this scenario is rarely encountered. The process can be used in a laboratory and at a crime scene, although it does create significant amounts of mess when used at scenes and subsequent scene clean-up may be an issue.

Basic Violet 3 is used worldwide for the development of fingermarks on adhesive surfaces (Haylock, 1979; Kent, 1980; Arima, 1981). It is not the most effective process in this application, powder suspensions and cyanoacrylate fuming both being capable of enhancing more marks, but it will consistently develop additional marks if used sequentially after both of these processes.

Basic Violet 3 can be used as the final stage of a sequential treatment for non-porous surfaces, where it can develop a small but significant number of additional marks. It can also be used on non-porous surfaces contaminated with grease or foodstuffs (Gaskell et al., 2013a, 2013b), but Solvent Black 3 is generally more effective in this application.

Oil Red O is beginning to be recommended as an alternative treatment to physical developer for fingermarks on wetted paper articles (Beaudoin, 2004; Rawji and Beaudoin, 2006) and in some countries is displacing it from use. It can potentially be used in sequences for wetted porous surfaces before physical developer because the two techniques target slightly different fingermark constituents (Guigui and Beaudoin, 2007; Salama et al., 2008). However, Oil Red O is usually less effective on older fingermarks and ideally should be used in combination with physical developer instead of replacing it. Nile Red has recently emerged as a fluorescent alternative to Oil Red O for the same range of applications (Braasch et al., 2013; Frick et al., 2014).

Some other lipid reagents also have niche applications that mean they find occasional operational use. Iodine solution (Haque et al., 1983) has been used as a treatment for porous wall surfaces at crime scenes (Pounds, 1989). The advantages of iodine solution are that it develops marks more rapidly than ninhydrin, and at scenes this is sometimes considered more important than developing more marks with a more sensitive reagent. Iodine solution is not in widespread use because it is less effective than other treatments, particularly on older marks. The flammability issues associated with the solvents also give cause for concern, although less flammable formulations have been evaluated and found effective in laboratory studies (Flynn et al., 2004; Tsala, 2014).

There is also a need for reagents that can enhance grease-contaminated marks on dark surfaces, where the dark products produced by Solvent Black 3 and Basic Violet 3 would be difficult to see. In these situations, europium chelate (Wilkinson, 1999) and Natural Yellow 3 (Gaskell et al., 2013a, 2013b; Perry and Sears, 2015) processes may offer a solution because the fluorescent reaction products they produce would be far easier to visualise.

RTX is used in some countries for a variety of applications (Mashiko and Miyamoto, 1998), including development of marks on adhesive tapes. It is also proposed as a technique for developing marks on live skin. The main barriers to wider implementation are the fact that the limited comparative studies that have been carried out do not show significant performance advantages for RTX, and there remain doubts about its safety (Blackledge, 1998; Mashiko, 1999). At best the toxicity of the substance has not been fully evaluated. Until this has been satisfactorily resolved, operational use may remain limited. The closely related osmium tetroxide process is no longer widely used because of the highly toxic nature of the substance.

11.3   Solvent Black 3 (Sudan Black)

11.3.1   Outline history of the process

1930s: Solvent Black 3 was first synthesised.

1935: Gérard proposed Solvent Black 3 as a biological stain for staining fats in animal tissues.

1980: Mitsui et al. reported the use of Solvent Black 3 dissolved in a mixture of ethylene glycol, ethanol and water as a method for enhancing fingermarks on wetted paper.

1981: Stone and Metzger compared Solvent Black 3 with black magnetic powders on wetted paper and concluded it to be inferior.

1982: Pounds et al. conducted a comparison of biological stains and proposed Solvent Black 3 for enhancement of fingermarks on non-porous surfaces.

1986: Pounds and Strachan conducted operational trials and concluded Solvent Black 3 to be inferior to small particle reagent and vacuum metal deposition for latent marks on non-porous surfaces.

1986: Solvent Black 3 was included in the Home Office Manual of Fingerprint Development Techniques as a process for enhancing grease-contaminated marks (Kent, 1986).

2005: Hart proposed a revised Solvent Black 3 formulation based on 1-methoxy-2-propanol with reduced flammability for application at crime scenes (Home Office, 2005).

2012: Cadd and Garrett conducted comprehensive studies of the ethanol and 1-methoxy-2-propanol-based formulations to establish their relative effectiveness and interactions with different contaminants (Cadd et al., 2013; Garrett and Bleay, 2013).

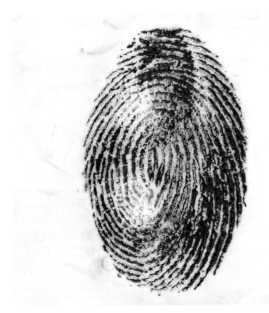

Figure 11.2 Mark contaminated with butter on a clean ceramic tile enhanced using Solvent Black 3.

Figure 11.2 shows a mark contaminated with butter enhanced using Solvent Black 3.

11.3.2 Theory

Solvent Black 3 is one of a class of compounds described as lysochromes, which are soluble dyes that are used for the staining of lipid materials including triglycerides and fatty acids that may be present in fingermarks. Most lysochromes are azo dyes that because of their structure have undergone molecular rearrangement, making them incapable of ionising. The structure of Solvent Black 3 is illustrated in Figure 11.3.

Lysochromes are mostly insoluble in strongly polar solvents, such as water, and somewhat more so in less polar solvents, such as ethanol. They are much more soluble in the non-polar triglyceride and fatty acid constituents of fingermarks. When Solvent Black 3 is used as a fingermark enhancement reagent, the dye is dissolved into solvents in which they have limited solubility. When the dye molecules in solution come into contact with the fingermark, the dye preferentially transfers into the lipidic constituents, often colouring them more strongly than the original solvent.

In addition to the primary staining action of Solvent Black 3 by dissolving into lipids, it can also stain materials ionically. This may result in some staining of

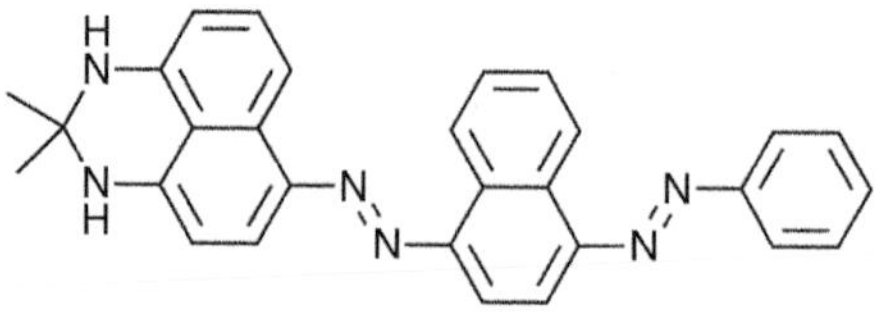

Figure 11.3   Structure of Solvent Black 3.

non-lipid materials in addition to strong colouration of the fingermark, which may give rise to background staining.

The staining of fingermarks by Solvent Black 3 is illustrated schematically in Figure 11.4.

For marks that are dominated by contaminants, the dyeing may be uniform across the entire ridge. For natural marks containing a more complex emulsion of constituents, dyeing may be specific to particular constituents, and on a microscopic scale dyeing may be inhomogeneous (Figure 11.5).

11.3.3   The Solvent Black 3 process

The process is a relatively simple one, utilising a single working solution. The original formulation based on ethanol (Kent, 1986) is:

Solvent Black 3	15 g
Ethanol	1 L
Distilled water	500 mL

The more recent reduced flammability formulation (Home Office, 2005) is:

Solvent Black 3	10 g
1-Methoxy-2-propanol	500 mL
Distilled water	500 mL

The roles of the constituents in these formulations are summarised in the following table:

Solvent Black 3	The role of Solvent Black 3 is to act as the dye for the fingermark. The concentration used is such that the limit of solubility in the ethanol/water solvent is almost exceeded, and some precipitation of Solvent Black 3 is occurring. These precipitating particles may also preferentially settle on fingermark ridges in addition to the dyeing action of Solvent Black 3 dissolving into the lipids.
Ethanol	The role of ethanol is to act as the initial solvent for Solvent Black 3, and the quantity used is capable of dissolving the quantity of dye outlined in the previous formulation.

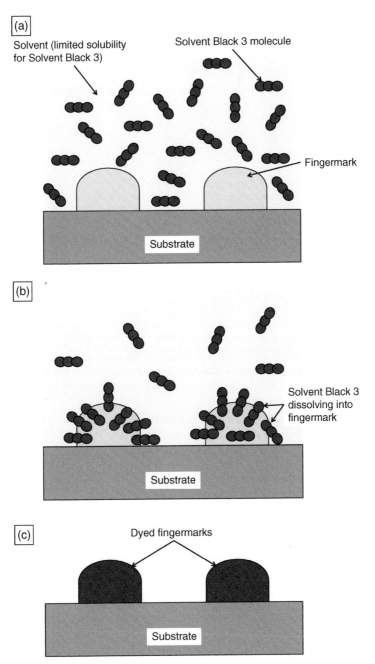

Figure 11.4 Schematic illustration of the Solvent Black 3 process. (a) Solvent Black 3 molecules in solvent with limited solubility, (b) lipophilic component of Solvent Black 3 molecule preferentially dissolving into lipids in fingermark ridges and (c) fingermark after drying, leaving dyed ridges.

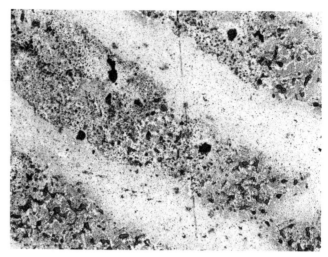

Figure 11.5 Optical micrograph of a natural (ungroomed) fingermark ridge dyed with Solvent Black 3, showing inhomogeneous staining of fingermark constituents. Reproduced courtesy of the Home Office.

Water	Solvent Black 3 is insoluble in water, and the addition of water reduces the solubility of the dye to the point where precipitation is beginning to occur and it becomes preferable for the dye to dissolve into the lipid constituents of the fingermark.
1-Methoxy-2-propanol	In the recent reformulation of Solvent Black 3, 1-methoxy-2-propanol fulfils the same role as ethanol whilst having a reduced flammability.

Articles are treated by dipping into the solution, or are drawn across the surface, and then rinsed with water. Staining takes place in seconds, although the surface may also absorb the dye, and the staining time should be adjusted to minimise the possibility of background staining obscuring the developed mark. The reagent can be applied to large articles or at scenes from a water wash bottle, washing the excess from the surface with copious amounts of water.

Marks enhanced using Solvent Black 3 are initially a deep blue-black colour but may fade and turn brown over time as they become oxidised to form polyazo derivatives.

11.4   Basic Violet 3 (Gentian Violet, Crystal Violet)

11.4.1   Outline history of the process

1860s: Basic Violet 3 was first synthesised as a one of a series of aniline dyes produced after the discovery of 'Mauve' in 1856.

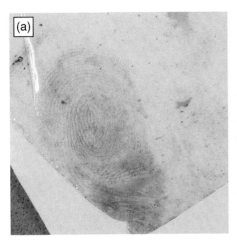 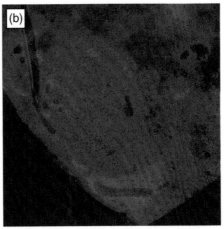

Figure 11.6   A mark on adhesive tape developed by Basic Violet 3, (a) viewed under white light and (b) using fluorescence examination.

1884: Gram utilised Basic Violet 3 as an integral part of the Gram stain for staining the cell walls of bacteria. It was subsequently adopted in a variety of microbiological staining applications.

Late 1960s: Basic Violet 3 was first used by the Italian police for enhancing marks on adhesive surfaces, primarily targeting epithelial cells pulled from the fingertip by the adhesive.

1979: Haylock published details of a phenol-based Basic Violet 3 formulation used in the United Kingdom during the 1970s.

1980: Kent published the transfer process for lifting marks enhanced using Basic Violet 3 from the adhesive surface of dark-coloured tapes using photographic paper.

1990: Hardwick et al. reported that marks enhanced using Basic Violet 3 are also fluorescent and can be excited by light in the green/yellow region of the spectrum.

2006: Hart published an alternative formulation of Basic Violet 3 using dioctyl sulfosuccinate sodium salt (DOSS) in place of phenol, giving reduced background staining on adhesive surfaces (Home Office, 2006).

Basic Violet 3 produces visible marks that are also fluorescent, examples being illustrated in Figure 11.6.

11.4.2   Theory

The exact mechanism by which Basic Violet 3 selectively dyes the lipid constituents of fingermarks is not known, nor has it been determined conclusively, which

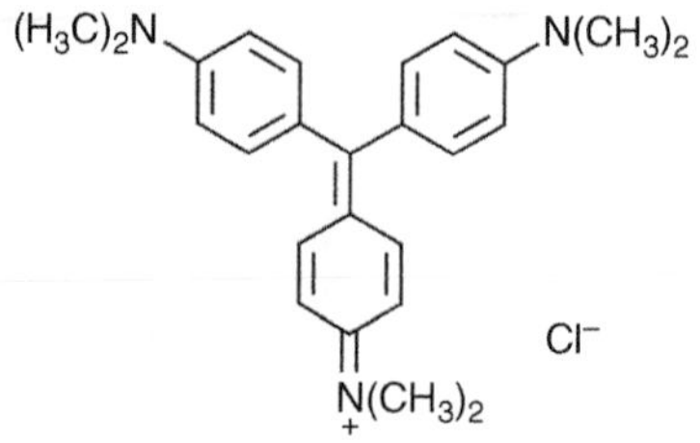

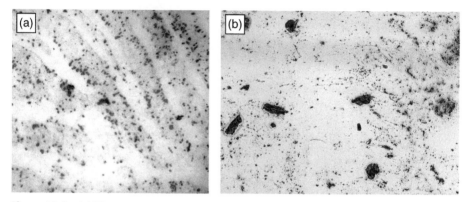

Figure 11.7   The Basic Violet 3 molecule.

Figure 11.8   (a) Photograph of adhesive side of tape sample treated with Basic Violet 3, show-ing violet staining of lipids in ridges and of epithelial cells in particular, and (b) higher magni-fication image of a mark on a glass microscope slide showing stained skin cells. Reproduced courtesy of the Home Office.

individual constituents are targeted by the dye. Gurr (1965) proposed that the basic groups of neutral dyes such as Basic Violet 3 could form a chemical union with the acidic group of the lipids being stained. The phenol and DOSS components of the two formulations described later also play a role in the staining process, making the actual mechanism complex to determine. Preferential solubility of the dye in the lipids, as described for Solvent Black 3, may also occur.

The Basic Violet 3 molecule is shown in Figure 11.7.

Lipids are not the only constituent of fingermarks that are stained by Basic Violet 3, which can also stain any skin cells shed from the fingertip. This is because basic dyes such as Basic Violet 3 are positively charged and are attracted to epithelial cells (which have a net negative charge), with the result that they may become strongly stained (Figure 11.8).

Fingermark development using Basic Violet 3 is essentially very similar in nature to that shown schematically for Solvent Black 3 in Figure 11.4, with the Basic Violet 3 molecules migrating to and dissolving into and/or binding with constituents in the fingermark.

The Basic Violet 3 molecule is fluorescent, but on non-porous surfaces, marks developed using Basic Violet 3 rarely exhibit fluorescence. Marks on adhesive tapes tend to exhibit much greater fluorescence, and weak marks that are very faint or not visible when examined under white light may be significantly enhanced by fluorescence examination. The stronger fluorescence observed on adhesive surfaces is attributed to the fact that binding occurs between the dye molecule and the adhesive, making it more rigid and creating more preferential conditions for fluorescence to occur (Taylor, 1975). The fact that weaker marks are more greatly enhanced during fluorescence examination than strongly developed, visible marks is attributed to 'self-quenching', that is, the reabsorption of the emitted fluorescence by the heavier dye deposits, whereas for more weakly coloured marks, the fluorescence is not reabsorbed and the marks are more readily detected.

11.4.3   The Basic Violet 3 process

Two formulations are in general use: one based on phenol (Bandey, 2014) and the other based on DOSS (Home Office, 2006).

The phenol-based formulation is produced by first mixing a stock solution:

Basic Violet 3	5 g
Phenol	10 g
96% ethanol	50 mL

A working solution is produced by measuring 1 mL of stock solution and progressively adding distilled water until the gold film formed on the surface of the solution disappears.

The role of each component in the formulation is outlined as follows:

Basic Violet 3	The role of the Basic Violet 3 in the formulation is to selectively stain the fingermarks. The quantity used is sufficient to produce a supersaturated solution of Basic Violet 3, thus promoting the transfer of the dye into the lipids in the fingerprint.
Phenol	The role of phenol in the formulation is not fully understood. The presence of phenol has been found to promote the staining ability of the Basic Violet 3 dye and appears to make it more specific to fingermark constituents. It is thought more likely that phenol acts by affecting the solution properties, either making it supersaturated or by changing its surface tension and increasing staining.
Ethanol	The ethanol component of the formulation provides a common solvent for both phenol and Basic Violet 3.
Water	Basic Violet 3 is insoluble in water, and the addition of water reduces the solubility of the dye to the point where precipitation is beginning to occur.

Development of fingermarks occurs by drawing the article to be treated across the surface of the Basic Violet 3 working solution and then rinsing the surface with water.

The DOSS formulation of Basic Violet 3 is produced by first producing a Basic Violet 3 stock solution:

Basic Violet 3	5 g
Absolute ethanol	50 mL

A separate 1% (w/v) DOSS solution is then produced by dissolving DOSS in distilled water, stirring for at least 12 h to allow the DOSS to dissolve.

A working solution is produced as follows:

Basic Violet 3 stock solution	1 mL
DOSS solution	25 mL

Similarly to phenol, the role of DOSS in the formulation is not fully understood. DOSS is an unusual detergent being preferentially soluble in non-polar solvents and forming reverse micelles. One theory is that Basic Violet 3 molecules could become contained within the reverse micelles, which are in turn preferentially soluble in the fingermark lipids compared with the polar water/ethanol solution and carry the Basic Violet 3 molecules into the fingermark.

The principal advantage of the DOSS-based formulation is that it is considerably less likely to cause background staining on adhesive surfaces that utilise acrylic-based adhesives than the phenol-based formulation. This issue does not occur for surfaces with rubber-based adhesives and difference in the performance of the two formulations on adhesive tapes with acrylic-based adhesives is illustrated in Figure 11.9.

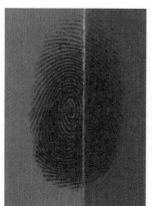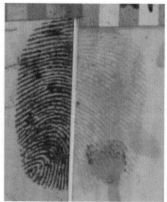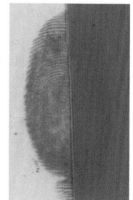

Figure 11.9 Photographs of different adhesive tapes, showing difference in fingermark enhancement between phenol (right-hand side) and DOSS-based (left-hand side) Basic Violet 3 formulations. Reproduced courtesy of the Home Office.

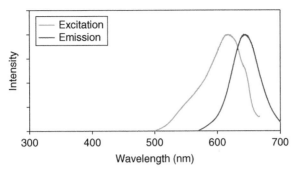

Figure 11.10 Measured excitation and emission spectra for Basic Violet 3.

Marks enhanced using Basic Violet 3 are a characteristic violet in colour, although the intensity of staining can vary significantly and some weakly stained marks may not be readily visible to the unaided eye. Basic Violet 3 is also fluorescent and additional marks can be found by fluorescence examination. It has a broad range of excitation wavelengths with a maximum at approximately 615 nm and emission in the red and infrared regions of the spectrum with a maximum at approximately 640 nm (Figure 11.10).

Fluorescence examination is conducted using excitation wavelengths in the green-yellow or yellow regions of the spectrum in conjunction with a red viewing filter such as the Schott glass RG610.

11.5 Oil Red O (Solvent Red 27)

11.5.1 Outline history of the process

1926: Oil Red O was reported as a stain for fatty constituents in biological samples (French, 1926).

2002: Castello et al. studied Oil Red O as a forensic method for enhancing lip prints.

2004: Beaudoin proposed Oil Red O as a novel method for enhancing fingermarks on wetted surfaces.

2007: Guigui and Beaudoin investigated the sequential use of Oil Red O with physical developer.

2012: Frick et al. issued a simplified formulation for Oil Red O, with more rapid processing times at the expense of some loss in effectiveness.

An example of a mark on a white paper surface developed using Oil Red O is shown in Figure 11.11.

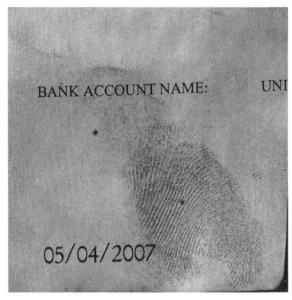

Figure 11.11   A fingermark developed on paper using Oil Red O. Reproduced courtesy of the
Home Office.

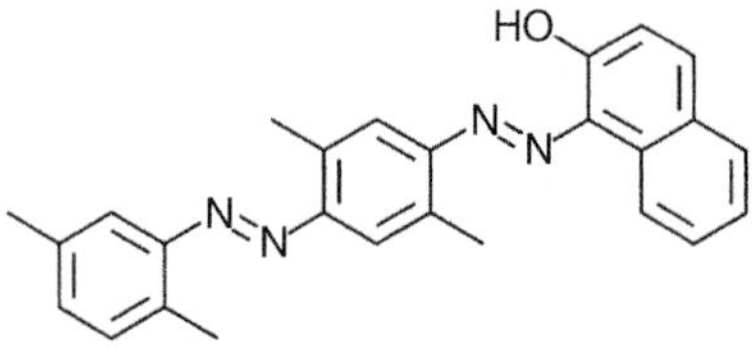

Figure 11.12   Structure of Oil Red O (Solvent Red 27).

11.5.2 Theory

Similarly to Solvent Black 3, Oil Red O (colour index name Solvent Red 27) is a
lysochrome, and the theory of lipid staining using Oil Red O is the same as that
outlined for Solvent Black 3 in the previous section. The principal difference
between the two formulations described in this chapter is that Solvent Black 3 has
been formulated for developing fingermarks on non-porous surfaces, whereas Oil
Red O is formulated for use on porous surfaces.

   Oil Red O is more strongly hydrophobic than some earlier dyes used for staining
lipids, and it is thought that this makes it more effective in staining applications
(Horobin, 1981). The structure of Oil Red O is shown in Figure 11.12.

11.5.3   The Oil Red O process

The Oil Red O formulation first proposed by Beaudoin in 2004 consists of three separate immersion stages: a staining solution, a buffer solution and a water wash.

Stain solution

Solution A	
Oil Red O	1.54 g
Methanol	770 mL
Solution B	
Sodium hydroxide	9.2 g
Water	230 mL

The staining solution is produced by adding solution A to solution B, mixing and filtering before use.

Buffer solution

Sodium carbonate	26.5 g
Water	2 L
Concentrated nitric acid	18.5 mL
Make to 2.5 L with water	

In the staining solution, the Oil Red O is the active dye component and methanol the principal solvent. Sodium hydroxide creates a basic environment that facilitates the staining process. The water constituent reduces the solubility of Oil Red O in the water/methanol mixture and makes its migration into the lipid components of the fingermark preferable.

The purpose of the buffer solution is to neutralise the base side of the staining solution and stabilise the developed marks.

Articles to be treated are immersed in the stain bath for up to 90 min until the fingermarks become strongly coloured, then removed, drained and placed in the buffer solution. Finally the articles are rinsed in distilled water and allowed to dry.

Marks enhanced using Oil Red O are a deep pink/red and are readily visible.

11.6   Iodine solution

11.6.1   Outline history of the process

1862: Coulier noted that traces of fingermarks can be enhanced on paper by iodine vapour (Quinche and Margot, 2010).

1983: Haque et al. published a method for applying iodine in a solution based on cyclohexane in combination with α-naphthoflavone fixative.

1989: Pounds reported the operational use of a two-part iodine formulation based on iodine dissolved in non-flammable 1,1,2-trichlorotrifluoroethane, with the α-naphthoflavone fixative dissolved in dichloromethane applied as a separate solution.

2004: Following the banning of the use of CFCs under the Montreal protocol, Flynn et al. proposed an alternative non-flammable iodine formulation based on HFC-4310mee.

11.6.2 Theory

The theory associated with visualisation of fingermarks by iodine solution is essentially the same as that for iodine fuming, except the means of delivering the iodine into the mark is different. In iodine solution the iodine is dissolved into a solvent and is bound into the fingermark by the same reactions that occur for iodine fuming. As the solvent evaporates, the iodine is fixed by the α-naphthoflavone that is also present in the solution.

11.6.3 The iodine solution process

A flammable iodine solution formulation developed for use in comparative work by the UK Home Office (Sears, 1999) is given as follows. It consists of two solutions that are mixed together immediately before use:

Solution A

Iodine	0.4 g
Heptane	194 mL

Solution B

α-Naphthoflavone	0.6 g
Dichloromethane	6 mL

In this formulation, the heptane is the principal solvent for the iodine and evaporates rapidly from the surface, allowing the interaction between iodine and the fingermark to occur. Dichloromethane acts as the solvent for the α-naphthoflavone fixative, which functions as outlined in the theory section for the iodine fuming process (Section 7.5.2).

Immediately prior to application, solutions A and B are mixed together and stirred well. Precipitation of the α-naphthoflavone begins almost immediately, so the solution is filtered through fast-run filter paper before being applied to the surface with a soft brush.

The reduced flammability iodine solution formulation described by Flynn et al. (2004) also utilises two solutions:

Solution A

Iodine	0.1 g
Methanol	10 mL
HFC4310mee	90 mL

Solution B

α-Naphthoflavone	1.2 g
Dichloromethane	10 mL

The working solution is produced by mixing 2 mL of solution B with 100 mL of solution A, allowing the mixture to stand for 5 min prior to filtration and then use.

Marks enhanced using iodine solution would normally be brown in colour, but because the solution contains α-naphthoflavone fixative, they are almost instantaneously converted to a dark blue product. Even with fixing, marks may fade and ultimately disappear with time as the reaction product breaks down and iodine resublimes from the mark.

11.7 Ruthenium tetroxide

11.7.1 Outline history of the process

1920s: RTX was first reported as a fingermark enhancement process using ruthenium crystals heated in a water bath at temperatures not exceeding 50°C. This process was dangerous to use because explosions could occur if heating was too rapid or the temperature exceeded 50°C (Olsen, 1975).

1991: Mashiko et al. proposed a safer chemical method for generating RTX vapours.

1998: Mashiko and Miyamoto introduced a RTX solution using tetradecafluorohexane solvent that can be applied by spraying onto surfaces.

2005: Mashiko published an alternative, safer formulation of RTX solution designed for spray application.

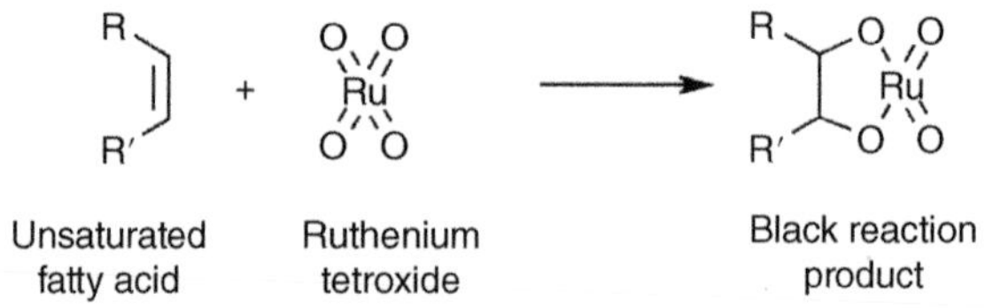

Figure 11.13 Reduction of ruthenium tetroxide by reaction with unsaturated fatty acids.

RTX is used in a variety of applications and is capable of enhancing marks on both porous and non-porous surfaces. However, there has been ongoing debate about the safety of the process because the toxicity of RTX remains at best undetermined (Blackledge, 1998; Mashiko, 1999). This has probably limited the wider uptake of the process.

11.7.2 Theory

RTX (and the closely related process osmium tetroxide) develops fingermarks by reacting across the carbon double bonds present in the unsaturated fatty acid constituents. The reaction product is a black hydrous oxide bound to the lipid constituents of the fingermark that that allows it to be visualised (Figure 11.13).

The same reaction will occur whether RTX is applied by fuming or in solution.

11.7.3 The ruthenium tetroxide process

A formulation published by Flynn et al. (2004) and utilised in comparative trials consists of:

1% aqueous ruthenium chloride solution	25 mL
5% ceric ammonium nitrate solution	25 mL
Carrier solvent (HFC4310mee or HFE7100)	125 mL

The three liquids are mixed in a separating funnel for 10 min. This produces two layers, a black (aqueous) upper layer and a yellow (organic) bottom layer. The yellow layer is collected and dried over anhydrous sodium sulphate for 24 h prior to use as a spray reagent. The solution is stored in the dark to increase its shelf life.

Marks enhanced using RTX are dark grey.

11.8 Osmium tetroxide

11.8.1 Outline history of the process

Late 1800s: Osmium tetroxide was first proposed for fingermark enhancement (Forgeot, 1891).

1920: Mitchell described two application processes for osmium tetroxide: 'osmic acid', a 1% aqueous solution of osmium tetroxide applied by brush to porous surfaces, and osmium tetroxide fuming, using the vapours generated by a boiling 1% aqueous solution.

1978: Olsen outlined an alternative fuming method, adding ethyl ether or carbon tetrachloride to osmium tetroxide crystals in a small, shallow glass dish within a fuming cabinet.

1978: Kerr proposed a revised, safer formulation using pre-prepared ampoules of osmium tetroxide within a fuming cabinet and pre-treatment with vapours of a sensitising chemical (5-norbornene-2-carbonyl chloride) to produce additional linkages for the osmium tetroxide to react with.

The known toxicity of osmium tetroxide has meant that it is no longer in operational use, and comparative studies in the 1980s indicated that it was less effective than alternative processes then available.

11.8.2 Theory

The theory associated with the osmium tetroxide is identical to that described for RTX and illustrated in Figure 11.13 (Olsen, 1975).

11.8.3 The osmium tetroxide process

A comparative study between osmium tetroxide, radioactive sulphur dioxide and vacuum metal deposition was conducted on fingermarks deposited on a range of fabrics (Albinson, 1984). In this study, osmium tetroxide was used as a fuming reagent and in solution. When used as a fuming process, fabrics were contained in a sealed enclosure similar to that illustrated in the section on iodine fuming and exposed to fumes from 0.1 mg of osmium tetroxide for 14 days. A further experiment utilised 0.2 mg of osmium tetroxide and an exposure time of 24 days.

The osmium tetroxide solution was 1.4 wt% in water, and articles were immersed until the fabric was fully wetted and then allowed to dry at ambient temperature.

The fuming process was found superior to solution dipping, but both processes were inferior to other methods being investigated at the time.

Marks enhanced using osmium tetroxide are dark grey to black.

11.9   Europium chelate

11.9.1   Outline history of the process

1990: Menzel and Mitchell first suggested europium salts as complexing agents for the post-treatment of marks developed using ninhydrin, utilising the large Stokes shift of the fluorescence to minimise background fluorescence.

1993: Europium chelates were suggested as dyes for marks developed using cyanoacrylate fuming, the dyes being dissolved in methyl ethyl ketone or petroleum ether (Misner et al., 1993; Wilkinson and Watkin, 1993).

1997: Allred et al. published the first europium chelate formulation designed to directly enhance fingermarks.

1999: Wilkinson published a simpler one-step europium chelate formulation that developed bright fluorescent marks on both porous and non-porous items.

Europium chelate has not found widespread use because the effectiveness of the process falls off rapidly as fingermarks age, and results observed in laboratory trials were not replicated when the technique was applied to casework. Marks developed using the process are colourless but fluoresce deep red when illuminated with ultraviolet light (Figure 11.14).

11.9.2   Theory

The theory associated with the europium chelate reagent relies on the transfer of europium complexes from the working solution into the lipids present in the fingermark. Wilkinson (1999) suggested that the methanol component of the working solution plays a part in this transfer process because it partially dissolves in the lipid constituents. The europium complex formed in the working solution is water insoluble and prefers the hydrophobic environment of the lipids; therefore some of the complex is transferred with the methanol. Once in the lipid environment, there is displacement of the water molecules attached to the europium complex followed by replacement by various lipid-based ligands to produce a biological fluorophore (Figure 11.15).

The bulky fluorophore structure protects the europium from the aqueous environment of the biological medium (in this case the water present in the fingermark residue).

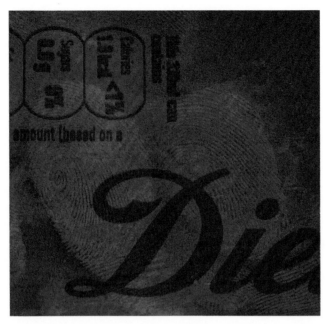

Figure 11.14   Marks developed using europium chelate on a drinks can, viewed using fluorescence examination. Reproduced courtesy of the Home Office.

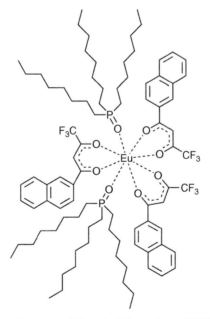

Figure 11.15   Structure of biological fluorophore (Wilkinson, 1999).

11.9.3 The europium chelate process

The formula proposed by Wilkinson (1999) is a two-part system and is made as follows:

Solution A

Europium chloride hexahydrate	23 mg
Distilled water	300 mL
Tergitol 7 (nonylphenol ethoxylate)	2 mL

Solution B

Thenoyltrifluoroacetone	42 mg
Trioctylphosphine oxide	50 mg
Methanol	700 mL

The two solutions are then mixed together for 30 min to produce a working solution.

In this formulation, europium chloride provides the europium ions that form the basis of the fluorescent complex. Thenoyltrifluoroacetone and trioctylphosphine oxide provide molecules that contribute to the formation of the fluorescent complex, and the Tergitol 7 detergent is added to further isolate the europium ion from the water molecules and stabilise the complex. As described in the theory section, methanol may aid the transfer process of the europium complex from solution into the fingermark as it partially dissolves in the lipid constituents.

Gaskell et al. (2013a, 2013b) replaced Tergitol 7 with DOSS and methanol with ethanol in the formulation, without apparent detriment to performance.

The articles to be treated are immersed in the working solution for 5 s, then washed in water and allowed to dry. The developed marks do not have a visible colour, but are fluorescent. Europium and other lanthanide series elements can form fluorescent complexes with extremely large shifts between excitation and emission wavelengths. In the case of europium chelate, there are an excitation maximum at approximately 335 nm and an emission maximum at approximately 615 nm (Figure 11.16). Such large Stokes shifts can be beneficial in reducing background fluorescence that may otherwise obscure fluorescent fingermarks.

Fluorescence examination of marks developed using europium chelate involves excitation with long-wave ultraviolet radiation, with the red fluorescence viewed through a red filter such as the Schott glass RG610.

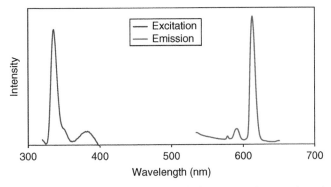

Figure 11.16   Measured excitation and emission spectra for europium chelate.

11.10   Natural Yellow 3 (curcumin)

11.10.1   Outline history of the process

1989: Stockert et al. reported the use of curcumin as a fluorescent stain for tissue sections.

2011: Garg et al. described how the natural spice turmeric (which contains curcumin as its principal active ingredient) can be used to develop fingermarks by a powdering process.

2013: Gaskell et al. proposed the use of Natural Yellow 3 (curcumin) in solution form for enhancing grease-contaminated marks on dark non-porous surfaces.

2015: Perry and Sears proposed a revised formulation of Natural Yellow 3 with reduced background staining.

An example of a grease-contaminated mark developed on a dark surface using Natural Yellow 3 is shown in Figure 11.17.

11.10.2   Theory

Natural Yellow 3 stains fingermarks by a similar mechanism to Solvent Black 3 and Oil Red O. The curcumin molecule (Figure 11.18) has very limited solubility in water but is highly soluble in fats. It therefore preferentially migrates into the fatty constituents of fingermarks from the staining solution.

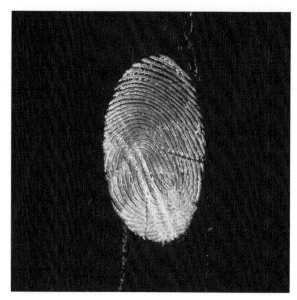

Figure 11.17 A fingermark contaminated with butter on a dark ceramic tile enhanced with Natural Yellow 3. Reproduced courtesy of the Home Office.

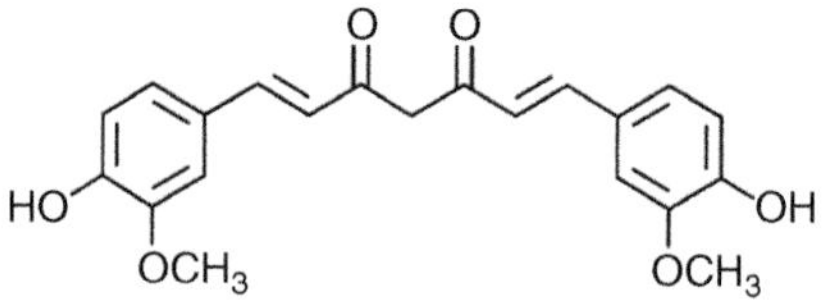

Figure 11.18 The chemical structure of Natural Yellow 3.

11.10.3 The Natural Yellow 3 process

The formulation published by Gaskell et al. (2013a, 2013b) was adapted from the ethanol-based formulation for Solvent Black 3 described earlier, but because the solubility of Natural Yellow 3 in water is lower, the dye content was reduced. Otherwise, the roles of the constituents in the formulation were the same as those described for Solvent Black 3:

Natural Yellow 3	0.9 g
Ethanol	100 mL
Distilled water	50 mL

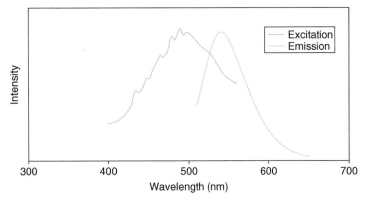

Figure 11.19   Measured excitation and emission spectra for Natural Yellow 3.

The roles of the constituents in the formulation were the same as those they perform for Solvent Black 3.

The refined formulation produced by Perry and Sears (2015) is as follows:

Natural Yellow 3	5.0 g
1 methoxy-2-propanol	500 mL
1% sodium chloride solution in water	250 mL
1% DOSS solution in water	250 mL

The sodium chloride assists in maintaining a neutral pH for the solution, and the DOSS detergent assists in clearing the dye that has not been absorbed by the fingermarks out of the background.

Articles are treated by dipping into the solution, or are drawn across the surface, and then rinsed with water. Staining takes place in seconds.

Marks enhanced using this formulation can be seen as faint yellow ridges on light surfaces, but fluorescence examination is required for most marks to be seen. Excitation of Natural Yellow 3 occurs in the blue-green region of the spectrum, with an excitation maximum at approximately 490 nm. Emission is predominantly in the green and yellow regions of the spectrum with a maximum at approximately 540 nm (Figure 11.19). Optimum fluorescence conditions require illumination in the blue to blue-green region of the spectrum using a yellow-orange Schott glass GG530 viewing filter. The colour of the fluorescence produced has been observed to be modified by the pH of the environment that the Natural Yellow 3 molecule is in and can range from green-yellow to orange-red in colour.

11.11   Nile Red and Nile Blue A

11.11.1   Outline history of the process

1985: Greenspan et al. proposed Nile Red as a fluorescent biological stain for intracellular lipids.

1996: Day and Bowker suggested the use of Nile Red as a stain for marks enhanced using cyanoacrylate fuming.

2013: Braasch et al. published revised Nile Red formulations as a direct stain for the lipid constituents of fingermarks on paper.

2014: Frick et al. proposed aqueous Nile Blue A as a lower toxicity, cheaper alternative to Nile Red, the dye undergoing conversion to the fluorescent Nile Red form during staining of the fingermarks.

Nile Red is being actively researched as an alternative lipid reagent to Oil Red O, particularly for use on wetted papers.

11.11.2   Theory

Nile Red stains fingermarks because the molecule (Figure 11.20) is more soluble in the fats of the fingermark than in the solvent system in which it is applied. It therefore migrates into the fats present in the fingermark due to preferential solubility. Nile Red is not generally fluorescent in the polar solvent system, but once in a neutral, lipid-rich environment (such as the triglyceride constituents of the fingermark), it can become intensely fluorescent. As a consequence, it is only the fingermark that becomes fluorescent when treated with Nile Red, with any dye retained in the porous surfaces remaining non-fluorescent.

The Nile Blue A stain can form salt linkages with the acidic constituents present in sebaceous sweat, including phospholipids and fatty acids, to give a blue colouration to the fingermark. Nile Blue A can also undergo spontaneous hydrolysis to Nile Red (Frick et al, 2014) in aqueous solution, and thus neutral lipids are stained red (and become fluorescent) due to the action of the Nile Red constituent when Nile Blue A is used as a reagent.

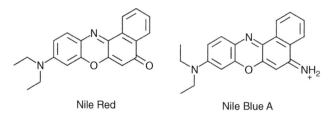

Nile Red   Nile Blue A

Figure 11.20   The chemical structures of Nile Red and Nile Blue A.

11.11.3 The Nile Red and Nile Blue A processes

The Nile Red process described as follows is that published by Braasch et al. (2013), consisting of a stock solution mixed with sodium hydroxide solution to form a working solution:

Nile Red stock solution

Nile Red	0.1 g
Methanol	1 L

Sodium hydroxide solution

Sodium hydroxide	0.1 g
Deionised water	1 L

Working solution

Nile Red stock solution	250 mL
Sodium hydroxide solution	250 mL

To process items using Nile Red, the item is first immersed in deionised water for approximately 5 min, agitating to remove any air pockets. It is then drained and then immersed in the Nile Red working solution for up to an hour, agitating periodically. The item is then given a final rinse in deionised water and allowed to dry.

Marks enhanced using Nile Red may be visible as pale red ridges but are best viewed using fluorescence examination (Figure 11.21).

The aqueous Nile Blue A formulation proposed by Frick et al. (2014) is as follows:

Nile Blue A	5 mg
Deionised water	100 mL

Processing is conducted by immersing articles in the Nile Blue solution for 20 min, followed by rinsing with deionised water. Developed marks may occasionally be seen as blue ridges against a paler blue background but are also fluorescent under the same conditions as Nile Red (Figure 11.21).

Optimum illumination for fluorescence examination is achieved using a light source outputting in the green region of the spectrum, with the fluorescence being viewed through an orange filter such as the Schott glass OG570. The excitation and emission spectra are shown in Figure 11.22.

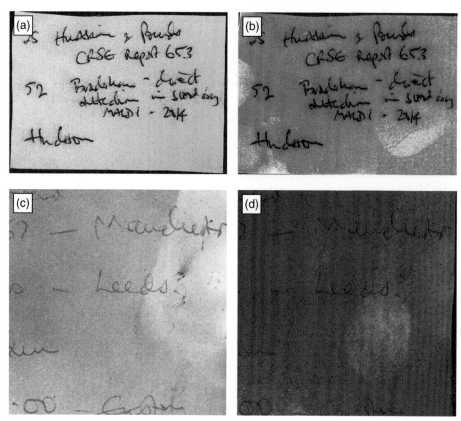

Figure 11.21 Articles processed using Nile Red and Nile Blue A. (a) Nile Red processed article viewed under white light and (b) viewed using fluorescence examination and (c) Nile Blue A processed article viewed under white light and (d) viewed using fluorescence examination.

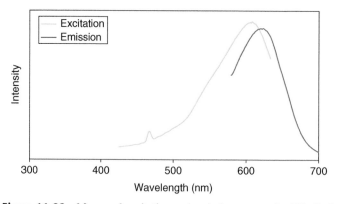

Figure 11.22 Measured excitation and emission spectra for Nile Red.

11.12   Basic Violet 2

11.12.1   Outline history of the process

1850s: The dye mixture magenta was first synthesised, which includes Basic
  Violet 2 (new fuchsin) as one of its four principal constituents.

Early 1900s onwards: Basic Violet 2 investigated as a stain for various types of
  biological tissue, both singly and in combination with other compounds (Chance,
  1953; Fullmer and Lillies, 1956).

2003: Miller conducted a comparative study of Basic Violet 2 with Basic Violet 3,
  examining the relative effectiveness of the dyes in developing visible marks on
  adhesive tapes.

2013: Garrett and Bleay re-evaluate Basic Violet 2, investigating its fundamental
  reactions with fingermark constituents and considering the fluorescence of the
  marks in addition to their visible appearance.

Basic Violet 2 has potential advantages over Basic Violet 3 in that the fluorescent
marks produced are easier to detect. It was originally investigated as a replacement
for Basic Violet 3 because this dye had been identified as a known carcinogen,
although similar concerns have since been raised about Basic Violet 2 and there may
be little benefit in selecting the dye on this basis.

11.12.2   Theory

Basic Violet 2 (Figure 11.23) is a very similar molecule to Basic Violet 3.
    It is a basic dye, and the mechanism by which it stains fingermarks is the same as
that described for Basic Violet 3 in Section 11.4, with chemical binding interactions
thought to occur between the basic amine groups of the dye molecule and acid
groups present on the fingermark lipid constituents.

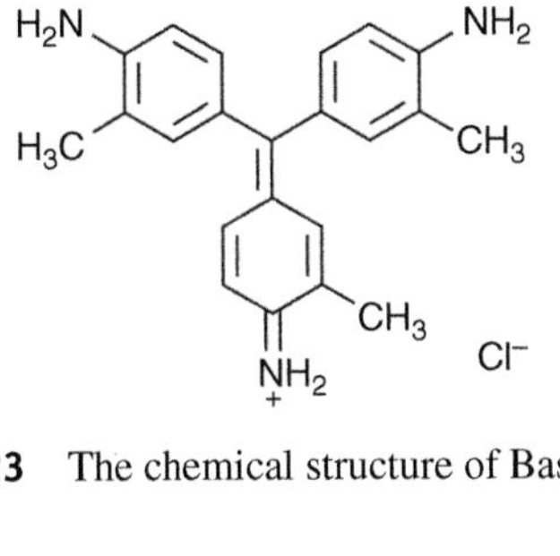

Figure 11.23   The chemical structure of Basic Violet 2.

11.12.3   The Basic Violet 2 process

The formulation developed by Miller (2003) for comparative studies with Basic Violet 3 on adhesive tapes consists of a stock solution diluted with water to give a working solution prior to use:

Stock solution

Basic Violet 2	1 g
Ethanol	50 mL
Benzoic acid	6.46 g

Working solution

Stock solution	1 mL
Water	30 mL

Development of fingermarks occurs by drawing the article to be treated across the surface of the Basic Violet 2 working solution and then rinsing the surface with water. Developed marks are magenta in colour (Figure 11.24) but are also fluorescent (Figure 11.25).

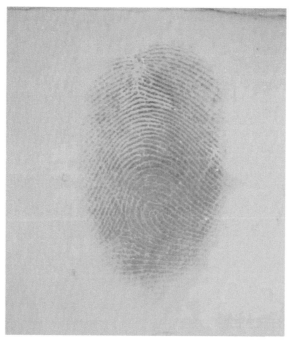

Figure 11.24   Fingermark developed on brown packaging tape using Basic Violet 2. Reproduced courtesy of the Home Office.

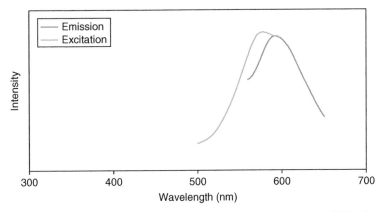

Figure 11.25 Measured excitation and emission spectra for Basic Violet 2.

The optimum excitation is in the green region of the spectrum, with the emission being in the orange region. This generally makes fluorescent marks potentially easier to detect than the fluorescence in the red-infrared region produced by Basic Violet 3, although the visible magenta staining colour produced by Basic Violet 2 is less intense than the violet of Basic Violet 3.

11.13   Rubeanic acid–copper acetate

11.13.1   Outline history of the process

1959: Holczinger proposed the rubeanic acid–copper acetate as a stain for labelling fatty acids.

1973: Vincent investigated rubeanic acid–copper acetate as a means of enhancing fingermarks on fabrics.

The process had not been further investigated since 1973 until recent research at Loughborough University. Although results indicate that it is probably less sensitive than direct stains such as Oil Red O and Nile Red, interest in the use of rubeanic acid as a means of enhancing metal ion contaminants in fingermarks has led to further work for these applications (Bleay et al., 2014; Davis et al., 2016).

11.13.2   Theory

The structures of the rubeanic acid and copper acetate molecules are illustrated in Figure 11.26.

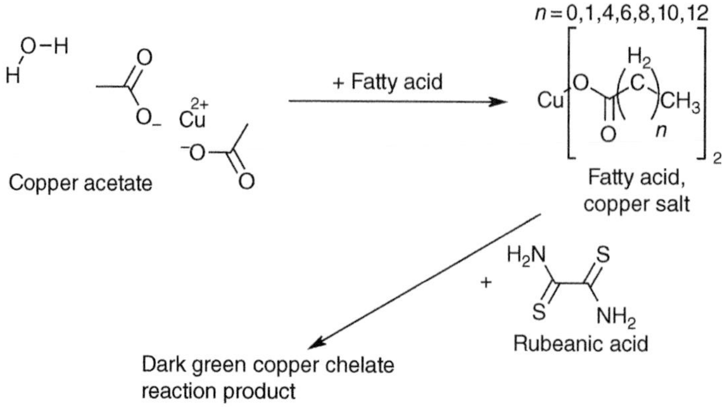

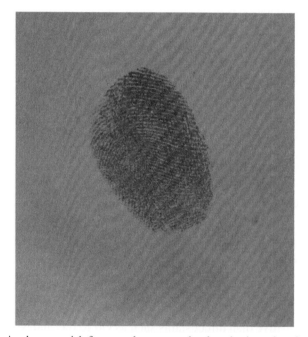

$n = 0, 1, 4, 6, 8, 10, 12$

Copper acetate

+ Fatty acid

Fatty acid, copper salt

+

Rubeanic acid

Dark green copper chelate reaction product

Figure 11.26 The reaction path for fingermark visualisation using rubeanic acid and copper acetate.

Figure 11.27 A sebaceous-rich fingermark on paper developed using rubeanic acid and copper acetate. Reproduced courtesy of the Home Office.

The theory associated with enhancement of fingermarks using rubeanic acid–copper acetate is that the copper(II) acetate initially binds strongly to the fatty acids present in the mark, reacting to form insoluble copper salts of fatty acids. Rubeanic acid is subsequently applied as a solution and undergoes a further reaction with the copper(II) ions to give a dark green chelate (Figure 11.27).

11.13.3   The rubeanic acid–copper acetate process

The rubeanic acid–copper acetate process utilises two separate solutions, as outlined as follows:

Copper (II) acetate solution

Copper (II) acetate	2 g
Distilled water	20 mL

This solution is then diluted to 1 L using distilled water.

Rubeanic acid solution

Rubeanic acid	0.1 g
Ethanol	1 L

Items are processed by being immersed in copper (II) acetate solution for approximately 10 min, agitating the solution occasionally. The item is then transferred to a water wash tank for 30 min before being immersed in rubeanic acid solution until fingermarks develop. The item is then given a final wash in deionised water before being left to dry.

For the enhancement of fingermarks suspected to contain copper ions, the copper acetate treatment stage is omitted and the rubeanic acid solution applied directly to the white gelatin lifter that has been used to lift the marks from the surface.

11.14   Phosphomolybdic acid

11.14.1   Outline history of the process

1952: Phosphomolybdic acid was proposed as an indicator for steroids (Kritchevsky and Kirk, 1952).

1973: Vincent included phosphomolybdic acid in a study of spray reagents capable of enhancing fingermarks on fabrics.

The process had not been further investigated since 1973 until recent research by Shah (2013). These tests have shown that phosphomolybdic acid has a wider range of potential applications beyond porous surfaces and its relatively rapid development time may make it suitable for spray application to some metal surfaces.

11.14.2   Theory

Phosphomolybdic acid (Figure 11.28) is a yellow-green compound that is readily soluble in water and polar organic solvents such as ethanol. One of its applications

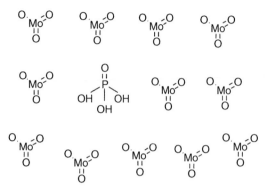

Figure 11.28   The chemical structures of phosphomolybdic acid.

is as a reagent in thin-layer chromatography where it is used to stain a variety of substances including phenolics, hydrocarbon waxes, alkaloids and steroids.

Phosphomolybdic acid develops fingermarks by reacting with unsaturated compounds in sweat, such as unsaturated fatty acids. These reactions reduce phosphomolybdic acid to a reduced heteropolymolybdate complex (molybdenum blue). The colour of the reaction product increases in intensity as the number of double bonds in the compounds being stained increases (Burstein, 1953).

On metals the reaction is more akin to the mechanisms described for electrochemical development processes in Chapter 14. The phosphomolybdic acid reacts with certain metal elements present in the metal surface (e.g. iron) to form coloured salts, giving a coloured background. The fingermark acts as a mask on the surface and protects the metal from the acid, thus giving a different appearance in the regions where the ridges are present. For many metals the reaction with phosphomolybdic acid can proceed without heating at room temperature. The outcome of the reaction between phosphomolybdic acid and a range of metals has been described (Lo and Chu, 1944).

11.14.3   The phosphomolybdic acid process

Recent work has been conducted by Shah (2013) to re-evaluate the phosphomolybdic acid reagent for fingermark development, investigating variations in concentration, heating temperature and heating time. The optimum process was found to be as follows:

Phosphomolybdic acid: 10% (w/v) solution in ethanol

Items are either briefly immersed in this solution or sprayed with it. For porous items development is achieved by heating for 5 min at 100°C. On certain surfaces, such as metals, development may occur more rapidly without the application of heat.

References

Albinson R A, 'The Development of Latent Fingerprints on Fabric', Draft HO SRDB Report No. 72/84 (unpublished) (1984).

Allred C E, Murdock R H, Menzel E R, 'New Lipid-Specific, Rare Earth-Based Chemical Fingerprint Detection Method', J Forensic Identif, vol 47(5), (1997), p 542–556.

Arima T, 'Development of Latent Fingerprints on Sticky Surfaces by Dye Staining or Fluorescent Brightening', Identif News, vol 31, (1981), p 9–10.

Bandey H (ed.), 'Fingermark Visualisation Manual', Home Office, London, 2014.

Beaudoin A, 'New Technique for Revealing Latent Fingerprints on Wet, Porous Surfaces: Oil Red O', J Forensic Identif, vol 54(4), (2004), p 413–421.

Blackledge R D, 'Re: "Latent Print Processing by the Ruthenium Tetroxide Method", JFI 48(3)', J Forensic Identif, vol 48(5), (1998), p 557–559.

Bleay S M, Grove L E, Kelly P F, King R S P, Mayse K, Shah B C, Wilson R, 'Non-invasive Detection and Chemical Mapping of Trace Metal Residues on the Skin', RSC Adv, vol 4(37), (2014), 19525–19528.

Braasch K, de la Hunty M, Deppe J, Spindler X, Cantu A A, Maynard P, Lennard C, Roux C, 'Nile Red: Alternative to Physical Developer for the Detection of Latent Fingermarks on Wet Porous Surfaces?', Forensic Sci Int, vol 230, (2013), p 74–80.

Burstein S, 'Reduction of Phosphomolybdic Acid by Compounds Possessing Conjugated Double Bonds', Anal Chem, vol 25 (3), (1953), p 422–424.

Cadd S J, Bleay S M, Sears V G, 'Evaluation of the Solvent Black 3 Fingermark Enhancement Reagent: Part 2, Investigation of the Optimum Formulation and Application Parameters', Sci Justice, vol 53(2), (2013), p 131–143.

Castello A, Alvarez M, Miquel M, Verdu F, 'Long Lasting Lipsticks and Latent Prints', Forensic Sci Commun, vol 4(2), (2002a). https://archives.fbi.gov/archives/about-us/lab/forensic-science-communications/fsc/april2002/verdu.htm (accessed 29 October 2017).

Chance H L 'A Bacterial Cell Wall Stain', Stain Technol, vol 28(4), (1953), p 205–207.

Davis L W L, Kelly P F, King R S P, Bleay S M, 'Visualisation of Latent Fingermarks on Polymer Banknotes Using Copper Vacuum Metal Deposition: A Preliminary Study', Forensic Sci Int, vol 266, (2016), p e86–e92.

Day K, Bowker W, 'Enhancement of Cyanoacrylate Developed Latent Prints Using Nile Red', J Forensic Identif, vol 46(2), (1996), p 183–187.

Flynn K, Maynard P, Du Pasquier E, Lennard C, Stoilovic M, Roux C, 'Evaluation of Iodine-Benzoflavone and Ruthenium Tetroxide Spray Reagents for the Detection of Latent Fingermarks at the Crime Scene', J Forensic Sci, vol 49(4), (2004), p 707–715.

Forgeot, R, 'Étude Medico-Légale des Empreintes peu Visibles ou Invisibles et Révélées par des Procédés Spéciaux', Arch Anthrop Crim (French), vol 6, (1891), p 387–404.

French R W, 'Notes on Technique: Fat Stains', Stain Technol, vol 1, (1926), p 78.

Frick A A, Fritz P, Lewis S W, Van Bronswijk W, 'A Modified Oil Red O Formulation for the Detection of Latent Fingermarks on Porous Substrates', J Forensic Identif, vol 62(6), (2012), p 623–641.

Frick A A, Busetti F, Cross A, Lewis S W, 'Aqueous Nile Blue: A Simple, Versatile and Safe Reagent for the Detection of Latent Fingermarks', Chem Commun (Camb), vol 50(25), (2014), p 3341–3343.

Fullmer H M, Lillie R D, 'A Selective Stain for Elastic Tissue (orcinol-new fuchsin)', Stain Technol, vol 31(1), (1956), 27–29.

Garg R, Kumari H, Kaur R, 'A New Technique for the Visualisation of Latent Fingerprints on Various Surfaces Using Powder from Turmeric: A Rhizomatous Herbaceous Plant (*Curcuma longa*)', Egypt J Forensic Sci, vol 1(1), (2011), p 53–57.

Garrett H J, Bleay S M, 'Evaluation of the Solvent Black 3 Fingermark Enhancement Reagent: Part 1, Investigation of Fundamental Interactions and Comparisons with Other Lipid-specific Reagents', Sci Justice, vol 53(2), (2013), p 121–130.

Gaskell C, Bleay S M, Ramadani J, 'Natural Yellow 3: A Novel Fluorescent Reagent for Use on Grease-Contaminated Fingermarks on Nonporous Dark Surfaces', J Forensic Identif, vol 63(3), (2013a), p 274–285.

Gaskell C, Bleay S M, Willson H, Park S, 'Enhancement of Fingermarks on Grease-Contaminated, Nonporous Surfaces: A Comparative Assessment of Processes for Light and Dark Surfaces', J Forensic Identif, vol 63(3), (2013b), p 286–319.

Gérard P, 'Sur la reaction plasmale', Bull Histol Appl Physiol Pathol Tech Microsc (French), vol 12 (1935), p 274.

Gram C, 'Ueber die isolirte Farbung der Schizomycetenin Schnitt-und Trockenpraparaten', Fortschr Med (German), vol 2, (1884), p 185–189.

Greenspan P, Mayer E P, Fowler S D, 'Nile Red: A Selective Fluorescent Stain for Intracellular Lipid Droplets', J Cell Biol, vol 100, (1985), p 965–973.

Guigui K, Beaudoin A, 'The Use of Oil Red O in Sequence with Other Methods of Fingerprint Development', J Forensic Identif, vol 57(4), (2007), p 550–581.

Gurr E, 'The Rational Use of Dyes in Biology and General Staining Methods', Leonard Hill, London, 1965.

Haque F, Westland A, Kerr M F, 'An Improved Non-Destructive Method for Detection of Latent Fingerprints on Documents with Iodine-7,8-Benzoflavone', Forensic Sci Int, vol 21, (1983), p 78–83.

Hardwick S A, Kent T, Sears V G, 'Fingerprint Detection by Fluorescence Examination: A Guide to Operational Implementation', Home Office Police Scientific Development Branch, Publication No. 3/90, 1990.

Haylock S E, 'Carbolic Gentian Violet Solution', Fingerprint Whorld, vol 4(15), (1979), p 82–83.

Holczinger L, 'Histochemischer Nachweis freier Fettsäuren', Acta Histochem (Jena), vol 8, (1959), p 167–175.

Home Office, 'Fingerprint Development and Imaging Newsletter', HOSDB Newsletter, Publication No. 20/05, April 2005.

Home Office, 'Additional Fingerprint Development Techniques for Adhesive Tapes', HOSDB Newsletter, Publication No. 23/06, March 2006.

Horobin R W, 'Structure-Staining Relationships in Histochemistry and Biological Staining: Part 3, Some Comments on the Intentional and Artifactual Staining of Lipids', Acta Histochem Suppl, vol 24, (1981), p 237–246.

Kent T, 'A Modified Gentian Violet Development Technique for Fingerprints on Black Adhesive Tape', HO PSDB Tech. Memo 1/80, 1980.

Kent T (ed.), 'Manual of Fingerprint Development Techniques', 1st ed., Home Office, London, 1986, ISBN 0-86252-230-7.

Kerr F M, 'Using Osmium Tetroxide to Develop Latent Fingerprints', RMCP Gaz, vol 40(3), (1978), p 28–29.

Kritchevsky D, Kirk M R, 'Detection of Steroids in Paper Chromatography', Arch Biochem Biophys, vol 35, (1952), p 346.

Lo C-P, Chu L J-Y, 'Qualitative Study of Color Reaction of Phosphomolybdic Acid', Ind Eng Chem Anal Ed, vol 16(10), (1944), p 637.

Mashiko K, 'Letter – Re: "Latent Print Processing by the Ruthenium Tetroxide Method", JFI 48(3)', J Forensic Identif, vol 49(2), (1999), p 111–112.

Mashiko K, 'Safe New Formulation for Ruthenium Tetroxide (RTX)', Fingerprint Whorld, vol 31(121), (2005), p 144–146.

Mashiko K, Miyamoto T, 'Latent Fingerprint Processing by the Ruthenium Tetroxide Method', J Forensic Identif, vol 48(3), (1998), p 279–290.

Mashiko K, German E R, Motojima K, Colman C D, 'RTX: A New Ruthenium Tetroxide Fuming Procedure', J Forensic Identif, vol 41(6), (1991), p 429–436.

Menzel E R, Mitchell K E, 'Intramolecular Energy Transfer in the Europium-Ruhemann's Purple Complex: Application to Latent Fingerprint Detection', J Forensic Sci, vol 35(1), (1990), p 35–45.

Miller E I, 'Fingerprint Development on Adhesive Tapes', PSDB Student Placement Report, 2003.

Misner A, Wilkinson D, Watkin J, 'Thenoyl Europium Chelate: A New Fluorescent Dye with a Narrow Emission Band to Detect Cyanoacrylate Developed Fingerprints on Non-porous Substrates and Cadavers', J Forensic Identif, vol 43(2), (1993), p 154–165.

Mitchell C A, 'The Detection of Fingerprints on Documents', Analyst, vol 45, (1920), 122–129.

Mitsui T, Katho H, Shimada K, Wakasugi Y, 'Development of Latent Prints Using a Sudan Black B Solution', Identif News, August 1980, p 9–10.

Olsen R D, 'The Oils of Latent Fingerprints', Fingerprint Identif Mag, vol 56(7), (1975), p 3–12.

Olsen R D Sr, 'Scott's Fingerprint Mechanics', Charles C Thomas, Springfield, 1978, ISBN 0-398-06308-7.

Perry H, Sears V G, 'The Use of Natural Yellow 3 (Curcumin) for the Chemical Enhancement of Latent Friction Ridge Detail on Naturally Weathered Materials', J Forensic Identif, vol 65(1), (2015), p 46–66.

Pounds C A, 'The Use of Iodine Solution to Reveal Latent Fingerprints on Wallpaper and Emulsion Painted Walls', Home Office Forensic Science Service CRSE Report No. 694, 1989.

Pounds C A, Strachan J M, 'The Use of Biological Dyes for Revealing Latent Fingerprints: Part 2, Operational Trials to Compare Performance of Sudan Black B with Metal Deposition and Small Particle Reagent on Plastic Surfaces', Home Office CRE Report no. 595, 1986.

Pounds C A, Jones R J, Hall S, 'The Use of Biological Dyes for Revealing Latent Fingerprints: Part 1, Selection of Suitable Dye and Laboratory Comparison with Metal Deposition on Plastic Surfaces', Home Office CRE Report no. 9, 1982.

Quinche N, Margot P, 'Coulier, Paul-Jean (1824–1890): A Precursor in the History of Fingermark Detection and Their Potential Use for Identifying Their Source (1863)', J Forensic Identif, vol 60(2), (2010), p 129–134.

Rawji A, Beaudoin A, 'Oil Red O Versus Physical Developer on Wet Papers: A Comparative Study', J Forensic Identif, vol 56(1), (2006), p 33–52.

Salama J, Aumeer-Donovan S, Lennard C, Roux C, 'Evaluation of the Fingermark Reagent Oil Red O as a Possible replacement for Physical Developer', J Forensic Identif, vol 58(2), (2008), p 203–237.

Sears V G, 'Iodine Solution for the Development of Latent Fingerprints', Unsubmitted journal paper, 1999 (presented in part at International Symposium of Fingerprint Detection Chemistry, Ottawa, Canada, 25–28 May 1999).

Shah B C, 'Novel Fingerprint Development Processes', PhD thesis, Loughborough University, 2013, https://dspace.lboro.ac.uk/2134/12533 (accessed 25 October 2017).

Stockert J C, Del Castillo P, Testillano P S, Risueño M C, 'Fluorescence of Plastic Embedded Tissue Sections After Curcumin Staining', Biotech Histochem, vol 64(4), (1989), p 207–209.

Stone R S, Metzger R A, 'Comparison of Development Techniques (Sudan Black B solution/ Black Magna Powder) for Water-Soaked Porous Items', Identif News, January 1981, p 13–14.

Taylor R J, 'A Unilever Educational Booklet: Fluorescence', Unilever, London 1975.

Tsala M, 'Validation of an Alternative Formulation of Iodine Solution for Development of Latent Fingerprints', Fingerprint Whorld, vol 40(152), (2014), p 44–58.

Vincent S E, 'Finger-Print Detection on Cloth', Final Year Project Report, Department of Chemical Physics, University of Surrey, June 1973.

Wilkinson D, 'A One-Step Fluorescent Detection Method for Lipid Fingerprints; Eu(TTA)3.2TOPO', Forensic Sci Int, vol 99, (1999), p 5–23.

Wilkinson D A, Watkin J E, 'Europium Aryl-β-Diketone Complexes as Fluorescent Dyes for the Detection of Cyanoacrylate Developed Fingerprints on Human Skin', Forensic Sci Int, vol 60, (1993), p 67–79.

Further reading

Allred C E, Menzel E R, 'A Novel Bio-conjugate Method for Latent Fingerprint Detection', Forensic Sci Int, vol 85, (1997), p 83–94.

Bramble S K, 'Deep Red to Near Infra-Red (NIR) Fluorescence of Gentian Violet-Treated Latent Prints', J Forensic Identif, vol 50(1), (2000), p 33–50.

Caldwell J P, Henderson W, Kim N D, 'Luminescent Visualisation of Latent Fingerprints by Direct Reaction with a Lanthanide Shift Reagent', J Forensic Sci, vol 46(6), (2001), p 1332–1341.

Castello A, Alvarez M, Verdu F, 'A New Chemical Aid for Criminal Investigation: Dyes and Latent Prints', Color Technol, vol 118, (2002b), p 316–318.

Frick A A, Fritz P, Lewis S W, Van Bronswijk W, 'Sequencing of a Modified Oil Red O Development Technique for the Detection of Latent Fingermarks on Paper Surfaces', J Forensic Identif, vol 63(4), (2013), p 369–385.

Gray A C, 'Measurement of the Efficiency of Lipid Sensitive Fingerprint Reagents', SCS Report No. 520, AWRE, 1978.

Horobin R W, Kiernan J A, 'Conn's Biological Stains', 10th ed., BIOS Scientific Publishers, Oxford, 2002, p 129–130.

Li C, Li B, Yu S, Gao J, Yao P, 'Study on the Direct Developing of a Latent Fingerprint Using a New Fluorescent Developer', J Forensic Identif, vol 54(6), (2004), p 653–659.

Lock E R A, Mazella W D, Margot P, 'A New Europium Chelate as a Fluorescent Dye for Cyanoacrylate Pretreated Fingerprints – EuTTAPhen: Europium ThenoylTrifluoroAcetone Ortho-Phenanthroline', J Forensic Sci, vol 40(4), (1995), p 654–658.

Wilson B L, McCloud V D, 'Development of Latent Prints on Black Plastic Tape using Crystal Violet Dye and Photographic Paper', Identif News, vol 32, (1982), p 3–4.

Wood M A, James T, 'ORO: The Physical Development Replacement?', Sci Justice, vol 49(4), (2009), p 272–276.

12

Liquid phase selective deposition techniques

Stephen M. Bleay

Home Office Centre for Applied Science and Technology, Sandridge, UK

Key points

- Liquid phase selective deposition processes all utilise solid particles held in aqueous suspensions.

- The stability of the particles in the suspension and their specificity for fingermark constituents are controlled by the addition of detergents.

- All liquid phase selective deposition processes are capable of developing marks on surfaces that have been wetted.

12.1 Introduction

There are several fingermark enhancement processes that function by the selective deposition of solid material from an aqueous medium onto fingermark ridges. All of these processes operate on a similar principle, the initial formation of a suspension of solid phase particles in an aqueous medium. Some of these suspensions may be designed to be only momentarily stable, whilst others may have long-term stability unless disrupted by an external stimulus (such as the presence of a fingermark). The stability of all of these systems is controlled by the addition of detergents, which contribute to the formation of micelle structures around the solid particles. In some cases (e.g. small particle reagent), the formulation is designed to be unstable and the particles to rapidly settle from solution. In this case the detergent molecules may play a role in binding the particle to the fingermark. In other cases (e.g. physical

---

Fingerprint Development Techniques: Theory and Application, First Edition.
Stephen M. Bleay, Ruth S. Croxton and Marcel de Puit.

developer), the micelle structure holds silver nanoparticles in a stable suspension until the item is immersed in the working solution. All of the liquid phase selective deposition techniques described in this chapter are capable of developing marks on surfaces that have been wetted.

The first liquid phase selective deposition processes, small particle reagent and physical developer, were first proposed for fingermark enhancement in the early mid-1970s and introduced operationally by the end of that decade. Small particle reagent (Morris et al., 1978) used fine, solid particles in a water/detergent mixture that were agitated in a dish containing the item to be processed to give an even suspension that rapidly became unstable. As these particles settled on the item, they could preferentially deposit and bind to the fingermark ridges. Small particle reagent could also be applied to fixed surfaces at crime scenes by spraying a dilute mixture over the surface and was found to be suitable for enhancing fingermarks on surfaces that were still wet, such as external windows (Pounds et al., 1981a, 1981b). However, it was recognised that spray application of small particle reagent was less effective than dish development and that its use at scenes should be restricted to surfaces that could not be recovered to a laboratory.

Although the small particle reagent could be used on porous surfaces, physical developer was more appropriate for this type of surface, and therefore small particle reagent was mostly used for enhancing marks on non-porous surfaces.

Physical developer (Fuller and Thomas, 1974; Morris and Goode, 1974) was adopted from processes developed for the photographic industry (Jonker et al., 1969a, 1969b). The working solution contained a fine suspension of silver nanoparticles within a redox solution. These were selectively precipitated on the fingermark ridges and subsequently grew to reveal the mark as dark grey ridges. A range of processes were subsequently proposed for enhancing the contrast of the developed mark with the background (Phillips et al., 1990; Home Office, 2003, 2004) by making it lighter, making it darker, changing its colour or converting to a radioactive mark that could be imaged by autoradiography (Knowles et al., 1976).

Multi-metal deposition was adapted from formulations used for protein-staining biological sections and was first proposed for fingermark enhancement in the late 1980s (Saunders, 1989). It is another liquid phase technique that utilised aspects of physical developer and vacuum metal deposition by first selectively depositing clusters of a nucleating metal on the fingermark ridges and then using a physical developer solution to grow a second, more visible metal on these metal nuclei. The process is recognised to be sensitive, applicable to a wide range of surfaces and also capable of enhancing marks on surfaces that have been wetted. However, the relative complexity of the early formulations and the high degree of control required over parameters such as temperature and pH limited the number of laboratories using it routinely. Research effort has since been directed into developing novel multi-metal deposition techniques, including work to produce simpler, more robust formulations (Stauffer et al., 2007; Durussel et al., 2009; Moret and Bécue, 2015) and attempts to impart additional functionality (e.g. fluorescence) to the particles being deposited (Becue et al., 2008).

The powder suspension process was also proposed in the early 1990s and was adapted from small particle reagent by increasing the powder concentration and changing the particle type to those with greater affinity for other constituents of fingermarks. Initially, modified formulations of this type were introduced for use on the adhesive side of tapes (Burns, 1994), but it was subsequently observed that the process was also applicable to a wider range of non-porous surfaces (Auld, 2004), including those that had been wetted (Nic Daeid et al., 2008). It has also been shown to develop marks in blood (although it cannot be used to confirm blood is present) and can be used sequentially after other blood enhancement processes using Acid Black 1 and Acid Yellow 7 to recover additional marks (Bergeron, 2003; Au et al., 2011).

Another more recent development has been the publication of reagents designed to give preferential deposition on the paper background, but not on fingermark ridges (Jaber et al., 2012; Shenawi et al., 2013), using gold nanoparticles functionalised to preferentially bind to cellulose. The potential advantages of these formulations are to reduce the variability seen in development between marks from different donors. Such reagents have not yet found widespread operational use.

12.2   Current operational use

Small particle reagent is routinely used worldwide, and several commercial, pre-mixed solutions are available. In many cases it is the only practical method that is capable of developing fingermarks on non-porous surfaces that are known to have been wetted, especially those in crime scenes. Although originally investigated for enhancing marks on both porous and non-porous surfaces, small particle reagent has mainly been used operationally for marks on non-porous surfaces. However, recent research has indicated that the more concentrated powder suspension formulations are more effective in many of the scenarios for which small particle reagent is currently used, and it is anticipated that the use of this solution will decline. There are still some surfaces where using small particle reagent continues to be amongst the most effective processes, such as wax and waxed surfaces.

Powder suspensions have been routinely used as an enhancement process for fingermarks on adhesive tapes for nearly 20 years and continues to be effective in this role with several premixed products commercially available.

The operational use of powder suspensions is anticipated to increase significantly following the observation that it is highly effective on non-porous surfaces, even those that have been wetted (Nic Daeid et al., 2008; Downham et al., 2012; Goldstone et al., 2015). It has shown to be effective when used sequentially after powders in crime scenes and also to have the potential to develop more marks than ninhydrin and iodine solution when applied to painted walls. However, the process is messy to apply, and its use under uncontrolled conditions at crime scenes will be limited unless better application and clean-up procedures can be identified. As the technique is evaluated fully across a wider range of surface types, it is anticipated that its operational use will increase further.

An important difference between small particle reagent and powder suspensions is that the former targets lipid constituents within the fingermark, while the latter appears to target other (possibly eccrine) constituents. This means that the processes are actually complementary and could potentially be used in sequence on wetted surfaces to maximise the number of marks recovered.

Physical developer is used in many countries around the world, but the stages involved and the time associated with its use mean that it is not routinely used except on items associated with serious crime or in other exceptional circumstances.

The principal application of physical developer is at the final stage of the sequential treatment process for porous items, paper in particular or untreated wood. It has been repeatedly demonstrated that physical developer targets different constituents within the fingermark to DFO, 1,2-indandione and ninhydrin and will frequently develop additional marks if used sequentially after them. It should not be used before DFO, 1,2-indandione and ninhydrin in a sequence because the aqueous solutions used will dissolve the amino acids targeted by these processes. Physical developer is not generally used on its own because it is less effective than all of the commonly used amino acid reagents, unless the item is known or suspected to have been wetted. Because physical developer targets insoluble components of the fingermark residue (or possibly soluble components retained within an emulsion of insoluble components), it is capable of developing fingermarks after long periods of immersion in water (Knowles et al., 1977, 1978).

Physical developer technique is a process that can still be applied when it is known that an item has been exposed to extreme conditions. It has been shown to develop marks on exhibits exposed to temperatures in excess of 200°C (Bradshaw et al., 2008; Dominick et al., 2009), providing evidence that the components targeted by the process are resilient to adverse conditions. This is supported by other experiments that showed physical developer could develop marks on items known to be nearly 60 years old (Fitzgerald, 2005) and after exposure to gamma radiation (Ramotowski and Regen, 2005). Examples of marks developed in some of these extreme circumstances are shown in Figure 12.1.

Physical developer method is not a process suited to application at scenes of crime, although there are occasions where improvisations known have been made, such as half-fish tanks pressed against walls and filled with each treatment solution in turn.

It has been shown that the lipid-specific reagent Oil Red O can also develop fingermarks on wetted surfaces (Beaudoin, 2004) and has been considered as a replacement for physical developer. However, subsequent tests indicate that physical developer remains more effective under typical operational conditions and can in fact be used in sequence with it (Salama et al., 2008).

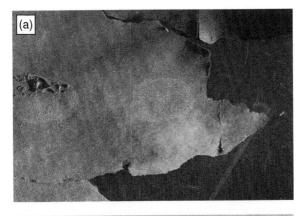

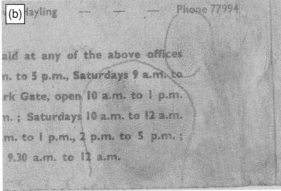

Figure 12.1 Photographs of marks developed on articles exposed to extreme conditions using physical developer: (a) marks on charred paper and (b) mark on invoice nearly 60 years old. Reproduced courtesy of the Home Office.

Use of the multi-metal deposition (and the closely related single-metal deposition) process is not widespread and has been limited to surfaces where it has been proven to give operational advantages. This is because the process is difficult to carry out effectively compared to many other existing processes. Some of the published formulations require siliconised glassware; all equipment used in the process must be kept scrupulously clean, and it may be necessary to constantly monitor temperature and pH whilst carrying out initial colloidal gold deposition. There are also many stages to the process, and some of these may be time consuming, even more so than the physical developer process.

However, in recent comparative studies (Fairley et al., 2012; Charlton et al., 2013), a modified multi-metal deposition process proved significantly more effective than any other technique on cling film, even where drug contamination was present, and it has since been proposed for operational use on such surfaces.

12.3 Small particle reagent

12.3.1 Outline history of the process

Mid 1970s: Researchers at AWRE investigating cheaper alternatives to physical developer noted that finely divided silver powder in the presence of water and a surfactant could develop fingermarks, and their work focused on identifying optimum particle and surfactant formulations. Morris and Wells filed a provisional patent application in 1976.

1978: It was found that formulations containing small (~1 μm) particles in concentrations of between 1 and $10\,g\,L^{-1}$ were most effective. Morris et al. published a small particle reagent formulation based on molybdenum disulfide (Goode et al., 1978; Morris et al., 1978).

1979: Reynoldson and Reed conducted the first operation trials of the process, comparing it to vacuum metal deposition for developing marks on polyethylene. Small particle reagent was found less effective than vacuum metal deposition in this application.

1981: Pounds et al. conducted further operational trials on paper, polyethylene, and glass and also investigated methods for its application at crime scenes. Small particle reagent is adopted for operational use.

Early 1990s: The original surfactant in the formulation Tergitol 7 (3,9-diethyl-6-tridecanol hydrogen sulfate sodium salt) became unavailable because of its potentially harmful impact to the environment, and a revised formulation was developed by based on dioctyl sulfosuccinate, sodium salt (DOSS).

An example of a mark developed on an expanded polystyrene surface using small particle reagent is shown in Figure 12.2.

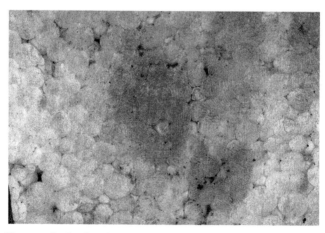

Figure 12.2   Fingermarks developed on an expanded polystyrene tile using small particle reagent.

12.3.2 Theory

The mechanism by which small particle reagent is thought to develop fingermarks is shown schematically in Figure 12.3.

The surfactant present in small particle reagent forms stable micelles around the MoS_2 particles, holding them momentarily in suspension. As the particles begin to settle, they come into close proximity to the surface and the fingermark. As the separation decreases, an interaction can occur between the fatty constituents in the fingermark and the hydrophobic tails of the surfactant in the micelles around the particles. This interaction preferentially binds the fine MoS_2 particles to the fingermarks and does not occur on the regions of the surface where fingermarks are not present. Subsequent washing with water removes excess, unbound particles and reveals the fingermark.

It is also thought that the hydrophilic head of the surfactant molecule can also react with the metal salt in the particle to give a black precipitate, hence giving the developed fingermark more contrast than what would be obtained with the light grey particles alone.

12.3.3 The small particle reagent process

Several premixed small particle reagent solutions are commercially available, but their compositions are not always known. The formulation described in the Fingermark Visualisation Manual (Bandey, 2014) is described hereafter because it enables a discussion of the roles of its constituent chemicals. This formulation consists of a concentrated solution that is diluted according to the method of development (dish development or spray application) being employed.

Concentrated solution

Surfactant solution (10% dioctyl sulfosuccinate, sodium salt in water)	7.5 mL
Water	500 mL
Molybdenum disulfide	50 g

Working solution (dish development)

Concentrated solution	500 mL
Water	4.5 L

Working solution (spray application)

Concentrated solution	500 mL
Water	3 L

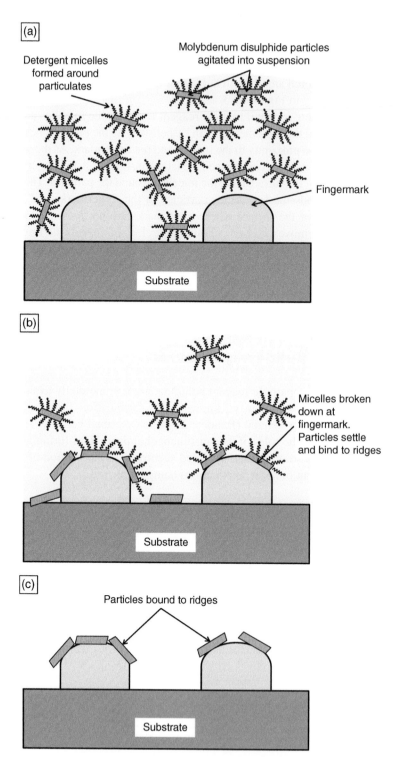

Figure 12.3 Schematic illustration of the small particle reagent process: (a) stable micelles formed around particles of molybdenum disulfide, (b) destabilisation of micelles by fingermark constituents leading to particles settling on ridges and (c) dried mark, leaving particles adhering to ridges.

The role of the constituents in the formulation is as follows.

Dioctyl sulfosuccinate, sodium salt (DOSS)	The role of the DOSS surfactant is to control the deposition of suspended particles so that it occurs onto the fingermark in preference to the background. The surfactant will form micelles around the suspended particles and although the nature (anionic, cationic, non-ionic) of the surfactant is not critical, there are properties that were found to be favourable in surfactant selection:

- The surfactant must be suitably soluble to achieve the optimum working concentration.
- The 'tail' of the surfactant should have an open carbon atom chain with no less than eight carbon atoms, with the optimum number in the chain being 12–17.

DOSS meets both these criteria. The concentration of DOSS used is not critical but must be controlled to be no greater than the critical micelle concentration (CMC). The optimum concentration range is between 1/3 and 1 of the CMC.

Molybdenum disulfide	The role of the MoS_2 is to preferentially deposit on the ridges and develop the mark. Several particulates can be used in this role but in general the best results are obtained with materials with a density of ~4 g cm^{-3} and a layered crystal lattice structure, both of which apply to MoS_2. There must be a sufficient quantity of MoS_2 in suspension for the particles to adhere to the fingermark ridges and give a clear mark. The quantity used in the formulation earlier is sufficient to give good development without excessive background staining.
Water	Water is the principal carrier liquid for the suspension. It also plays a role in diluting the formulation to its working concentration. Uniform wetting of the powder by the DOSS surfactant is difficult to achieve if the powder is directly added to the water/surfactant ratio used in the working solution, so the MoS_2 is added to a water/surfactant solution with a higher surfactant concentration. After dispersion of the particles, water is used to dilute small particle reagent to the working concentration.

The two application methods recommended for operational use using the formulations earlier are dish development and spray application. The dish development technique can be applied to non-porous surfaces such as plastic bags and packaging materials, waxed and plastic coated paper, small gloss painted or glass articles and expanded polystyrene articles such as drinking cups and packaging materials. Such items may be difficult to treat with conventional cyanoacrylate fuming, where uptake of the fluorescent dye by the expanded polymer makes any marks developed very difficult to visualise.

In dish development, a tray or tank of sufficient size for the item being processed is filled with a sufficient depth of working solution for full submersion of the item.

The working solution is then stirred to ensure all powder is in suspension before submerging the item with the surface of interest facing upwards. The article is then kept submerged and stationary for approximately 30 s, whilst the MoS_2 particles settle out of suspension across the surface being processed. Alternatively, working solution can be poured over the surface of items that are not suited to being submerged.

After processing, items are removed carefully from the dish, and the uniform grey deposit is carefully washed off by placing the surface of interest face downwards into a second dish of water and agitating it gently. The item should then be dried at room temperature. There are limits on the size of an item that can be treated in the laboratory using dish development, but for larger items or for use at scenes of crime, spray application can be used.

Spray application may be carried out on all types of non-porous surface, but it is primarily recommended for objects that are exposed to outside environments, awkwardly shaped, large or immovable. Although wet or damp surfaces can be processed, when working in an outside environment, the area being treated needs to be sheltered from direct rainfall.

For spray application a simple spray unit is used, set to produce a conical, fine spray of the working solution and with any filter unit removed to prevent it from clogging with the particulates. The working solution should be shaken to give an even particulate distribution, and the area to be processed should be sprayed liberally. As the liquid runs down the surface, fingermarks may begin to develop, and spraying should be continued until there is no further build-up of the grey deposit. A second spray unit is then used to provide a spray of water above the developed fingermarks before they have dried, which flows down across the marks and carries away excess particles. If marks are directly sprayed with water, they may be damaged. In cold weather, 200 mL of ethanol may be added per 1 L of working solution to prevent freezing on the surface.

The spray application method is much less effective than dish development and should only be used where dish development is not possible.

12.4   Powder suspensions

12.4.1   Outline history of the process

Late 1970s: Morris et al. (1978) considered alternative particulates as constituents in the small particle reagent, including amorphous carbon and graphite and the oxides of the magnetic elements cobalt and iron. These are not as consistently effective as molybdenum disulfide and are not pursued further.

1989: Haque et al. published details of a 'small particle suspension' based on iron oxide (Fe_3O_4) and state that it gave better results than the molybdenum disulfide-based small particle reagent. This is not widely adopted at the time.

1994: Burns reported on powder suspension formulations developed by researchers at the National Identification Centre, Tokyo Metropolitan Police as simple methods for developing fingermarks on the adhesive side of tapes. The consistency of these formulations was much thicker than the dilute suspensions used in small particle reagent and was commercialised as 'sticky-side powder'.

1996: Bratton and Gregus proposed an alternative black powder suspension formulation based on Lightning Black powder (predominantly carbon black) with Liquinox surfactant.

1996: Kimble investigated a wider range of powders and proposed a formulation with grey filler particles for use on dark-coloured adhesive tapes.

2002: Wade produced a white powder suspension based on titanium dioxide by concentrating an existing commercial small particle reagent formulation and adding Photoflo surfactant. The rutile form of titanium dioxide was found to give better performance than the anatase form.

2004: Auld observed that the powder suspension formulations used for enhancing marks on adhesive tapes are also more effective than small particle reagent when used to enhance marks on non-porous surfaces.

2010: UK Home Office published formulations for powder suspensions and incorporated them into processing flowcharts for non-porous and adhesive surfaces.

An example of marks developed on a dark-coloured, printed cardboard box using a white powder suspension is shown in Figure 12.4.

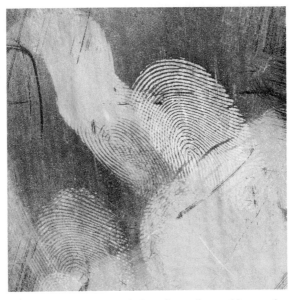

Figure 12.4 Fingermarks developed on a dark surface using a white powder suspension formulation.

12.4.2 Theory

The exact mechanism for development of marks using powder suspensions is unknown, and studies to establish which factors are most important in determining selective deposition are continuing. However, it is thought that the development process is very similar with that for small particle reagent, where micelles or a more random layer of surfactant is formed around the particles. Some component or property of the latent fingermark destabilises these micelles, causing the particulates to deposit preferentially on the ridges.

The effect of varying different constituents of the formulation on the effectiveness of iron oxide-based powder suspension has been extensively studied by Downham et al. (2017a, 2017b). It was found that surfactant concentration is an important factor in controlling deposition of the particles and can be varied to produce a regime where little powder deposition occurs at all, through a range from where selective deposition occurs on the fingermark, to concentrations where excessive deposition occurs on the background and to where marks are obscured. Surface topography is believed to be another factor contributing to particle deposition. Downham et al. (2017b) propose three possible models by which Triton X-100 stabilises iron oxide particles in suspension: by forming a micelle with aligned Triton X-100 molecules fully encapsulating the particle; by Triton X-100 molecules forming individual micelles that then surround the iron oxide particle; or by Triton X-100 forming a more random coating on the surface of the particle. It is not known which, if any, of the models operate in practice, but it is apparent that whatever stabilisation mechanism is in place can be broken down by some constituent of fingermarks.

By examining marks of different compositions (sebaceous, eccrine and 'natural', Figure 5.2) developed using black powder suspension, it is evident that the iron oxide particles of the powder suspension preferentially deposit on the regions where eccrine constituents are present. The fact that the process can still develop marks after the surface has been wetted implies that it cannot be the eccrine constituents exposed on the surface of the mark that interact, and therefore the constituents responsible may be those that are encapsulated within non-water-soluble constituents. It has also been observed that the process is less effective on freshly deposited fingermarks than on older marks or those that have been exposed to moderately elevated temperatures (Dominick et al., 2011). A possible explanation for this is that as the fingermark deposit dries out, the interaction distance between the encapsulated eccrine constituents and the particles in the suspension decreases, making deposition more likely. This is illustrated schematically in Figure 12.5.

Further support to the theory that the interaction that destabilises the micelles and results in particle deposition is electrical and proximity dependent comes from work conducted by Bacon et al. (2013) to investigate reasons for high background staining of certain substrates by black powder suspension. It was found that titanium dioxide pigment particles blended into the polymer substrate acted as preferential deposition sites for the carbon particles in the suspension, and this effect was not observed where the pigment particles were more than 30 nm below the surface.

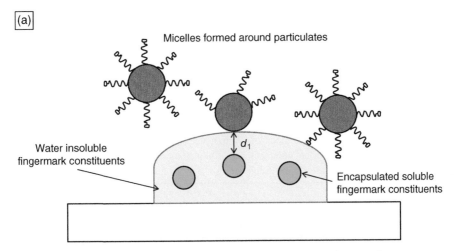

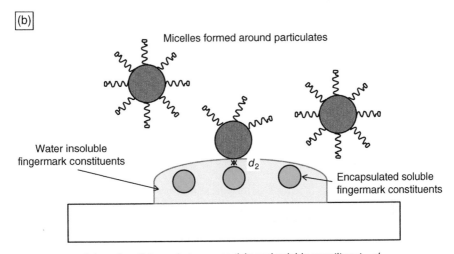

Figure 12.5 Schematic diagrams illustrating a proposed mechanism for powder suspensions and a possible explanation why the process is more effective on older, dried marks: (a) freshly deposited mark with relatively large interaction distance d$_1$ and (b) with significantly reduced interaction distance d$_2$.

The mechanism proposed earlier has not been conclusively demonstrated, and research is continuing in this area.

Powder suspension formulations contain far higher concentrations of powder than small particle reagent, and this, in addition to chemical differences in the particles used, may account for some of the differences in behaviour noted between the two processes.

Table 12.1   Variants of powder suspension in operational use and their principal applications.

Type	Application
Black, carbon based	Development of fingermarks on the adhesive side of adhesive tapes
Black, iron oxide based	Development of fingermarks on light, non-porous surfaces, including those known to have been wetted. Additional enhancement of blood contaminated marks on light surfaces after use of protein stains
White, titanium dioxide based	Development of fingermarks on dark, non-porous surfaces and dark adhesive tapes known to have been wetted Additional enhancement of blood contaminated marks on dark surfaces after use of protein stains

12.4.3   The powder suspensions process

Three slightly different powder suspensions are recommended for operational use; these are summarised in Table 12.1.

Carbon and titanium dioxide-based formulations are available as premixed suspensions, whereas the iron oxide-based formulation can be made from the following simple constituents:

Working solution

Precipitated magnetic iron oxide (Fe_3O_4/Fe_2O_3) powder	50 g
Stock detergent solution	50 mL

Stock detergent solution

Ethylene glycol	350 mL
Triton® X-100	250 mL
Water	400 mL

All three abovementioned formulations contain the same essential constituents: inorganic powder, surfactant and water. The role of each of these can be summarised as follows:

Powder	The role of the powder is to develop fingermarks by selectively depositing on them. The three powders used appear to have a greater affinity for fingermark residues than several other inorganic compounds investigated. The grade of powder used and its particle size distribution has been found to be important in producing an effective formulation (Downham et al., 2017a).

Triton X-100	The role of Triton X-100 is to act as the surfactant in the formulation. The surfactant stabilises the suspension (either by the formation of micelles or a more random surface layer) against indiscriminate precipitation over the entire surface, ensuring that it only deposits where constituents are present that can destabilise the micelles.
Ethylene glycol	Ethylene glycol does not appear to play a significant role as a surfactant but is required to dissolve the Triton X-100 into solution in a reasonable time.
Water	Water is added to dilute the powder suspension to the required consistency and to produce the required range of critical micelle concentration.

The ratio of powder to surfactant/distilled water mixture recommended in the formulations for application to adhesive tapes (Home Office, 2006) has been determined by laboratory tests. If there is excess surfactant/water present, a thinner suspension is produced that does develop marks although these are significantly fainter than those obtained with optimum formulations. If there is insufficient surfactant/water present, the suspensions do not flow, and clumps of powder may be left behind on the tape, obscuring developed marks. The influence of varying the thickness of the powder suspension has been extensively studied by Downham et al. (2017a, 2017b).

When powder suspensions are applied to non-porous surfaces, it has been observed that the formulation can be diluted from the thicker paste applied to adhesive tapes to make it easier to apply to large areas and still give effective results.

Powder suspensions are applied to the surface of interest using a soft, pre-wetted brush, ensuring that the brush is well loaded with the suspension mixture to avoid damage that could be caused to the fingermark by a dry brush and to avoid 'streakiness' in background development. The suspension should be stirred to achieve a paint-like consistency and painted onto the surface, left in situ for typically 10–15 s and then washed off using running water (either from a tap, hose or wash bottle). The temperature of the wash water has not been found to be important. The surface may also be wetted prior to application of the suspension, reducing the chances of the suspension drying out on the surface and any damage caused during application of the brush.

Marks can become over-developed if the suspension is left on the surface too long because the suspension starts to dry and fills in ridges. Powder suspensions can also be reapplied if necessary, and there is also evidence to suggest the different types of powder suspension can be applied in sequence and still develop additional marks.

The process is suited to application both in a laboratory and at scenes of crime, none of the constituents posing a significant health and safety issue. However, the process is messy to apply, and the implications for cleaning of the scene should be carefully considered before application.

12.5   Physical developer

12.5.1   Outline history of the process

Late 1800s onwards: Physical development processes were introduced for use in photography, developing images by converting silver ions from solution to metallic silver.

1969–1971: Jonker and co-workers at the Philips research laboratory in Eindhoven published a series of papers on physical developers when investigating methods for making printed circuit boards, including a stabilised physical developer formulation (Jonker et al., 1969a, 1969b, 1971). The potential for fingermark development was recognised by chance when fingermarks were accidentally developed during the processing of photographic plates.

1972–1974: Initial reformulation work on physical developer as a fingermark enhancement reagent was conducted by Morris and Goode. Tests indicated that marks can be developed on both non-porous and porous surfaces, but that the process is most effective on porous surfaces.

1976–1978: Knowles and co-workers conducted a series of operational trials on physical developer on wetted surfaces, including the use of a radioactive sulfide toner to assist in visualising marks on patterned surface.

1981: The process was operationally implemented throughout the United Kingdom and guidance into its use produced by Hardwick.

1990: Phillips et al. proposed a bleaching post-treatment method to improve the contrast of developed marks with the surface. A range of other bleaching and toning systems were subsequently proposed.

2003: Cantu et al. published a comprehensive review of the physical developer process and adaptations made to the original process.

An example of a mark developed using physical developer on a cheque is shown in Figure 12.6.

12.5.2   Theory

In conventional physical developer solutions, spontaneous, homogeneous nucleation of silver nuclei occurs by reduction of silver ions. These nuclei carry a negative charge and grow by progressive silver deposition onto them from the solution, the negative charge being maintained throughout their growth (Figure 12.7).

In stabilised physical developer solutions, such as the formulation used for fingermark enhancement, several other chemicals are added to suppress the reduction

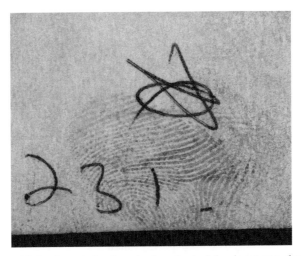

Figure 12.6 A mark developed using physical developer on a cheque.

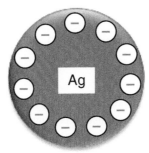

Figure 12.7 Schematic diagram of a negatively charged silver nucleus.

of silver ions to elemental silver in the absence of a suitable initiation site. During fingermark enhancement the initiation sites for the silver nuclei are provided by the fingermark ridges (although it has not been conclusively established that constituents in the ridges actually initiate deposition).

The essential element of the physical developer solution is the fine balance that is set up between silver and iron ions in the working solution. This contains both ferrous (Fe^{2+}) and ferric (Fe^{3+}) ions, setting up a ferrous/ferric couple reaction that acts as a reducing agent for the silver ions. The reversible reaction hereafter is set up:

$$Ag^+ + Fe^{2+} \rightleftharpoons Ag + Fe^{3+}$$

Addition of citric acid reduces the ferric ion concentration by the formation of ferric citrate, which releases three protons and essentially drives the overall reaction in the direction of suppressing elemental silver deposition.

$$Ag^+ + Fe^{2+} + H_3Cit \rightleftharpoons Ag + FeCit + 3H^+$$

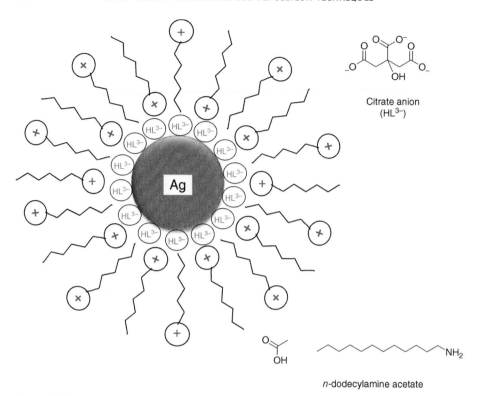

Citrate anion
(HL^{3-})

n-dodecylamine acetate

Figure 12.8   A schematic representation of the micelle formed around silver particle by cationic surfactant molecules (*n*-dodecylamine acetate) interacting with citrate anions (HL^{3-}) and the associated structures of the citrate anion and *n*-dodceylamine acetate molecule.

By adjusting the relative concentrations of each component, the reduction reaction can be finely balanced so that it only occurs on fingermark ridges (or other sites where initiators are present) rather than in solution. However, once silver nuclei have formed, they can act as a site for further silver deposition, and this will result in depletion of silver ions from solution unless the initiation capability of the nuclei is suppressed.

Surfactants are added to the formulation in order to inhibit the growth of the colloidal silver particles in solution. As stated previously, the silver nuclei formed in solution are negatively charged, attributed to the adsorption of the negatively charged citrate anions on the surface. A cationic surfactant is therefore added to suppress particle growth, with the molecules of the surfactant arranging themselves around the silver particle in a staggered fashion to form a micelle with a positive charge (Figure 12.8).

A further non-ionic surfactant is added to prevent the cationic surfactant being precipitated out of solution.

For physical developer to be able to enhance fingermarks, the stable structure of the micelles around the silver particles must be somehow disrupted in the vicinity of the ridge to favour deposition of the silver particle onto the ridge itself. Once this has occurred, the delicate balance between silver and iron ions in the solution around the ridge will favour further deposition of elemental silver, and the particles will grow.

It is thought that the essential factor in destabilising the micelles is that certain constituents of the fingermark become positively charged in the physical developer working solution, which is acidic (pH < 3) in nature. Possible reasons for the development of this positive charge are the protonation of amine groups and carbon–carbon double bonds in the constituents of the fingermark. Amine groups are present in amino acids and proteins, and carbon–carbon double bonds may be found in unsaturated fatty acids, so both eccrine and sebaceous constituents may contribute. Water-soluble amino acids and proteins may still contribute to this charging effect on surfaces that have been wetted, provided that they are fully encapsulated by an insoluble matrix. It should be noted that this encapsulation effect is very similar to that proposed to explain the development of wetted marks using powder suspensions (Section 12.4.2).

Studies (Gray, 1978; Wright, 2006) have failed to conclusively identify the individual fingermark constituents responsible for triggering nucleation. Wright (2006) showed that physical developer gave weak positive development with an amino acid mixture, a strong development with a lipid mixture and the strongest reaction with a mixture of lipids and amino acids. The mixed chemical environment within the fingermark residue may create a better environment for protonation and subsequent deposition to occur. More detailed work in this area was conducted by de la Hunty et al. (2015a, 2015b) who considered eccrine and sebaceous constituents separately and natural fingermarks containing a combination of the two. These studies also concluded that although eccrine constituents may be capable of triggering nucleation, they are washed away by the aqueous solutions used in physical developer unless protected by insoluble constituents, and a more complex mixture of both eccrine and lipid constituents may be required for deposition to occur.

Once the fingermark ridges have become positively charged, they will try to interact with any negatively charged silver particles in their vicinity. Although these are initially protected by positively charged micelles, there is competition from the positively charged components of the residue. In this environment the micelle may be destabilised, and the silver nucleus is deposited on the ridge, where it becomes neutralised. Once a metallic silver particle has been deposited, it can grow autocatalytically, resulting in a series of silver particles 10–40 μm in diameter deposited along the length of the fingermark ridge (Figure 12.9). Note that deposition of silver particles is occurring on the surface of the paper only, and not in the interior. This is not true of marks developed by amino acid reagents, which have been shown to interact with amino acids that have migrated into the porous substrate (see Chapter 4).

This localised deposition on the fingermark ridges will only occur if there are no other initiation sites present. In practice, alkaline filler particles such as calcium carbonate that are incorporated into many types of paper can also act as initiation sites, and silver deposition can occur over the entire surface (Ramotowski, 1996, 2000).

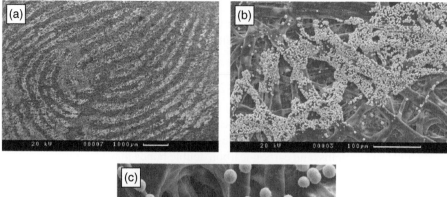

Figure 12.9 Scanning electron micrographs of a fingermark developed with physical developer: (a) low magnification showing fingermark ridge flow, (b) medium magnification showing fingermark ridge and (c) high magnification showing individual silver particles. Reproduced courtesy of the Home Office.

To overcome this, a pretreatment is used for paper items that is consists of an acid solution (Maleic, malic and nitric acid have all been used). This neutralises the filler particles according to the reaction hereafter, generating bubbles of carbon dioxide gas:

$$CaCO_3 + 2H^+ \rightarrow Ca^{2+} + H_2O + CO_2$$

12.5.3 The physical developer process

The process detailed in the Fingermark Visualisation Manual (Bandey, 2014) consists of three stages, an acid pre-wash, exposure to the physical developer solution and finally a water wash or stop solution.

Further detail of the solutions used in each stage and their constituents is given hereafter:

Maleic acid solution	
Maleic acid	25 g
Deionised water	1 L

The role of the maleic acid solution is summarised hereafter:

Maleic acid	The role of the maleic acid is to neutralise the calcium carbonate filler found in many papers. Maleic acid reacts with calcium carbonate to form calcium maleate, releasing bubbles of carbon dioxide. The reaction is considered to be complete when bubbles are no longer seen forming on the surface of the paper.

The physical developer working solution is produced by adding pre-mixed stock detergent solution and pre-mixed silver nitrate solution to a further redox solution containing the ferrous and ferric ions and citric acid. The formulations and roles of the constituents in each of the components of the working solution are summarised hereafter:

Stock detergent solution

N-Dodecylamine acetate	2.8 g
Deionised water	1 L
Synperonic N	2.8 g

The solution should be stored covered to present ingress of particles such as dust that may initiate unwanted nucleation.

N-Dodecylamine acetate	Acts as the cationic surfactant, forming micelles around any silver nuclei forming in the physical developer working solution.
Synperonic N	A non-ionic surfactant, primarily added to prevent precipitation of the cationic surfactant from solution although it is thought that it may have other functions in the development reactions. It is known that without the non-ionic surfactant being present, physical developer solutions do not work.

Silver nitrate solution

Silver nitrate	10 g
Deionised water	50 mL

The solution should be stored in a dark cupboard until required.

Silver nitrate	Silver nitrate is the source of the Ag^+ ions in the redox reaction leading to silver deposition.

Redox solution

Deionised water	900 mL
Iron (III) nitrate	30 g
Ammonium iron (II) sulfate	80 g
Citric acid	20 g

Iron (III) nitrate	Is the source of the Fe^{3+} ions for the redox reaction
Ammonium iron (II) sulfate	Provides the Fe^{2+} ions for the redox reaction
Citric acid	Acts as a buffer for the reaction, reducing pH to below 3 and suppressing formation of elemental silver. It also provides the acid environment required to protonate fingermark constituents so that they become initiation sites for silver deposition.

The working solution is produced by adding 40 mL of the stock detergent solution and all of the silver nitrate solution to the redox solution earlier. The concentrations of each component have been selected such that the redox reaction is balanced in favour of silver deposition on initiation sites amongst the fingermark residue, and not in solution.

It is essential that the resultant working solution is clear at this stage for optimum performance. Solutions may become cloudy if the temperature is too low (<17°C) or from contamination in one of the components, giving poor results. Both possible causes should be investigated if this issue begins to arise.

Physical developer is applied to articles by processing them through a series of shallow dishes, out of direct sunlight (Millington, 1978). The paper item is first placed into a dish containing the acid pre-wash to ensure that the substrate is neutralised and darkening of the background will not occur, agitating the dish gently until bubbles are no longer formed on the surface. This stage may be omitted if untreated wood is being processed or if the paper is known to be particularly fragile.

The item is then transferred to a dish containing the physical developer working solution that is rocked gently until optimum development of the marks has occurred. This typically takes 10–15 min, but may take longer.

Finally the paper is removed to a series of water wash baths, removing all traces of the physical developer solution and stopping the reaction. It is then allowed to dry in air on an absorbent surface. Once the article is dry and developed marks have been examined, a decision can be made about whether a re-treatment with physical developer is required or a post-treatment should be used to improve contrast. It is important to control the temperature during processing, with temperatures below 17°C inhibiting successful development by destabilising the developer solution. It is recommended that glassware used for all these treatment baths is kept scrupulously clean and scratch free to prevent silver depositing on surface imperfections or residual impurities such as dust particles. Alternatively, processing dishes may be lined with cling film or another disposable polymer liner.

It is possible to reduce the time taken for the washing stage of physical developer by introducing a fixing bath after treatment with physical developer. A commercial photographic fixing agent can be used for this purpose, following the manufacturer's instructions. This has the advantage of reducing the overall treatment time but means that it will not be possible to re-treat the exhibit with physical developer if faint marks are detected that could have benefited from a longer development time.

A range of post-treatments have been proposed for enhancing marks. One of the earliest treatments proposed was the treatment of developed marks with a radioactive toner, then using autoradiography to capture the marks. The principal application of this technique was to reveal developed marks that would otherwise be obscured by highly coloured or patterned backgrounds (Knowles et al., 1976, 1977, 1978). In the radioactive toning process, the item is treated with radioactive sodium sulfide. This converted the silver particles to silver sulfide, resulting in the radioactive sulfur being bound into the fingermark ridges. The treated exhibit was then sandwiched between sheets of film for several days, during which radiation emitted from the sulfur caused the film to selectively darken. On development the film revealed all the regions of the film that had become radioactive. The treatment was only effective if the underlying background, ink, or contamination had not also taken up the radioactive sulfur. The technique has not been used operationally for many years.

Sulfide toning can also be used without radioactive labelling as a two-stage process that utilises a ferricyanide-bromide 'bleach' solution that reacts with the silver in the mark and converts it to silver bromide. This is followed by a second treatment with an alkaline solution of thiourea that converts the silver bromide to the dark grey/black silver sulfide. The silver sulfide formed is darker in colour than the original light grey silver, and the contrast can be increased (Figure 12.10).

It is also possible to lighten physical developer marks, which may be useful on dark-coloured papers where the grey-coloured marks are difficult to visualise. This form of enhancement utilises a hypochlorite 'bleach' solution that first oxidises the silver to Ag_2O, which is a darker compound than silver metal. The hypochlorite solution may also bleach pigments in the background, so the contrast between the mark and the background may be improved by this step alone. The

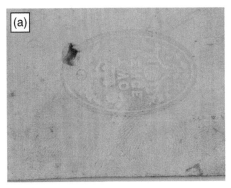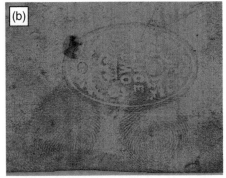

Figure 12.10   Marks developed using physical developer on an old receipt (a) after development and (b) after further enhancement with sulfide toning. Reproduced courtesy of the Home Office.

article is then treated with a potassium iodide solution, which converts Ag_2O to the white-yellow coloured silver iodide. The tri-iodide ions in the potassium solution may also react with any starch present in the paper to further darken the background and increase the contrast with silver iodide. An example of a lightened mark is shown in Figure 12.11.

Alternatively, developed marks can be treated with standard photographic colour toning solutions using the manufacturer's instructions to change the colour of the mark and enhance its contrast. Any silver deposited on the background will also be toned in this way. Figure 12.12 illustrates a mark that has been contrast enhanced using a blue toning solution.

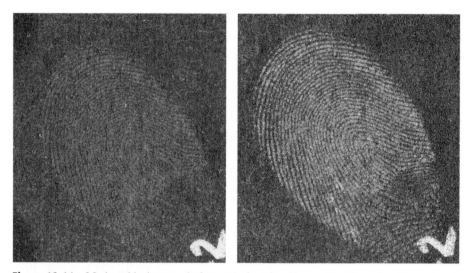

Figure 12.11   Mark on black paper, before and after bleaching and iodide toning. Reproduced courtesy of the Home Office.

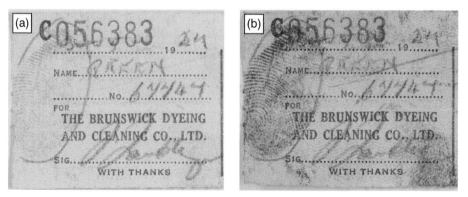

Figure 12.12   A mark developed using physical developer on an old receipt (a) after development and (b) after further enhancement with Fotospeed Blue Toner. Reproduced courtesy of the Home Office.

12.6 Multi-metal deposition

12.6.1 Outline history of the process

Mid 1980s: Silver enhancement methods for colloidal gold labelling of proteins were introduced (Birrell et al., 1986; Seopsi et al., 1986).

1989: Saunders proposed the multi-metal deposition process as a universal developing agent capable of enhancing fingermarks on porous, semi-porous and non-porous surfaces.

1992: Allman et al. at the Home Office Forensic Science Service Central Research and Support Establishment evaluated multi-metal deposition on a range of surfaces known to be difficult to treat, including cling film, plastic shotgun cartridges, masking tape and expanded polystyrene, and concluded that it has operational benefits.

2001: Schnetz and Margot re-evaluated the multi-metal deposition process and proposed an improved formulation offering increased reactivity, improved resolution and greater amplification selectivity.

2007: Stauffer et al. published details of a simpler, single-metal deposition process utilising gold deposition. This is subsequently optimised by Durussel et al. (2009) and claimed to have the advantages of reducing the number of treatment stages, reducing the number of different reagents used and their associated costs and utilising reagents with a longer shelf life.

2012: Fairley et al. conducted a comparison of multi- and single-metal deposition methods for enhancement of fingermarks on a range of substrates giving low fingermark yields in operational work, including cling film, leather and plasticised vinyl. Multi-metal deposition is found to be more effective than vacuum metal deposition and cyanoacrylate fuming on these substrates.

2013: Charlton et al. showed that multi-metal deposition remains effective on cling film in the presence of drug contamination and after prolonged immersion in water.

2015: Moret and Bécue published a simplified and more effective single-metal deposition formulation

12.6.2 Theory

Multi-metal deposition is essentially a two-phase development process, illustrated schematically in the Figure 12.13.

The item to be treated is immersed in an acidified solution containing colloidal gold particles (Frens, 1973; Slot and Gueze, 1985), which bind preferentially to the

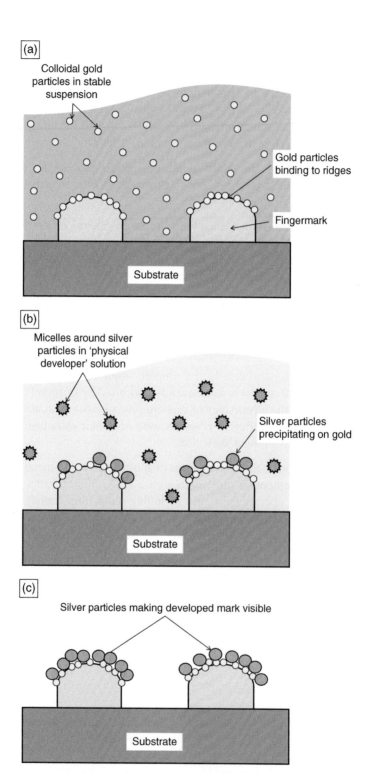

Figure 12.13 Schematic diagram illustrating the stages in the multi-metal deposition process: (a) colloidal gold binding to ridges, (b) preferential deposition of silver particles on pre-existing gold and (c) dried mark with contrast provided by silver particles.

amino acid, protein and peptide constituents of the fingermark. This stage alone generally gives poor contrast of the ridges, and therefore a second stage is used to deposit another metal that increases the contrast of the mark. This involves the use of a modified (less stable) physical developer solution, where surfactant-stabilised silver particles preferentially deposit on the colloidal gold thus turning the ridges dark grey to black in colour.

The colloidal gold particles are formed by the chemical reduction of tetrachloro-auric acid and are used because they are both negatively charged and hydrophobic. Binding between organic compounds and colloidal gold particles can occur by both electrostatic and hydrophobic reactions. The dominant binding mechanism varies with pH, with hydrophobic interactions dominating at high pH and electrostatic interactions dominating at low pH. Schnetz and Margot (2001) suggests that it is the electrostatic interactions that are responsible for the reaction with fingermark deposits and the pH of the treatment solution is kept low (pH 2.5–3) to facilitate this. Mildly acidic compounds such as amino acids, fatty acids and proteins carry a positive charge under these conditions (as discussed for physical developer earlier) and attract and bind to gold particles from solution.

The size of the gold particles is also regarded as important, with smaller particles claimed to result in higher specificity to the fingermark. A colloidal gold particle size of 5–15 nm is recommended, although some workers claim to have obtained equivalent results with 30 nm particles.

The physical developer solution is effectively a modification of the system used to develop fingermarks on paper, containing silver ions in the presence of a reducing system, the solution being stabilised by surfactants. The physical developer solution used in multi-metal deposition is less stable than conventional physical developer, and this accelerates the development of fingermarks. The gold particles bound to the ridges act as nucleation sites for silver nucleation and to catalyse the reduction of the silver.

Scanning electron micrographs showing the stages in a fingermark being developed using multi-metal deposition are shown in Figure 12.14.

12.6.3 The multi-metal deposition process

Multi-metal deposition is a relatively complex process to apply because of the number of individual solutions that need to be made up and mixed to produce the working solutions. However, many of these solutions have relatively long shelf lives, and if the solutions are made in advance and mixed together only when required, the time associated with the process can be significantly reduced.

The multi-metal deposition process described in this section is that adapted from the Saunders formulation by Fairley et al. (2012) and subsequently tested on cling film by Charlton et al. (2013). The principal solutions used in the process are

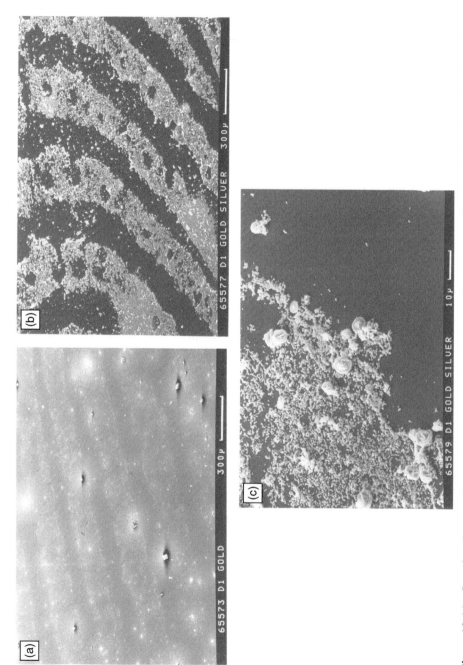

Figure 12.14 Scanning electron micrographs of marks developed using MMD: (a) low magnification showing fingerprint ridges after gold deposition stage only, (b) low magnification showing fingerprint ridges after silver deposition and (c) higher magnification of an area in (b) showing precipitated silver particles. Reproduced courtesy of the Home Office.

a colloidal gold working solution and a silver-based physical developer solution. These are produced as follows:

Colloidal gold working solution

Three solutions are required: a gold chloride stock solution (0.1 g/mL gold (III) chloride hydrate in distilled water), a sodium citrate solution (0.01 g/mL sodium citrate tribasic dihydrate in distilled water) and a 0.5 M citric acid solution. The working solution is prepared as follows:

Gold chloride stock solution	1 mL
Distilled water	1 L

This solution is then brought to boil. Infrared hotplate stirrers have been found to be more efficient than conventional hotplates for this purpose. Once boiling, the following is added:

Sodium citrate solution	10 mL

The solution is boiled for 10 min by which time it should progressively change from clear to black to a deep red/purple colour. The following is then added:

Tween® 20	5 mL

The solution is stirred and allowed to cool, followed by the addition of

0.5 M citric acid	(~18 mL)

Citric acid is added until pH is in the range 2.5–2.8. This can be monitored using a pH meter although approximately 18 mL is generally sufficient to achieve the required range.

The volume lost by boiling is then restored by adding distilled water to make the total volume of working solution up to 2 L.

The role of the constituents in the formulation are as follows:

Gold (III) chloride hydrate	Gold chloride is the source of the colloidal gold particles in the working solution.
Sodium citrate tribasic dihydrate	Sodium citrate provides negatively charged citrate ions to the solution, which surround the colloidal gold particles and have a residual negative charge. The gold particles repel each other electrostatically, and this assists in stabilising the solution.

| Tween® 20 | Tween 20 is a surfactant and also assists in stabilising the solution. |
| Citric acid | Citric acid reduces pH into the range 2.5–2.8 and provides the acid environment required to protonate fingermark constituents so that they become initiation sites for gold deposition. |

Physical developer working solution

The physical developer working solution is very similar to that used in the physical developer process, but has a reduced stability that results in more rapid deposition of silver from solution. It is produced by producing a redox solution and a silver nitrate solution and mixing them together immediately before use.

Redox solution	
Iron (II) nitrate nonahydrate	33 g
Ammonium Iron (II) sulfate hexahydrate	89 g
Citric acid	22 g
Tween® 20	1 mL
Distilled water	1 L

Silver nitrate solution	
Silver nitrate	2 g
Distilled water	10 mL

The role of the constituents in the formulation is as follows:

Iron (III) nitrate nonahydrate	Is the source of the Fe^{3+} ions for the redox reaction.
Ammonium iron (II) sulfate hexahydrate	Provides the Fe^{2+} ions for the redox reaction.
Citric acid	Acts as a buffer for the reaction, reducing pH to below 3 and suppressing formation of elemental silver. It also provides the acid environment required to protonate fingermark constituents so that they become initiation sites for silver deposition.
Tween 20	Acts as the cationic surfactant, forming micelles around any silver nuclei forming in the physical developer working solution.
Silver nitrate	Silver nitrate is the source of the Ag^+ ions in the redox reaction leading to silver deposition.

The multi-metal deposition process should be conducted out of direct sunlight and preferably under subdued lighting conditions.

The process is conducted in series of scratch free dishes filled with

Dish 1 – Distilled water

Dish 2 – Colloidal gold working solution

Dish 3 – Distilled water

Dish 4 – Physical developer solution (to be mixed and added to dish immediately before use)

Dish 5 – Distilled water

Processing is carried out by rinsing the item thoroughly in two changes of distilled water in dish 1 and then immersing it in the colloidal gold working solution in dish 2 for 45 min. The item is then rinsed again in two changes of distilled water in dish 3 and

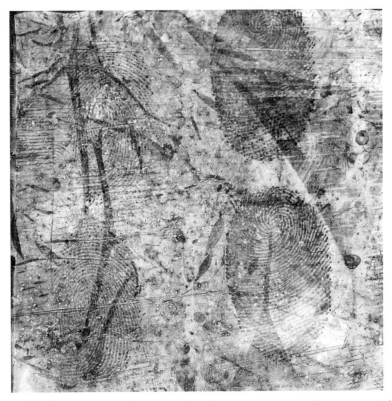

Figure 12.15   Fingermarks developed on a cling film test substrate used to wrap a sample of cannabis resin, showing the ability of the process to discriminate the ridge detail in the presence of contamination.

then incubated in physical developer working solution in dish 4 for approximately 10 min (or until development is seen). Finally the items are rinsed in two changes of distilled water in dish 5, hung to air dry and then any developed marks photographed.

An image of a mark developed on drug-contaminated cling film using multi-metal deposition is illustrated in Figure 12.15.

References

Allman D S, Maggs S J, Pounds C A, 'The Use of Colloidal Gold/Multi-metal Deposition for the Detection of Latent Fingerprints – A Preliminary Study', HO FSS CRSE Report No. 747, 1992.

Au C, Jackson-Smith H, Quinones I, Jones B J, Daniel B, 'Wet powder suspensions as an additional technique for the enhancement of bloodied marks', Forensic Sci. Int., vol 204(1–3), (2011), p 13–18.

Auld C, 'An Investigation into the Recovery of Latent Fingerprints From the Inner and Outer of Motor Vehicles', Final Year Project Report, BSc Forensic Science, University of Lincoln, April 2004.

Bacon S R, Ojeda J J, Downham R, Sears V G, Jones B J, 'The effects of polymer pigmentation on fingermark development techniques', J. Forensic Sci., vol 58(6), (2013), p 1486–1494.

Bandey H L (ed.), 'Fingermark Visualisation Manual', Home Office, London, 2014.

Beaudoin A, 'New technique for revealing latent fingerprints on wet, porous surfaces: oil red O', J. Forensic Identif., vol 54(4), (2004), p 413–421.

Becue A, Scoundrianos A, Champod C, Margot P, 'Fingermark detection based on the in-situ growth of luminescent nanoparticles: towards a new generation of multimetal deposition', Forensic Sci. Int., vol 179(1), (2008), p 39–43.

Bergeron J, 'Development of bloody prints on dark surfaces with titanium dioxide and methanol', J. Forensic Identif., vol 53(2), (2003), p 149–159.

Birrell G B, Habliston D L, Hedberg K K, Griffith O H, 'Silver-enhanced colloidal gold as a cell surface marker for photoelectron microscopy', J. Histochem. Cytochem., vol 34(3), (1986), p 339–345.

Bradshaw G, Bleay S, Deans J, Nic Daeid N, 'Recovery of fingerprints from arson scenes: part 1 – latent fingerprints', J. Forensic Identif., vol 58(1), (2008), p 54–82.

Bratton R, Gregus J, 'A black powder methods to process adhesive tapes', Fingerprint Whorld, vol 22(83), (1996), p 28.

Burns D S, 'Sticky-side powder: the Japanese solution', J. Forensic Identif., vol 44(2), (1994), p 133–138.

Cantu A A, Leben D, Wilson K, 'Some advances in the silver physical development of latent prints on paper', in 'Sensors and Command, Control, Communications and Intelligence (C3I) Technologies for Homeland Defense and Law Enforcement II', Carapezza E M (ed.), Proceedings of SPIE, vol 5071, (2003), p 164–167.

Charlton D T, Bleay S M, Sears V G, 'Evaluation of the multi metal deposition process for fingermark enhancement in simulated operational environments', Anal. Methods, vol 5, (2013), p 5411–5417.

Dominick A J, Nic Daeid N, Bleay S M, Sears V, 'Recoverability of fingerprints on paper exposed to elevated temperatures: part 1 – comparison of enhancement techniques', J. Forensic Identif., vol 59(3), (2009), p 325–339.

Dominick A J, Nic Daeid N, Bleay S M, 'The recoverability of fingerprints on nonporous surfaces exposed to elevated temperatures', J. Forensic Identif., vol 61(5), (2011), p 520–536.

Downham R P, Mehmet S, Sears V G, 'A pseudo-operational investigation into the development of latent fingerprints on flexible plastic packaging films', J. Forensic Identif., vol 62(6), (2012), p 661–682.

Downham R P, Ciuksza T M, Desai H J, Sears V G, 'Black iron (II/III) oxide powder suspension (2009 CAST formulation) for fingermark visualisation, part 1: formulation component and shelf life studies', J. Forensic Identif., vol 67(1), (2017a), p 118–143.

Downham R P, Ciukzsa T M, Desai H J, Sears V G, 'Black iron (II/III) oxide powder suspension (2009 CAST formulation) for fingermark visualisation, part 2: surfactant solution component investigations', J. Forensic Identif., vol 67(1), (2017b), p 145–167.

Durussel P, Stauffer E, Becue A, Champod C, Margot P, 'Single metal deposition: optimisation of this fingermark enhancement technique', J. Forensic Identif., vol 59(1), (2009), p 88–96.

Fairley C, Bleay S M, Sears V G, Nic Daeid N, 'A comparison of multi-metal deposition processes utilising gold nanoparticles and an evaluation of their application to "low yield" surfaces for finger mark development', Forensic Sci. Int., vol 217(1–3), (2012), p 5–18.

Fitzgerald L, 'Development of fingerprints on old documents', Presentation at International Fingerprint Research Group, 11–15 April 2005. Netherlands Forensic Institute, The Hague.

Frens G, 'Controlled nucleation for the regulation of the particle size in monodisperse gold suspension', Nat. Phys. Sci., vol 241, (1973), p 20–22.

Fuller A A, Thomas G L, 'The Physical Development of Fingerprint Images', PSDB Technical Memorandum 26/74, 1974.

Goldstone S L, Francis S C, Gardner S J, 'An investigation into the enhancement of sea-spray exposed fingerprints on glass', Forensic Sci. Int., vol 252, (2015), p 33–38.

Goode G C, Morris J R, Wells J M, 'Chemical Aspects of Fingerprint Technology: Report for April 1976 to April 1977 on PSDB Contract', SSCD Memorandum No. 510, AWRE, 1978.

Gray AC, 'Measurement of the Efficiency of Lipid Sensitive Fingerprint Reagents', SCS Report No. 520, AWRE, 1978.

Haque F, Westland A D, Milligan J, Kerr F M, 'A small particle (iron oxide) suspension for detection of latent fingerprints on smooth surfaces', Forensic Sci. Int., vol 41, (1989), p 73–82.

Hardwick S A, 'User Guide to Physical Developer – A Reagent for Detecting Latent Fingerprints', HO SRDB User Guide 14/81, December 1981.

Home Office, Fingerprint Development and Imaging Newsletter, November 2003, PSDB Publication No. 26/03.

Home Office, Fingerprint Development and Imaging Newsletter, April 2004.

Home Office, 'Additional Fingerprint Development Techniques for Adhesive Tapes', HOSDB Newsletter, March 2006, Publication No. 23/06.

de la Hunty M, Moret S, Chadwick S, Lennard C, Spindler X, Roux C, 'Understanding physical developer (PD): part I – is PD targeting lipids?', Forensic Sci. Int., vol. 257, (2015a), p 481–487.

de la Hunty M, Moret S, Chadwick S, Lennard C, Spindler X, Roux C, 'Understanding physical developer (PD): part II – is PD targeting eccrine constituents?', Forensic Sci. Int., vol 257, (2015b), p 488–495.

Jaber N, Lesniewski A, Gabizon H, Shenawi S, Mandler D, Almog J, 'Visualization of latent fingermarks by nanotechnology: reversed development on paper – a remedy to the variation in sweat composition', Angew. Chem. Int. Ed., vol 51(49), (2012), p 12224–12227.

Jonker H, Dippel C J, Houtman H J, Janssen C J G F, van Beek L K H, 'Physical development recording systems: I, general survey and photochemical principles', Photogr. Sci. Eng., vol 13(1), (1969a), p 1–8.

Jonker H, Molenaar A, Dippel C J, 'Physical development recording systems: III, physical development', Photogr. Sci. Eng., vol 13(2), (1969b), p 38–44.

Jonker H, van Beek L K H, Dippel C J, Janssen C J G F, Molenaar A, Spiertz E J, 'Principles of PD recording systems and their use in photofabrication', J. Photogr. Soc., vol 19, (1971), p 96–105.

Kimble G W, 'Powder suspension processing', J. Forensic Identif., vol 46(3), (1996), p 273–280.

Knowles A M, Jones R J, Clark L S, 'Development of Latent Fingerprints on Patterned Papers and on Papers Subjected to Wetting: An Evaluation of a New Reagent System – 35-SPD', PSDB Technical Memorandum 6/76, 1976.

Knowles A M, Lee D, Wilson D, 'Development of Latent Fingerprints on Patterned Papers and on Papers Subjected to Wetting: An Operational Trial of a New Reagent System – 35-SPD. Phase 1 Results', PSDB Technical Memorandum 12/77, 1977.

Knowles A M, Lee D, Wilson D, 'Development of Latent Fingerprints on Patterned Papers and on Papers Subjected to Wetting: An Operational Trial of a New Reagent System – 35-SPD', PSDB Technical Memorandum 5/78, 1978.

Millington S, 'The Influence of Light on the Performance of a Physical Developer System', PSDB Technical Memorandum 13/78, 1978.

Moret S, Bécue A, 'Single-metal deposition for fingermark detection – a simpler and more efficient protocol', J. Forensic Identif., vol 65(2), (2015), p 118–137.

Morris J R, Goode G C, 'The Detection of Fingerprints by Chemical Techniques – Report for Period April 1972 – March 1974', SSCD Memorandum No, 256, AWRE, 1974.

Morris J R, Wells J M, Hart P A, 'A Surfactant Controlled Small Particle Reagent for the Detection of Fingerprints', SSCD Memorandum No. 580, AWRE, 1978.

Nic Daeid N, Carter S, Laing K, 'Comparison of vacuum metal deposition and powder suspension for recovery of fingerprints on wetted nonporous surfaces', J. Forensic Identif., vol 58(5), (2008), p 600–614.

Phillips C E, Cole D O, Jones G W, 'Physical developer: a practical and productive latent print developer', J. Forensic Identif., vol 40(3), (1990), p 135–146.

Pounds C A, Jones R J, Sanger D G, 'The Use of Powder Suspensions for Developing Latent Fingerprints: Part 2, Assessment on Paper, Polythene and Window Glass Surfaces', HOCRE Fingerprint Report No. 5, January 1981a.

Pounds C A, Jones R J, Sanger D G, Strachan J, 'The Use of Powder Suspensions for Developing Latent Fingerprints: Part 3, Operational Trial at Scenes of Crime', HOCRE Fingerprint Report No. 8, February 1981b.

Ramotowski R, 'Importance of an acid prewash prior to the use of physical developer', J. Forensic Identif., vol 46(6), (1996), p 673–677.

Ramotowski R, 'A comparison of different physical developer systems and acid pre-treatments and their effects on developing latent prints', J. Forensic Identif., vol 50(4), (2000), p 363–383.

Ramotowski R S, Regen E M, 'The effect of electron beam irradiation on forensic evidence: 1, latent print recovery on porous and non-porous surfaces', J. Forensic Sci., vol 50(2), (2005), p 298–306.

Reynoldson T E, Reed F A, 'Operational Trial Comparing Metal Deposition with Small Particle Reagent for the Development of Latent Fingerprints on Polythene', Home Office SRDB Tech. Memo. 16/79, 1979.

Salama J, Aumeer-Donovan S, Lennard C, Roux C, 'Evaluation of the fingermark reagent oil red O as a possible replacement for physical developer', J. Forensic Identif., vol 58(2), (2008), p 203–237.

Saunders G C, 'Multimetal Deposition Method for Latent Fingerprint Development', Los Alamos National Laboratory Guidelines, 1989.

Schnetz B, Margot P, 'Technical note: latent fingermarks, colloidal gold and multimetal deposition (MMD): optimisation of the method', Forensic Sci. Int., vol 118, (2001), p 21–28.

Seopsi L, Larsson L-I, Bastholm L, Hartvig N M, 'Silver-enhanced colloidal gold probes as markers for scanning electron microscopy', Histochemistry, vol 86(1), (1986), p 35–41.

Shenawi S, Jaber N, Almog J, Mandler D, 'A novel approach to fingerprint visualization on paper using nanotechnology: reversing the appearance by tailoring the gold nanoparticles' capping ligands', Chem. Commun., vol 49, (2013), p 3688–3690.

Slot J, Gueze H, 'A new method of preparing gold probes for multiple-labelling cytochemistry', Eur. J. Cell Biol., vol 38, (1985), p 87–93.

Stauffer E, Becue A, Singh K V, Champod C, Margot P, 'Single metal deposition (SMD) as a latent fingermark enhancement technique: an alternative to multimetal deposition (MMD)', Forensic Sci. Int., vol 168(1), (2007), p 5–9.

Wade D C, 'Development of latent prints with titanium dioxide (TiO_2)', J. Forensic Identif., vol 52(5), (2002), p 551–559.

Wright S, 'Replacement of Synperonic-N within Physical Developer', HOSDB Student Placement Report, 2006.

Further reading

Becue A, Champod C, Margot P, 'Use of gold nanoparticles as molecular intermediates for the detection of fingermarks', Forensic Sci. Int., vol 168(2–3), (2007), p 169–176.

Burow D, 'An improved silver physical developer', J. Forensic Identif., vol 53(3), (2003), p 304–314.

Burow D, Seifert D, Cantu A A, 'Modifications to the silver physical developer', J. Forensic Sci., vol 48(5), (2003), p 1094–1100.

Goode G C, Morris J R, 'Latent Fingerprints: A Review of Their Origin, Composition and Methods of Detection', AWRE Report No. 22/83, 1983.

Gray M L, 'Sticky-side powder versus gentian violet: the search for the superior method for processing the sticky side of adhesive tape', J. Forensic Identif., vol 46(3), (1996), p 268–272.

Jones N, 'Metal Deposition Techniques for the Detection and Enhancement of Latent Fingerprints on Semi-porous Surfaces', PhD thesis, Centre for Forensic Science, University of Sydney, 2002.

LeRoy H A, 'Physical developer', Identif. News, December 1986, p 4.

Martin B L, 'Developing latent prints on the adhesive surface of black electrical tape', J. Forensic Identif., vol 49(2), (1999), p 127–129.

Morris J R, 'The Detection of Latent Fingerprints on Wet Paper Samples', SSCD Memorandum No. 367, AWRE, April 1975.

Parisi K M, 'Getting the most from fingerprint powders', J. Forensic Identif., vol 49(4), (1999), p 494–498.

Pounds C A, 'Developments in fingerprint visualisation', Forensic Sci. Prog., vol 3, (1988), p 93–119.

Pounds C A, Jones R J, 'Physiochemical techniques in the development of latent fingerprints', Trends Anal. Chem., vol 2(8), (1983), p 180–183.

Ramotowski R, Cantu A A, 'Recent latent print visualisation research at the US secret service', Fingerprint Whorld, vol 27(104), (2001), p 59–65.

Sneddon N, 'Black powder method to process duct tape', J. Forensic Identif., vol 49(4), (1999), p 347–356.

Williams N H, Elliot K T, 'Development of latent prints using titanium dioxide (TiO$_2$) in small particle reagent, white (SPR-W) on adhesives', J. Forensic Identif., vol 55(3), (2005), p 292–305.

13

Enhancement processes for marks in blood

Stephen M. Bleay

Home Office Centre for Applied Science and Technology, Sandridge, UK

Key points

- Blood is an important contaminant that may be encountered with crime scenes, and fingermark recovery needs to be integrated with recovery of other forms of blood-related forensic evidence.

- Blood can be enhanced using a wide range of processes, but there is usually a compromise between the sensitivity of the process and its specificity to blood.

- The most commonly used processes either target proteins (higher sensitivity) or the haem molecule present in blood (higher specificity).

13.1 Introduction

Fingermarks may be deposited with a number of contaminants at crime scenes, and of all these blood is the most commonly encountered. In these circumstances enhancement techniques that target the contaminant of interest, rather than the constituents of the latent fingermark, are required.

Blood is a contaminant that is generally of high operational significance because of its association with serious crimes. The selection of enhancement processes in situations where blood is suspected to be present can be complicated by the fact that fingermark evidence is only one element of the blood-related forensic examination that may need to be conducted, others including blood pattern analysis, recovery of

---

Fingerprint Development Techniques: Theory and Application, First Edition.
Stephen M. Bleay, Ruth S. Croxton and Marcel de Puit.
© 2018 John Wiley & Sons Ltd. Published 2018 by John Wiley & Sons Ltd.

footwear marks and DNA analysis. There may be conflicting requirements between the collection of these evidence types, and forensic strategies will need to take this into account.

The chemical processes that are utilised for enhancement of fingermarks contaminated with blood all target constituents that are known to be present in the blood and give different levels of specificity according to which constituents they interact with. To aid the understanding of blood enhancement processes, it is necessary to expand on what substances are present in the principal components of blood, plasma and blood cells, and these are summarised in Table 13.1.

Approximately 95% of the protein content in the red blood cells is made up of haemoglobin (Hb). This molecule is made of four protein subunits each containing a haem group, which is made of a flat porphyrin ring and a conjugated ferrous ion (Figure 13.1).

There are many processes that are capable of reacting with and enhancing the constituents of blood, but there is a conflict between the sensitivity of these processes and their specificity. In general, highly sensitive processes that are capable of enhancing the faintest traces do so by reacting with multiple constituents in the blood. However, this sensitivity comes at the expense of a loss of specificity because there are an increased number of related substances that can give false-positive reactions. A summary of the chemical processes that are available and the constituents that they can target is provided in Table 13.2.

Table 13.1 Summary of the constituents of blood.

Plasma (55%)	Blood cells (45%)
Water (91%) Plasma proteins • Albumins • Globulins • Fibrinogen Amino acids Nitrogeneous waste (lactic acid, uric acid, urea, metabolites) Nutrients (glucose, amino acids, fats, cholesterol, phospholipids, vitamins and minerals) Inorganic salts (Na^+, K^+, Ca^{2+}, Cl^-, HCO_3^-, HPO_2^{2-}) Gases (nitrogen, oxygen and carbon dioxide) Enzymes Hormones	Red blood cells (erythrocytes) 99% – Contain haemoglobin protein and surface specific proteins (agglutinogens) that determine blood group White blood cells (leukocytes) – Have a nucleus that contains DNA and are sub-divided into granulocytes (consisting of neutrophils, eosinophils and basophils) and agranulocytes (consisting of lymphocytes and monocytes) Platelets (thrombocytes) – Fragments of bone marrow cells

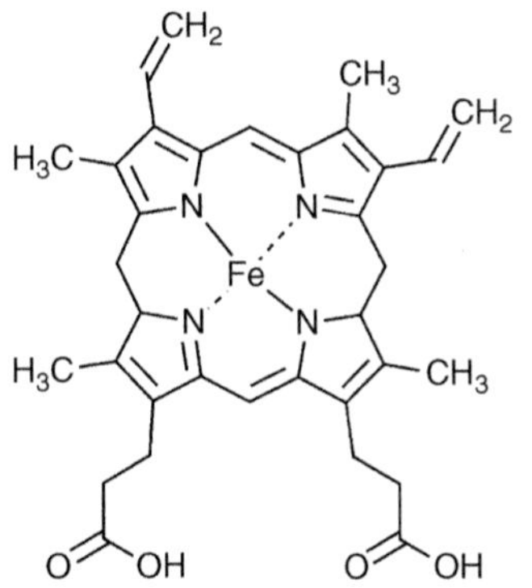

Figure 13.1 Chemical structure of the haem molecule.

Table 13.2 Summary of blood enhancement processes, confirmatory tests and their relative specificities to blood.

Process type (and examples)	Blood constituents targeted	Specificity to blood
Amino acid reagents (ninhydrin, DFO, 1,2 indandione)	Amine groups in proteins, amino acids and haem groups	Low: False positives include latent fingermarks, proteinaceous materials such as egg white, whey protein, body fluids such as saliva and semen
Protein stains (acid dyes: Acid Black 1, Acid Violet 17, Acid Yellow 7)	Proteins in plasma, haem groups and agglutinogens	Medium: False positives include proteinaceous materials such as egg white, whey protein and semen
Peroxidase reagents (Leuco Crystal Violet, Leuco Malachite Green, diaminobenzidine)	Haem groups	Medium–high: False positives may include other species with peroxidase functionality such as vegetable peroxidases (e.g. horseradish), also elemental iron and its oxides (rust)
Crystal tests (Takayama and Teichmann tests) – These require blood samples removed from the surface and are not suitable for in situ fingermark enhancement	Haem groups	High: False positives include haem groups from animal blood
Antibody tests Functionalised nanoparticles	Human Hb proteins	Very high: Specific to human blood

As a consequence of this potential conflict between sensitivity and specificity, it may be necessary to use processes in combination to both visualise faint traces of blood and confirm that the substance present is blood. For example, a highly specific confirmatory test can be used on an area not containing ridge detail, and a more sensitive process is speculatively performed on a larger area to reveal any marks that may be present.

DNA analysis is sometimes applied to marks that have been revealed by enhancement processes to confirm that blood is present. However, it should be noted that a positive reaction with an enhancement process and confirmation that DNA is present is still not conclusive evidence that a substance is blood, because other DNA-containing body fluids (e.g. semen) can also give positive reactions with some processes such as the protein stains.

In addition to the chemical processes outlined previously, there are several other processes described in other chapters of this book that are capable of enhancing fingermarks contaminated with blood, but none of these can be regarded as blood specific. Their use therefore needs to be accompanied by another confirmatory test including the following:

Multispectral imaging – Blood has a characteristic reflectivity spectrum that also changes in a well characterised way over time. Multispectral imaging has been proposed by several groups as a means of detecting faint traces of blood and determining the time since its deposition on the surface (Li et al., 2011, 2013; Edelman et al., 2012).

Vacuum metal deposition – Blood will form a thin film on the surface that will have different chemical and physical properties from the surface it has been deposited on. This may enable the film of the blood to be discriminated from the background during subsequent metal deposition.

Powder suspensions – Powder suspensions preferentially deposit particles on some blood constituents, possibly proteins (Au et al., 2011).

In addition to these non-specific processes, the feasibility of using analytical techniques to detect molecules specific to blood has been explored. MALDI has been used to confirm the presence of Hb molecules in a fingermark previously enhanced with Acid Black 1 and also to show that it may be possible to discriminate human Hb from the equivalent molecule in animal blood (Bradshaw et al., 2014; Patel et al., 2016). This approach may find increasing application in future.

The other issue that can be associated with enhancement of blood-contaminated fingermarks is establishing the particular scenario that results in the formation of the mark. Marks may be deposited by a blood-contaminated finger touching a clean surface, a clean finger making contact with blood that is already on the surface or blood running down over a pre-existing mark in a substance such as grease. It is important to establish which of these scenarios applies, but the enhancement process will not determine this, and additional examination by an expert in blood pattern analysis may be required. Several studies have been conducted in this area (Jaret et al., 1997; Huss et al., 2000; Langenburg, 2008), but this is a subject that would benefit from further research.

13.2 Current operational use

The two generic types of processes that are most widely used for enhancement of marks in blood are the protein stains (e.g. Acid Black 1, Acid Violet 17, Acid Yellow 7, Hungarian Red, Coomassie Blue) and the peroxidase reagents (e.g. Leuco Crystal Violet, Leuco Malachite Green and diaminobenzidine).

Both types of blood enhancement processes are routinely used by fingermark development laboratories worldwide, with protein stains being more widely used when development of fingermarks is required and the area where they may be present is well defined. Protein dyes are more sensitive than peroxidase reagents in detecting faint traces of blood because the haem targeted by peroxidase reagents is only a small component of the total amount of proteinaceous material available to interact with the protein dyes.

There will be circumstances where the use of peroxidase reagents will be preferable, for example, where there is another proteinaceous contaminant present and a more specific dye will more clearly identify the blood. Peroxidase reagents are also more suited to speculative searching of scenes and can be more easily spray applied. However, this approach is more suited to footwear mark development and blood pattern analysis than to fingermarks.

Of the protein stains, Acid Black 1 (Amido Black) was the first introduced for operational use (Godsell, 1963) and is by far the most widely used. It is suitable for use on both porous and non-porous surfaces, and several different formulations have been developed, both in flammable solvents such as methanol and in non-flammable solvents such as water (Sears and Prizeman, 2000). Acid Black 1 is suited for use on light-coloured surfaces because it stains the proteins present in blood a dark blue-black colour. The other protein stains that are in regular use are Acid Violet 17, Coomassie Blue (Acid Blue 83) and Crowles Double Stain (a combination of Acid Blue 83 and Acid Red 71) (Norkus and Noppinger, 1986; Sears et al., 2001). All of these stain proteins dark colours such as violet and blue.

Where dark surfaces are encountered, the marks enhanced by the abovementioned processes will not be readily visible, and therefore fluorescent dyes are required. The most widely used dye for these situations is Acid Yellow 7, which stains proteins a pale yellow colour that produces a strong yellow fluorescence when illuminated with blue light (Sears et al., 2005). Acid Yellow 7 is used on non-porous surfaces, but not recommended for porous surfaces because it produces strong background staining that can be difficult to wash out. Another protein stain that is in operational use and suitable for use on both light and dark surfaces is Hungarian Red (Acid Violet 19), which produces a visible violet stain that also produces an orange fluorescence when illuminated with green light.

A wide range of peroxidase reagents have been used for blood enhancement, but several of these (including benzidine and *o*-tolidine) have now been classified as carcinogens and are no longer used. Of those that are still in use, most are either known or suspect carcinogens and need to be used under carefully controlled conditions.

The most widely used of these reagents is Leuco Crystal Violet (Bodziak, 1996), which has been shown to be an effective treatment for marks in blood, albeit less sensitive than the protein stains. It is in widespread operational use at crime scenes but the purple-coloured form crystal violet (Basic Violet 3) is now classified a known carcinogen that makes large-scale spraying at scenes undesirable. Leuco Malachite Green is also routinely used in several countries for enhancement of marks in blood both at crime scenes and in laboratories. It can be applied as a non-flammable formulation. It is less sensitive than protein stains and does not produce as vivid a colour change (clear to green-blue) as some other reagents studied. It has also been found to be less consistent in performance than Leuco Crystal Violet (Theeuwen et al., 1998).

Other peroxidase reagents that are in use to a lesser extent include diaminobenzidine (Hussain and Pounds, 1989; Allman and Pounds, 1992), which forms a brown reaction product with blood. This can be similar in appearance to dried blood and therefore not ideal for enhancement of bloody fingermarks. There are also reports on the suspected carcinogenic activity of diaminobenzidine, but it continues in operational use although this is increasingly within the controlled confines of laboratories rather than speculative searching at crime scenes. Some laboratories also use 3,3′,5,5′ tetramethylbenzidine (Garner et al., 1976; Hussain and Pounds, 1989), although there are also concerns about tetramethylbenzidine being a possible carcinogen and mutagen, and its use is therefore reducing.

In common with protein stains, there are also peroxidase reagents that give fluorescent or chemiluminescent reaction products. The principal reagents used for these purposes are fluorescein (Acid Yellow 73), which produces a fluorescent product (Cheeseman and DiMeo, 1995), and luminol, which gives a characteristic blue chemiluminescence when it reacts with blood (Grodsky et al., 1951).

Fluorescein has been found to be lower in sensitivity to most of the other dyes outlined in this section and is not commonly used for fingermark enhancement. It also has a relatively complex formulation compared to some of the alternative reagents.

Luminol is a highly sensitive reagent for detection of blood because, if properly dark adapted, the human eye can detect the chemiluminescence from even very faint traces. However, luminol and related compounds are not recommended for fingermark detection because they are spray applied and do not contain blood-fixing agents. Because luminol relies on a chemiluminescent reaction to produce blue fluorescence that fades with time, multiple applications may be required to first locate and then photograph any fingermarks. However, it has been demonstrated that repeat applications will ultimately cause diffusion of ridge detail, particularly on non-porous surfaces (Figure 13.2), and therefore use of a reagent giving a coloured or conventionally fluorescent mark is preferred. The reagent is more widely used for location of footwear marks and blood patterns at crime scenes.

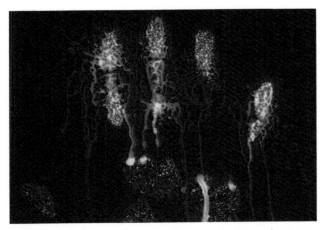

Figure 13.2 Part of a palm mark in blood on glass, with ridge detail diffused by excessive spraying. Reproduced courtesy of the Home Office.

13.3 Protein stains

13.3.1 Outline history of the process

1963: Godsell presented the use of Amido Black (Acid Black 1) as a protein stain for enhancing marks in blood.

1986: Norkus and Noppinger published formulations using Coomassie Blue (Coomassie Brilliant Blue R250, Acid Blue 83) and Crowles Double Stain (a mixture of Coomassie Blue and Crocein Scarlet 7B, Acid Red 71), based on formulations already in use for staining proteins in forensic serology and overcame the need to fix marks with heat before treatment. Both these formulations utilised de-staining solution to remove excess dye from the surface.

1988: Barnett et al. evaluated water soluble protein stains for enhancing footwear marks in blood and first reported the use of Acid Violet 19 (Hungarian Red, fuchsin acid).

2000: Sears and Prizeman re-evaluated Acid Black 1 and proposed a revised formulation based on water/acetic acid/ethanol solvent as an alternative to the water- and methanol-based formulations then in use.

2001: Further work by Sears et al. demonstrated that Acid Violet 17 is a highly effective protein stain and can be used as an alternative to Acid Black 1.

2005: Sears et al. evaluated a range of fluorescent dyes and ultimately proposed Acid Yellow 7 as a fluorescent protein stain for enhancing marks in blood on dark coloured surfaces.

13.3.2 Theory

The enhancement of blood using protein stains is a three-stage process. Firstly the marks are fixed. If acid dye formulations are applied directly to fingermarks in blood without a fixing stage, the blood will begin to dissolve, and ridges may either become diffused or be completely washed away. Fixing can be achieved in several ways including by applying heat, using methanol or using an acidic fixing solution. Both heat and methanol fix blood proteins by dehydrating the blood but are less regularly utilised (methanol only being recommended instead of an acid fixing solution when methanol-based staining solutions are used). In most cases a solution of 5-sulphosalicylic acid in water is used as the fixative; this precipitates the basic proteins and thus prevents diffusion of the marks and any associated loss of detail.

The marks are then treated with a protein stain that dyes the precipitated basic proteins to give a coloured product. The protein stains that are used can all be described as acid dyes. The particular class of acid dyes that are used to stain blood proteins are often characterised by the presence of one or more sulphonate ($-SO_3^-$) groups, usually the sodium (Na^+) salt. These groups function in two ways: by providing solubility in water or alcohol, the solvents that are most commonly used for application of these dyes and because they have a negative charge (i.e. they are anionic). If acidic conditions are used in the staining solution (acetic acid being the favoured option to provide this), the protein molecules present in the blood become positively charged (making them cationic), and this attracts the acid dye anions. Hydrogen bonding and other physical forces such as van der Waals bonds may also play a part in the affinity of acid dyes to protein molecules (Christie et al., 2000).

The final stage in the process is the application of a de-staining solution. This functions by re-dissolving and removing excess dye that has not become bound to the proteins whilst retaining the intensity of colour of the dye in the fingermark. A similar solvent mix to that used for the dyeing process is generally most effective in this application.

13.3.3 The protein-staining process using acid dyes

The acid dye process described is that outlined in the Home Office *Fingermark Visualisation Manual* (Bandey, 2014) and consists of three solutions: a fixing solution, a staining solution and a de-staining solution. These are formulated as follows:

Fixing solution

5-Sulphosalicylic acid dihydrate	46 g
Water	1 L

The role of the constituents is as follows:

5-Sulphosalicylic acid dihydrate	Precipitates basic proteins from the blood

Staining solution

Acid dye (Acid Black 1, Acid Violet 17 or Acid Yellow 7)	1 g
Distilled water	700 mL
Ethanol	250 mL
Acetic acid	50 mL

The roles of the constituents are as follows:

Acid dye (see in the succeeding text)	Stains the proteins with the desired coloured and/or fluorescent species. Dye concentrations of <0.1 w/v give less effective staining (Sears and Prizeman, 2000), and therefore the dye concentration used in the formulation is selected to minimise dye content yet retain staining effectiveness.
Distilled water	The use of water as the major solvent gives the solution a flash point of around 30°C enabling this formulation, containing water, ethanol and acetic acid, to be used at scenes of crime with a few simple precautions.
Ethanol	The presence of a short-chain alcohol in the dyeing solution helps to prevent the blood from diffusing during the dyeing stage. Ethanol is preferred as this offers lower toxicity and flammability than methanol.
Acetic acid	Creates acidic conditions, meaning that the blood protein molecules acquire a positive charge (cationic) that subsequently attracts the acid dye anions.

Three acid dyes (Acid Black 1 [Naphthalene Black, Naphthol Blue Black, CI 20470], Acid Violet 17 [Coomassie Brilliant Violet R150, CI 42650] and Acid Yellow 7 [Brilliant Sulpho Flavine, CI 56205]) are recommended for use in this formulation.

Acid Black 1 is a diazo dye (Figure 13.3) that stains the proteins present in blood to give a blue-black colour (Figure 13.4). It can be absorbed by some porous surfaces so an area away from the mark needs to be tested first to establish the level of background staining liable to occur.

Acid Violet 17 is a triarylmethane dye (Figure 13.5), which stains proteins to give a bright violet product (Figure 13.6). It can also be absorbed by some porous surfaces; therefore an area of substrate away from the target enhancement area should be tested to assess background staining.

Acid Yellow 7 is an amino ketone dye (Figure 13.7) that stains proteins to give a pale yellow product that fluoresces bright yellow when illuminated with blue light sources (Figure 13.8). The haem group acts as an energy sink that improves the enhancement of lighter deposits of blood. Acid Yellow 7 is only recommended for use on dark non-porous surfaces because it cannot easily be washed out from the background of porous surfaces.

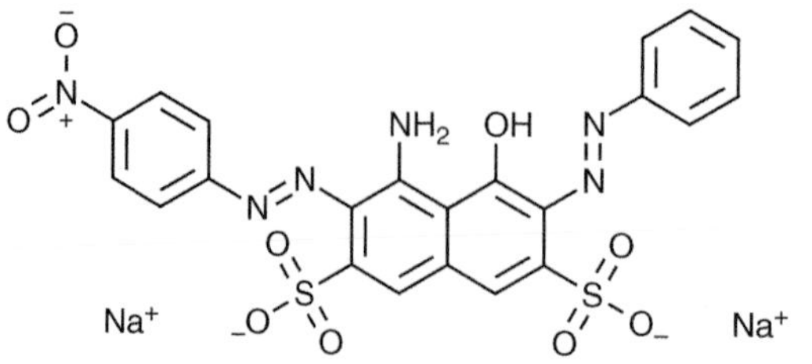

Figure 13.3 Structure of Acid Black 1.

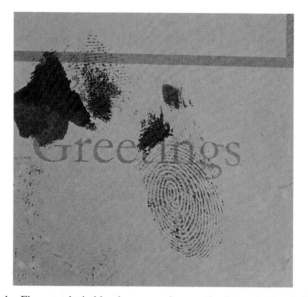

Figure 13.4 Fingermarks in blood on a greetings card enhanced using Acid Black 1.

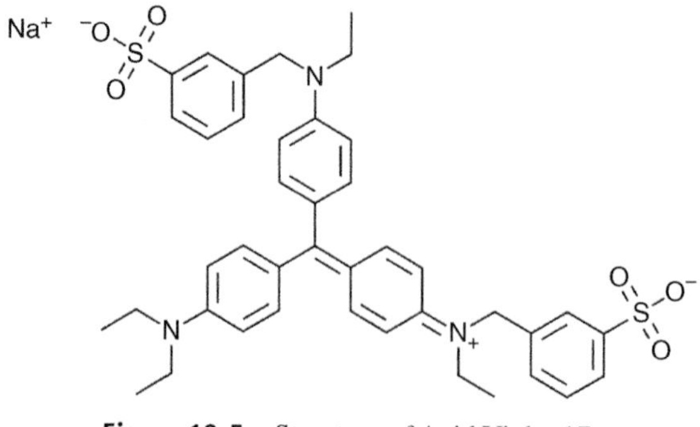

Figure 13.5 Structure of Acid Violet 17.

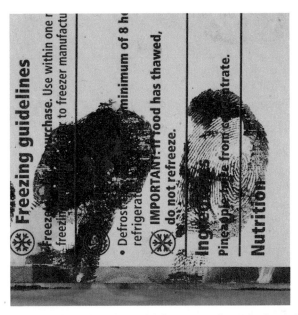

Figure 13.6 Fingermarks in blood on a drinks carton enhanced using Acid Violet 17.

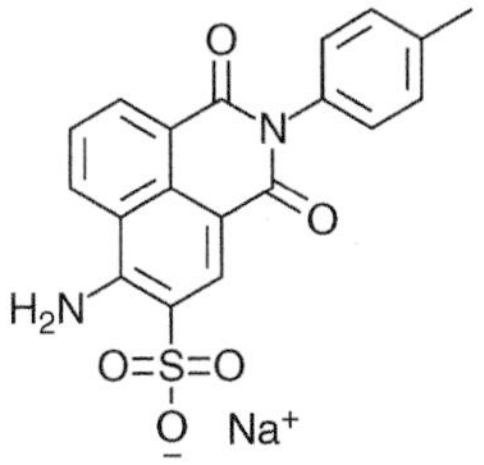

Figure 13.7 Structure of Acid Yellow 7.

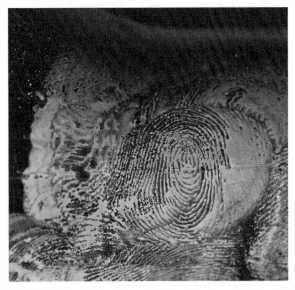

Figure 13.8 Fingermarks in blood on a dark bottle enhanced using Acid Yellow 7.

De-staining solution

Acid dye (Acid Black 1, Acid Violet 17 or Acid Yellow 7)	1 g
Distilled water	700 mL
Ethanol	250 mL
Acetic acid	50 mL

The de-staining solution utilises the same constituents as the staining solution, but without the dye molecule being present. It is designed to re-dissolve any residual dye molecules that are not bound to the proteins.

When items that are suspected to be contaminated with blood are processed using the acid dyes, they are first fixed for at least 5 min using the fixing solution of 5-sulphosalicylic acid. If immersion is not possible, the surface should be kept wetted for an equivalent period of time by pouring the solution over the surface. Alternative methods, such as the application of a wetted absorbent tissue over the area of interest, can also be used.

Once the blood has been fixed, it is either immersed in the staining solution or kept wetted with the staining solution in the ways outlined previously. For Acid Black 1 and Acid Violet 17, staining time should be at least 3 min, and for Acid Yellow 7 longer staining times (~5 min) should be used. Staining times should also be extended if particularly heavy deposits of blood are present.

Finally, the items are immersed in or kept wetted with the de-staining solution until all excess dye has been removed from the surface. Ethanol-containing staining or de-staining solutions should never be sprayed in environments without adequate extraction or ventilation because this lowers the flash point by at least 100°C, making it impossible to work without creating a flammable atmosphere.

Marks enhanced using Acid Black 1 and Acid Violet 17 are strongly coloured and visible to the eye. Marks enhanced using Acid Yellow 7 are a pale yellow and are best visualised using fluorescence examination. The excitation and emission spectra for Acid Yellow 7 are illustrated in Figure 13.9.

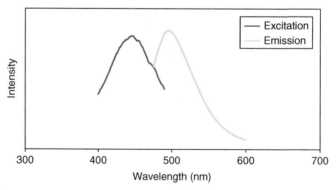

Figure 13.9   Measured excitation and emission spectra for Acid Yellow 7.

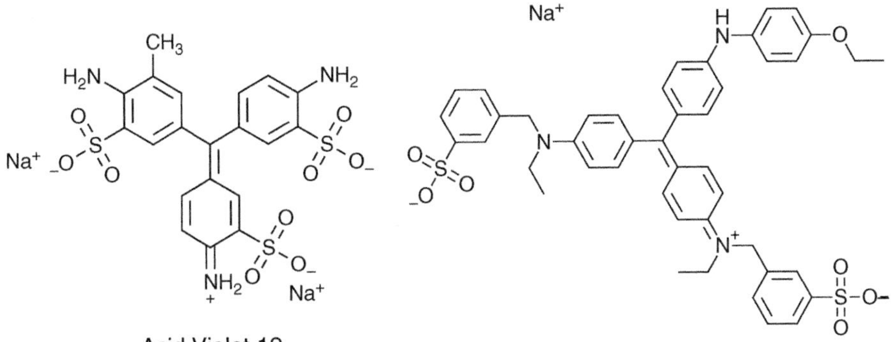

Figure 13.10 The structures of Acid Violet 19 and Acid Blue 83, used as dyes in alternative protein stain formulations for enhancing marks in blood.

To view this fluorescence, marks are excited using blue (420–485 nm) light, although broadband blue light sources outputting 400–500 nm may be more effective. The resultant yellow fluorescence from the stained mark is viewed through a yellow or yellow-orange filter. The maxima of the excitation and emission spectra are known to vary slightly in position according the thickness of the blood present. The intensity of fluorescence emitted from heavy deposits of blood can be reduced because the haem group can both absorb the excitation wavelengths and reabsorb light that is emitted as fluorescence.

It has also been observed that Acid Violet 17 has weak fluorescence in the deep red and near-infrared regions of the spectrum when excited with green-yellow and yellow wavelengths, and this fluorescence could also be utilised to view developed marks.

The structure of other acid dyes that have been used for enhancement of blood is illustrated in Figure 13.10.

13.4 Peroxidase reagents

13.4.1 Outline history of the process

1853: Teichmann proposed the first crystal confirmatory test for the presence of blood.

1901: Kastle and Shedd proposed phenolphthalein as a presumptive test for blood, producing a pink reaction product when blood was present.

1904: Benzidine and Leuco Malachite Green are evaluated by Alder and Alder and proposed as reagents that utilise the peroxidase activity of haem to enhance blood, turning from colourless to dark blue and blue-green, respectively, in the presence of blood.

1912: Ortho-tolidine (closely related structurally to benzidine) first was suggested by Ruttan and Hardisty as an alternative process for blood enhancement.

1937: Specht proposed luminol as a chemiluminescent method for the enhancement of blood.

1974: Holland et al. investigate safer alternatives to benzidine. It was suggested that the participation of ortho-hydroxy derivatives of aromatic amines contributed to the carcinogenic action observed for benzidine and o-tolidine. Holland et al. proposed the use of 3,3′,5,5′-tetramethylbenzidine (TMB), where ortho-hydroxylation is impossible.

1989: Hussain and Pounds proposed diaminobenzidine as an alternative peroxidase reagent with high specificity for blood enhancement. The pH of the DAB reaction (~pH 7) was high enough to prevent cross reactions with vegetable peroxidase and no 'false-positive' reactions with iron or rust were seen.

1995: Cheeseman and DiMeo published a formulation for fluorescein as a blood enhancement reagent, producing green-yellow fluorescent marks.

1996: Bodziak proposed Leuco Crystal Violet as a method for enhancing footwear marks in blood.

13.4.2 Theory

All of the peroxidase reagents used for blood enhancement rely on the peroxidase activity of the haem group, that is, the ability to reduce hydrogen peroxide to water and oxygen. This reaction may then be coupled to the oxidation of colourless reduced dyes, such as Leuco Crystal Violet, tetramethylbenzidine and fluorescein, which form their coloured counterparts when oxidised according to the general reaction:

$$H_2O_2 + \text{colourless reduced dye} \rightarrow H_2O + \text{coloured oxidised dye}$$

The means by which the different types of peroxidase reagents react to reveal traces of blood does differ.

For reagents related to benzidine, such as diaminobenzidine and tetramethylbenzidine, the oxidised dye reaction product then combines to form a coloured polymer or dimer (Figure 13.11).

In the case of Leuco dyes such as Leuco Crystal Violet and Leuco Malachite Green, the oxidation reaction results in a minor structural rearrangement producing the coloured form (Figure 13.12).

The fluorescein process also utilises a minor structural rearrangement between the reduced and oxidised forms (Figure 13.13) to enhance traces of blood. The reduced fluorescin molecule is colourless, but in the presence of blood associated

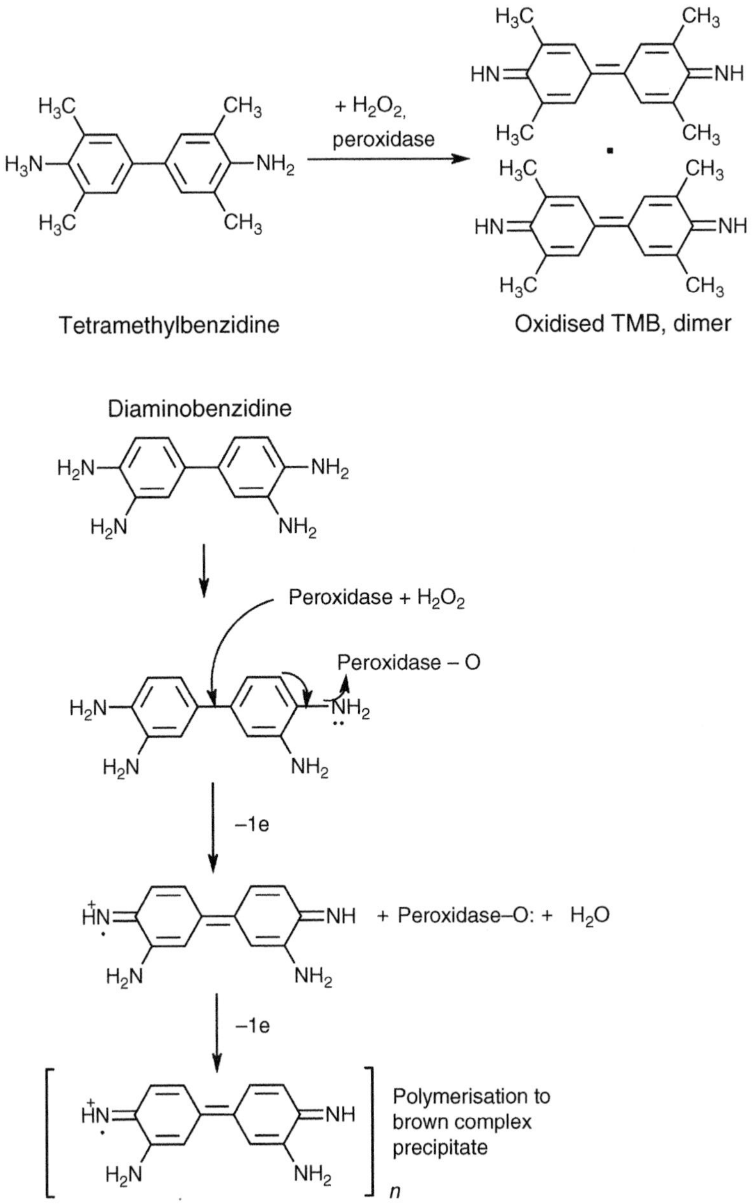

Figure 13.11 Peroxidase reactions for tetramethylbenzidine and diaminobenzidine, showing how they become oxidised from the colourless form to coloured polymers/dimers.

proteins and iron ions found in the Hb molecule and hydrogen peroxide, it is oxidised into a coloured/fluorescent product.

The luminol test also relies on the peroxidase activity of the haem group but may use sodium perborate instead of hydrogen peroxide to catalyse the reaction.

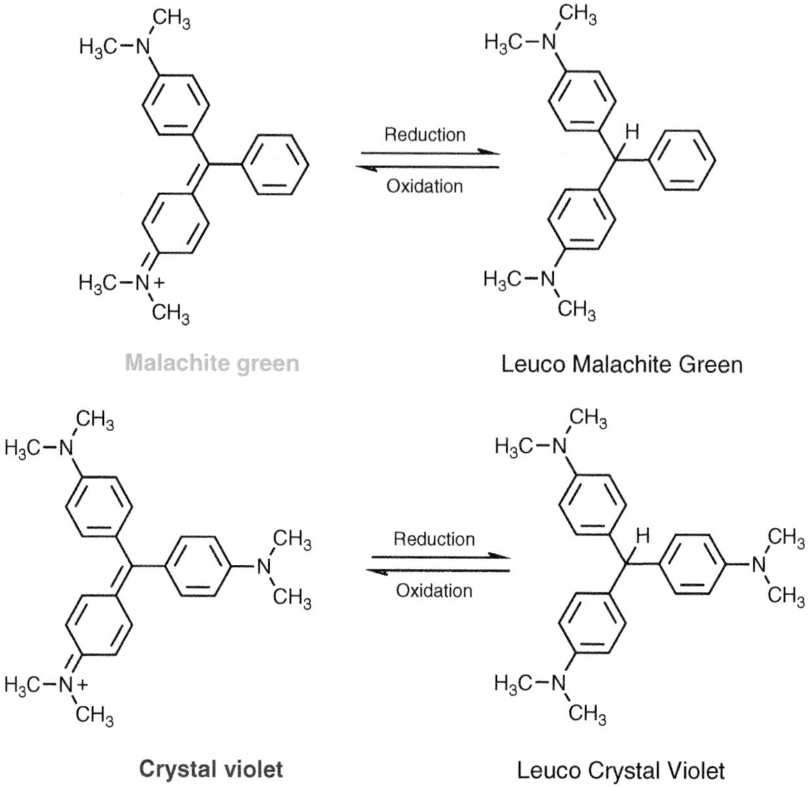

Figure 13.12   The coloured and colourless forms of the dyes Leuco Crystal Violet and Leuco Malachite Green.

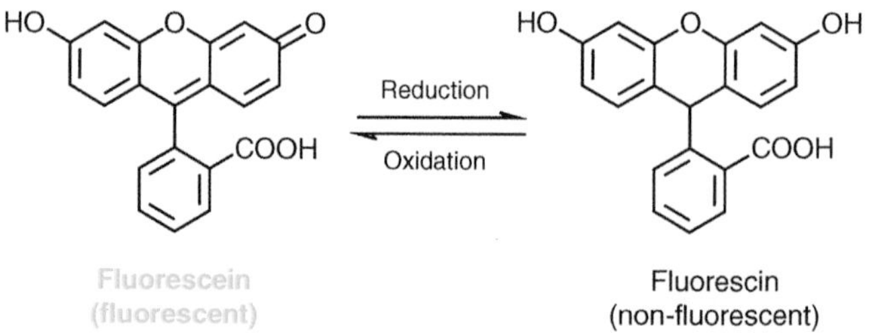

Figure 13.13   The chemical structures of the fluorescent, coloured fluorescein molecule, and the non-fluorescent, colourless reduced form fluorescin.

The hydrogen peroxide/sodium perborate and the luminol react in alkaline conditions to produce a blue chemiluminescence, with the reaction being catalysed by the iron present in Hb.

In the resultant oxidation reaction (Figure 13.14), the luminol molecule loses nitrogen and hydrogen atoms and gains oxygen atoms, resulting in a compound called 3-aminophthalate. The reaction leaves the 3-aminophthalate in an excited

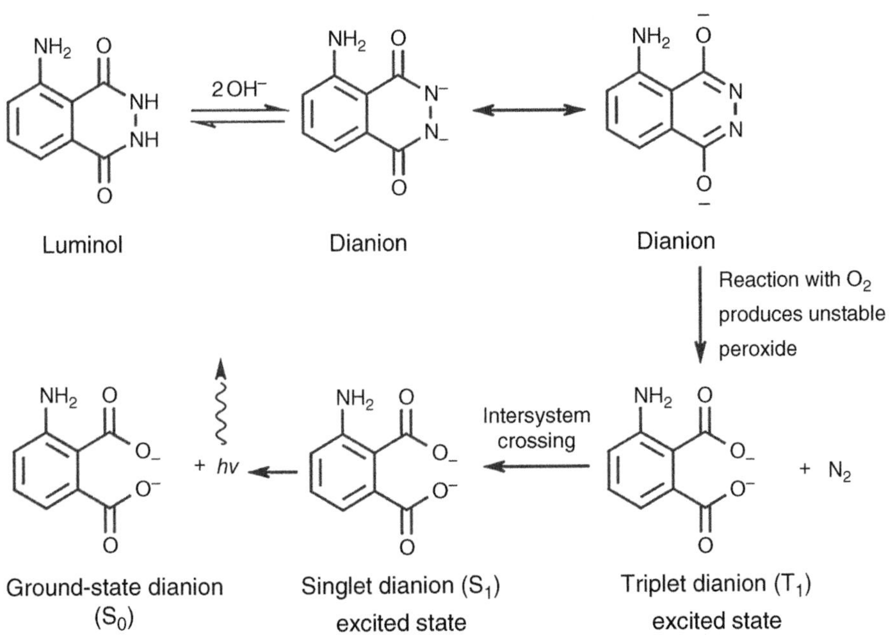

Figure 13.14 Schematic diagrams showing the mechanisms associated with the chemiluminescent reaction between luminol and blood.

state with the electrons in the oxygen atoms being promoted to higher energy levels. The electrons quickly fall back to a lower energy level, emitting the extra energy as a light photon.

Peroxidase reagents are more specific to blood than protein stains, although there are still a range of compounds that can produce false-positive reactions (Cox, 1991). These include chemical oxidants and vegetable peroxidase examples including salts of heavy metals such as copper, nickel and iron, and the peroxidases present in horseradish and numerous root vegetables (Préstamo and Manzano, 1993). To overcome some of these issues, peroxidase reagents are sometimes applied in two stages. The reduced colourless dye is applied to the surface where blood is suspected to be present, and if a colour change is observed, this may be indicative of a false-positive reaction. If no colour change is observed, a second solution containing hydrogen peroxide is applied, and a colour change that occurs at this stage is more likely to indicate the presence of blood.

It is generally accepted that a negative result with a peroxidase reagent proves the absence of blood; however strong reducing agents such as ascorbic acid (Ponce and Pascual, 1999) and active oxygen cleaning products (Castelló et al., 2009) may inhibit such tests and conceal the fact that blood is present.

13.4.3   Peroxidase reagent processes

13.4.3.1   *Diaminobenzidine*

This peroxidase reagent is a derivative of benzidine and reacts with the haem molecule turning marks in blood to a dark brown. The reaction is initiated by hydrogen peroxide. It can be used for enhancing marks in blood on both porous and nonporous surfaces.

The formulation originally proposed by Hussain and Pounds (1989) consists of a fixing solution and a working solution that is produced immediately before use by the addition of a phosphate buffer working solution to an aqueous solution of diaminobenzidine.

Fixing solution

5-Sulphosalicylic acid dihydrate	20 g
Distilled water	1 L

The role of the constituents is as follows:

5-Sulphosalicylic acid dihydrate	Precipitates basic proteins from the blood

The working solution is produced by first producing a buffer solution and an aqueous solution of diaminobenzidine:

Buffer solution

1 M potassium phosphate buffer (pH 7.4)	100 mL
Distilled water	100 mL

Diaminobenzidine solution

3,3′-Diaminobenzidine tetrahydrochloride	1 g
Distilled water	100 mL

These are then mixed immediately before use to form the working solution:

Working solution

Buffer solution	180 mL
Diaminobenzidine solution	20 mL
30% hydrogen peroxide	1 mL

The roles of the constituents are as follows:

1 M potassium phosphate buffer (pH 7.4)	Keeps the pH of the working solution in a range that favours 'true' reactions with haem molecules and inhibits false-positive reactions, thus increasing specificity of the reagent
3,3'-Diaminobenzidine tetrahydrochloride	The active colourless dye constituent, oxidised during the peroxidase reaction to give a molecule that then polymerises to give a dark brown-coloured product
Hydrogen peroxide	Acts as the catalyst for the peroxidase reaction with the haem molecule

Articles to be processed using diaminobenzidine are fixed for approximately 3 min by immersion in the fixing solution of 5-sulphosalicylic acid. In common with the protein dyes, the fixing solution may be applied by alternative methods such as pouring, spraying or application of soaked tissues if immersion is not possible.

Once any traces of blood have been fixed, the item is exposed to the working solution for 3–4 min and then rinsed in water to remove excess unreacted dye.

13.4.3.2   Leuco Malachite Green

This Leuco dye is oxidised to form a deep green coloured product (Basic Green 4) in a reaction catalysed by the haem group in blood.

There are several published formulations of Leuco Malachite Green in the literature, some using methanol as a fixative prior to application of a working solution (Frégeau et al., 2000) and others incorporating the fixative in a single working solution (Jaret et al., 1997). For optimum results the reagent must be prepared immediately prior to use, regardless of the formulation.

The formulation described hereafter is that used by the Royal Canadian Mounted Police and is adapted from that utilised by Frégeau et al. (2000):

Fixing solution

Methanol	
Methanol fixes the haem (and other blood proteins) by dehydrating the blood	

Working solution

Leuco Malachite Green	0.2 g
Sodium perborate	0.67 g
Glacial acetic acid	33 mL
Methanol	67 mL
HFE7100	300 mL

The roles of the constituents in the working solution are as follows:

Leuco Malachite Green	The active colourless Leuco dye constituent, oxidised during the peroxidase reaction to give the green-coloured form of the dye
Sodium perborate	Fulfils an equivalent role to hydrogen peroxide and acts as the catalyst for the peroxidase reaction with the haem molecule
Acetic acid	Acts as a solvent for Leuco Malachite Green
Methanol	The presence of a short-chain alcohol in the dyeing solution helps to prevent the blood from diffusing during the dyeing stage
HFE7100	Acts as the principal carrier solvent for the working solution, having the advantages of low toxicity and low flammability. It also evaporates rapidly from the surface being treated

To fix any marks in blood present, the item is first immersed in methanol for 5 min. Once fixing is complete, the item is exposed to the working solution by immersion or pouring and then allowed to air dry. The green colour develops rapidly as the item dries.

13.4.3.3   *Leuco Crystal Violet*

This Leuco dye is converted from its colourless Leuco form to the purple/violet coloured form (Basic Violet 3) on contact with blood.

Most Leuco Crystal Violet formulations use a single working solution. A commonly used formulation originally proposed for enhancing footwear marks in blood (Bodziak, 1996) is given hereafter:

Working solution

5-Sulphosalicylic acid	10 g
3% Hydrogen peroxide	500 mL
Sodium acetate	3.7 g
Leuco Crystal Violet	1 g

The roles of the constituents in the working solution are as follows:

5-Sulphosalicylic acid	Acts as the fixing agent and operates by precipitating basic proteins from the blood
Hydrogen peroxide	Acts as the catalyst for the peroxidase reaction with the haem molecule
Sodium acetate	Provides alkali conditions that increase the specificity of Leuco Crystal Violet reaction with blood over potential false-positive reactions
Leuco Crystal Violet	The active colourless Leuco dye constituent, oxidised during the peroxidase reaction to give the violet coloured form of the dye

Leuco Crystal Violet is generally applied to the enhancement area via a spray method, sprayers giving a fine, even mist being preferable. Alternatively, items can be immersed into the working solution in a dish.

13.4.3.4 *Luminol*

The two most widely published formulations for luminol (3-aminophthalhydrazide) are those proposed by Grodsky et al. (1951) and Weber (1966) in the following text, and proprietary pre-prepared products are also available. The formulations given by Grodsky and Weber are summarised hereafter:

Grodsky et al. (1951):

Working solution

Sodium perborate	3.5 g
Distilled water	500 mL
Luminol	0.5 g
Sodium carbonate	25 g

The roles of the constituents in the formulation are as follows:

Sodium perborate	Acts as the catalyst for the peroxidase reaction with the haem molecule
Luminol	The active constituent of the reagent, producing a blue chemiluminescence when reacting with haem
Sodium carbonate	Provides alkali conditions that are required for the chemiluminescent luminol reaction to occur with the haem present in blood

The solution earlier is left to stand for 5 min after mixing and then used immediately.

Weber (1966):

A working solution is produced from three stock solutions:

Sodium hydroxide solution:	
Sodium hydroxide	8 g
Distilled water	500 mL
Hydrogen peroxide solution:	
30% Hydrogen peroxide	10 mL
Distilled water	490 mL
Luminol solution:	
Luminol	0.354 g
Sodium hydroxide solution	62.5 mL

Make up to final volume of 500 mL with distilled water

The roles of the constituents in the formulation are as follows:

Sodium hydroxide	Provides alkali conditions that are required for the chemiluminescent luminol reaction to occur with the haem present in blood
Hydrogen peroxide	Acts as the catalyst for the peroxidase reaction with the haem molecule
Luminol	The active constituent of the reagent, producing a blue chemiluminescence when reacting with haem

The working solution is produced by mixing a 10 mL sodium hydroxide solution with 10 mL of hydrogen peroxide, 10 mL of luminol solution and 70 mL distilled water.

Both formulations of luminol are applied to the area being treated via a spray method. In common with other spray reagents, sprayers giving a fine, even mist give the best results and minimise diffusion of detail.

The bluish-white chemiluminescence that results from a positive reaction with blood is faint and must be viewed in the dark by an operator who is fully dark adapted to obtain the best results. Even with careful application of luminol the fine detail of blood-contaminated fingerprints may be easily damaged by diffusion (Figure 13.2), because the formulations do not contain a fixative. For this reason the process is not recommended for fingermarks where the retention of the fine detail is essential.

13.4.3.5 *Fluorescein*

Fluorescein is used in another presumptive test for blood that utilises the peroxidase activity of the haem group. It is usually applied in a two-step process. The application of fluorescein alone will develop the yellow colouration; however an overspray of hydrogen peroxide is also used to reduce the occurrence of background fluorescence and false-positive reactions.

The preparation of fluorescein is not a trivial process and can be time-consuming. The solution containing the reduced form fluorescin has a very short shelf life, and it is recommended that it is used within 24 h. The original formulation (Cheeseman and DiMeo, 1995) is as follows:

Fluorescein solution	
Fluorescein	1.0 g
Sodium hydroxide	10 g
Deionised water	100 mL
Zinc powder	10.0 g

The water and sodium hydroxide should be mixed first, and then the fluorescein is added, whilst the solution is gently heated and stirred. It should then be heated to a gentle boil when zinc powder is added. The solution should be allowed to cool then be decanted to remove undissolved zinc.

Thickening solution

Xanthan gum	4.75 g
Deionised water	950 mL

The working solution is produced by mixing 50 mL fluorescein solution with 950 mL of the thickening solution. This reagent must then be kept in dark glassware. The roles of the constituents in the formulation are as follows:

Fluorescein	The active dye constituent of the reagent. Reduced to the colourless, non-fluorescent fluorescin form in the working solution and converted back to the fluorescent fluorescein form in the presence of haem
Sodium hydroxide	Provides alkali conditions that increase the specificity of fluorescein reaction with blood over potential false-positive reactions
Deionised water	The common, non-flammable solvent for fluorescein and sodium hydroxide
Zinc powder	Acts as the reducing reagent in the working solution, converting the fluorescein dye to the reduced fluorescin form
Xanthan gum	Acts as a thickening agent for the working solution

The process is carried out in two stages, the second stage requiring a hydrogen peroxide overspray solution:

Hydrogen peroxide overspray solution

30% Hydrogen peroxide	100 mL
Deionised water	200 mL

Hydrogen peroxide	Acts as the catalyst for the peroxidase reaction with the haem molecule

The fluorescein working solution is applied to the surface of interest using a fine spray unit, using no more than two applications to minimise diffusion of detail. It is then oversprayed with the hydrogen peroxide solution. The developed marks are detected using fluorescence examination, with excitation using a light source with output between 425 and 485 nm and viewing through a yellow-orange barrier filter.

A potential drawback of this formulation is that it is caustic and can cause damage to some substrates that may be treated, for example, aluminium. Alternative formulations have been proposed to overcome this (Di Benedetto et al., 2004).

References

Alder O, Alder R, 'Über das Verhalten gewisser organischer Verbindungen gegenüber Blut mit besonderer Berücksichtigung des Nachweises von Blut', Z Physiol Chem (Germ), vol 41, (1904), p 59.

Allman D, Pounds C A, 'The specificity of diaminobenzidine for the detection of blood', Technical Note, Central Research and Support Establishment, The Forensic Science Service, April 1992.

Au C, Jackson-Smith H, Quinones I, Jones B J, Daniel B, 'Wet powder suspensions as an additional technique for the enhancement of bloodied marks', Forensic Sci Int, vol 204(1–3), (2011), p 13–18.

Bandey H L (ed.), 'Fingermark Visualisation Manual', Home Office, London, 2014.

Barnett K G, Bone R G, Hall P W, Ide R H, 'The use of water soluble protein dye for the enhancement of footwear impressions in blood on non-porous surfaces part 1', Forensic Science Service UK, Tech Note No 629, July 1988.

Bodziak W J, 'Use of Leuco-Crystal Violet to enhance shoeprints in blood', Forensic Sci Int, vol 82, (1996), p 45–52.

Bradshaw R, Bleay S, Clench M R, Francese S, 'Direct detection of blood in fingermarks by MALDI MS profiling and Imaging', Sci Justice, vol 54(2), (2014), p 110–117.

Castelló A, Francés F, Corella D, Verdú F, 'Active oxygen doctors the evidence', Sci Nat, vol 96(2), (2009), p 303–307.

Cheeseman R, DiMeo L A, 'Fluorescein as a field-worthy latent bloodstain detection system', J Forensic Identif, vol 45(6), (1995), p 631–646.

Christie R M, Mather R R, Wardman R H, The Chemistry of Colour Application, Blackwell Science Ltd, Oxford, 2000, p 19–20.

Cox M, 'A study of the sensitivity and specificity of four presumptive tests for blood', J Forensic Sci, vol 36, (1991), p 1503–1511.

Di Benedetto J, Kyle K, Boan T, Marie C, 'Method and compositions for detecting of bloodstains using fluorescin-fluorescein reaction', Patent US 6692967 B1, Publication date 17 February 2004.

Edelman G, van Leeuwen T G, Aalders M C, 'Hyperspectral imaging for the age estimation of blood stains at the crime scene', Forensic Sci Int, vol 223(1–3), (2012), p 72–77.

Frégeau C J, Germain O, Fourney R M, 'Fingerprint enhancement revisited and the effects of blood enhancement chemicals on subsequent Profiler Plus™ fluorescent short tandem repeat DNA analysis of fresh and aged bloody fingerprints', J Forensic Sci, vol 45(2), (2000), p 354–380.

Garner D D, Cano K M, Peimer R S, Yeshion T E, 'An evaluation of tetramethylbenzidine as a presumptive test for blood', J Forensic Sci, vol 21(4), (1976), p 816–821.

Godsell J, 'Fingerprint techniques', J Forensic Sci Soc, vol 3(2), (1963), p 79–87.

Grodsky M, Wright K, Kirk P L, 'Simplified preliminary blood testing: an improved technique and comparative study of methods', J Am Inst Crim Law Criminol, vol 42, (1951), p 95–104.

Huss K, Clark J, Chisum W J, 'Which was first – fingerprint or blood?', J Forensic Identif, vol 50(4), (2000), p 344–350.

Hussain J I, Pounds C A, 'The enhancement of marks made in blood with 3,3′,4,4′-tetraaminobiphenyl', Forensic Science Service UK, Central Research and Support Establishment Report 653, March 1989.

Jaret Y, Heriau M, Donche A, 'Transfer of bloody fingerprints', J Forensic Identif, vol 47(1), (1997), p 38–41.

Kastle J H, Shedd O M, 'Phenolphthalin as a reagent for the oxidizing ferments', Am Chem J, vol 26, (1901), p 526.

Langenburg G, 'Deposition of bloody friction ridge impressions', J Forensic Identif, vol 58(3), (2008), p 255–289.

Li B, Beveridge P, O'Hare W T, Islam M, 'The estimation of the age of a blood stain using reflectance spectroscopy with a microspectrophotometer, spectral pre-processing and linear discriminant analysis', Forensic Sci Int, vol 212(1), (2011), p 198–204.

Li B, Beveridge P, O'Hare W T, Islam M, 'The age estimation of blood stains up to 30 days old using visible wavelength hyperspectral image analysis and linear discriminant analysis', Sci Justice, vol 53(3), (2013), p 270–277.

Norkus P, Noppinger K, 'New reagent for the enhancement of blood prints', Identif News, vol 26(4), (1986), p 5.

Patel E, Cicatiello P, Deininger L, Clench M R, Marino G, Giardina P, Langenburg G, West A, Marshall P, Sears V, Francese S, 'A proteomic approach for the rapid, multi-informative and reliable identification of blood', Analyst, vol 141, (2016), p 191–198.

Ponce A C and Pascual F A V, 'Critical revision of presumptive tests for bloodstains', Forensic Sci Commun, vol 1(2), (1999). https://archives.fbi.gov/archives/about-us/lab/forensic-science-communications/fsc/july1999/ponce.htm (accessed 29 October 2017).

Préstamo G, Manzano P, 'Peroxidases of selected fruits and vegetables and the possible use of ascorbic acid as an antioxidant', Hort Sci, vol 28(1), (1993), p 48–50.

Ruttan R F, Hardisty R H M, 'A new reagent for detecting occult blood', Can Med Assoc J, vol 2(11), (1912), p 995–998.

Sears V G, Prizeman T M, 'The enhancement of fingerprints in blood – part 1: the optimization of Amido Black', J Forensic Identif, vol 50(5), (2000), p 470–480.

Sears V G, Butcher C P G, Prizeman T M, 'The enhancement of fingerprints in blood – part 2: protein dyes', J Forensic Ident, vol 51(1), (2001), p 28–38.

Sears V G, Butcher C P G, Fitzgerald L, 'Enhancement of fingerprints in blood – part 3: reactive techniques, Acid Yellow 7 and process sequences', J Forensic Identif, vol 55(6), (2005), p 741–763.

Specht W, 'Die Chemiluminescenz des Hämins, ein Hilfsmittel zur Auffindung und Erkennung forensisch wichtiger Blutspuren,' Angew Chem, vol 50(8), (1937), p 155–157.

Teichmann L, 'Ueber die Krystallisation des Orpnischen Be-standtheile des Blutes', Z Ration Med, vol 3, (1853), p 375–388.

Theeuwen A B, van Barneveld S, Drok J W, Keereweer I, Limborgh J C, Naber W M, Velders T, 'Enhancement of footwear impressions in blood', Forensic Sci Int, vol 95(2), (1998), p 133–151.

Weber K, 'Die andwendung der chemiluminescenz des Luminols in der gerichtlichenmedizin und toxicology. I. Der nachweis van blutspuren', Dtsch Z Gesamte Gerichtl Med, vol 57, (1966), p 410–423.

Further reading

Caldwell J P, Kim N D, 'Extension of the colour suite available for chemical enhancement of fingerprints in blood', J Forensic Sci, vol 47(2), (2002), p 332–340.

Gershenfeld L, 'Orthotolidine and orthotoluidine tests for occult blood', Am J Pharm, vol 111, (1939), p 17.

Hochmeister M N, Budowle B, Sparkes R, Rudin O, Gehrig C, Thali M, Schmidt L, Cordier A, Dirnhofer R, 'Validation studies of an immunochromatographic 1-step test for the forensic identification of human blood', J Forensic Sci, vol 44(3), (1999), p 597–602.

Holland V R, Saunders B C, Rose F L, Walpole A L, 'A safer substitute for benzidine in the detection of blood', Tetrahedron, vol 30, (1974), p 3299–3302.

Hoppe F, 'Ueber das Verhalten des Blutfarbstoffes in Spectrum des Sonnenlichtes', Arch Pathol Anat Physiol Klin Med, vol 23(4), (1862), p 446.

Johnston E, Ames C E, Dagnell K E, Foster J, Daniel B E, 'Comparison of presumptive blood test kits including hexagon OBTI', J Forensic Sci, vol 53(3), (2008), p 687–689.

Kastle J H, Amoss H L, 'Variations in the Peroxidase Activity of the Blood in Health and Disease', US Hygienic Laboratory, Bulletin No 31, US Public Health and Marine Hospital Service, US Govt. Printing Office, Washington, DC, 1906.

Lee H C, 'Benzidine or O-tolidine?', Identif News, January 1984, p 13.

Medinger P, 'Zum Nachweis minimalster Blutspuren', Dtsch Z Gesamte Gerichtl Med, vol 20, (1933), p 74.

Meyer E, 'Beiträge zu rLeukocyten frage', Munch Med Wochenschr, vol 50(35), (1903) p 1489.

Olsen R D, 'Sensitivity comparison of blood enhancement techniques', Identif News, August 1985, p 10–14.

Schönbein C F, 'Ueber das Verhalten des Blutes zum Sauerstoff', Verh Naturforsch Ges Basel, vol 3, (1863), p 516.

Shipp E, Fassett M, Wright R, Togneri E, 'Tetramethylbenzidine to the rescue', J Forensic Identif, vol 44(2), (1994), p 159–164.

Sorby H C, 'On the application of spectrum analysis to microscopical investigations, and especially to the detection of bloodstains', Q J Sci, vol 2, (1865), p 198.

Soret J L, 'Analyse spectrale: sur le spectre d'absorption du sang dans la partie violette et ultraviolette', CR Acad Sci, vol 97, (1883), p 1269.

Stokes G G, 'On the reduction and oxidation of the colouring matter of the blood', Proc R Soc Lond, vol 13, (1864), p 355.

Takayama M, 'A method for identifying blood by hemochromogen crystallization', Kokka Igakkai Zasshi, vol 306, (1912), p 463.

Van Deen J, 'Tinctura guajaci und ein Ozontrager, als reagens auf sehr geringe Blutmengen, nämentlich in medico-forensischen fallen', Arch Holland Beitr Naturkd Heilk, vol 3(2), (1861), p 227–230.

14

Electrical and electrochemical processes

Stephen M. Bleay

Home Office Centre for Applied Science and Technology, Sandridge, UK

Key points

- The principal application of electrical and electrochemical processes is in the enhancement of fingermarks on metal surfaces.

- Most processes in the general group utilise the ability of the fingermark to act as a mask on the metal surface, resulting in different rates of material growth or etching between ridges and background.

- There is the potential to tailor processes for use on different types of metal.

- Some processes in this group operate by enhancing the residual effect of the fingermark on the surface, as opposed to constituents or properties of the mark itself. They may therefore continue to be effective when marks have been wiped from the surface.

14.1 Introduction

The principal application of electrical and electrochemical processes is in the enhancement of fingermarks on metal surfaces. Whilst the majority of non-porous substrates received in laboratories are effectively chemically inert, in the case of metals there is the potential for chemical reactions to occur between the metal and either the chemicals in the fingermark or those used in the enhancement process. Both these possible modes of reaction can be utilised to enhance fingermarks on metal surfaces.

Fingerprint Development Techniques: Theory and Application, First Edition.
Stephen M. Bleay, Ruth S. Croxton and Marcel de Puit.
© 2018 John Wiley & Sons Ltd. Published 2018 by John Wiley & Sons Ltd.

It has been discussed in Chapter 3 how reactions can occur between constituents of the fingermark (e.g. salts) and the metal surface. In extreme circumstances this can result in a permanent record of the fingermark being etched into the metal surface (e.g. Figure 4.14), and it has been shown that heating metals may be used as a means of promoting this corrosion mechanism and visualising marks (Bond, 2008a, 2008b; Wightman and O'Connor, 2011). However, the interactions that occur are very dependent on the metals present and the particular constituents in the fingerprint, and reactions will only occur if conditions are favourable. In many cases the metal will be alloyed with other elements to inhibit such corrosion reactions occurring, for example, 'stainless' steel.

Even if the corrosion of the metal does not proceed to the extent that the fingermark becomes visible, the fact that corrosion has been initiated can still be exploited. Such exploitation may still be possible even where the fingermark deposits have been wiped from the surface, because although the physical deposits have been removed, the residual corrosion signature left by them on and beneath the metal surface remains. Chemical etching processes can be used to selectively etch the surface in the regions where corrosion has already been initiated, thus increasing the contrast between the ridges and the background. Other researchers have proposed using alternative means to image the residual corrosion signature, including scanning the surface to produce a map of Volta potential (Williams et al., 2001; Williams and McMurray, 2007) and charging the surface then using cascade toner powder to develop an electrostatic image of the corroded areas (Bond, 2008a).

When sebaceous marks are deposited on metals, corrosion reactions are less likely to occur between the fingermark and the surface. However, sebaceous marks can still be enhanced on metals using similar methods to those outlined previously but using different mechanisms. Because sebaceous fingermarks contain many water-insoluble constituents, they effectively act as a 'mask' and protect the metal surface from aqueous etching solutions and vapours. As a consequence, etching solutions (or fumes) will attack the exposed metal surface, but not the protected areas under the fingermark, providing sufficient contrast for the mark to be visualised (Given, 1976; Cantu et al., 1998). The sebaceous material can also behave as a thin insulating layer giving local modification of the Volta potential on the surface, enabling the mark to be revealed by scanning processes (Williams et al., 2001; Williams and McMurray, 2007).

In addition to etching techniques, where material is selectively dissolved from the surface and into solution, electrodeposition processes have been proposed for fingermark enhancement (Belcher, 1977; Migron and Mandler, 1997; Beresford and Hillman, 2010). In electrodeposition, metal (or polymer) is deposited from solution onto the surface, and if the presence of the fingermark constituents inhibits (or accelerates) growth of the deposit on the ridges relative to the rate of growth on the background, contrast between the two regions will again be enhanced. Most commonly, the presence of the fingermark constituents acts as a mask, and preferential deposition occurs on the exposed metal surface, although both types of behaviour may be observed.

Because of the wide range of different types of metal and alloy that may be encountered, there is no single electrical or electrochemical process that is capable of enhancing marks on all of them. There is, however, the potential to optimise processes for particular types of metal so that the most appropriate process can be selected once the type of metal surface present has been identified.

14.2 Current operational use

The untreated metal surface of most operational relevance is brass, particularly when encountered in the form of cartridge cases. These items have always presented a problem for fingermark enhancement because of the conditions they are exposed to during the firing process. High temperatures, abrasion and deposition of propellant residue all reduce the chances of recovering fingermarks (Wiesener et al., 1995), and operational success rates are very low. As a consequence, a variety of processes continue to be considered and evaluated for this application. Other commonly encountered metals such as stainless steel and aluminium are more chemically inert, and results obtained using conventional processes (such as cyanoacrylate fuming), which are described in other chapters, are reasonable. However, it is possible that that improved performance could be obtained using processes more optimised to the metal type present, although more research would be required to establish which processes were most suited to different metal types.

In general, etching processes are less effective than those involving electrodeposition of metals or polymers, and they are not widely used.

There are two processes that utilise the residual corrosion signature left on the metal surface by the fingermark, the scanning Kelvin probe (SKP) and the cartridge electrostatic recovery apparatus (CERA). The SKP process is not currently in routine use on casework. The process is in theory non-destructive, for subsequent fingermark enhancement techniques, DNA recovery and examination of firing and rifling marks. The process is relatively slow, taking several hours to scan a single cartridge casing at high resolution, but for serious cases may provide valuable information. It has been applied to a limited number of operational cases, and although some ridge detail and other features of interest have been detected, no identifiable fingermarks have been imaged.

The CERA technique has been applied to several operational cases, and in some of these cases some ridge detail has been developed (Bond and Heidel, 2009). The early reported effectiveness of the technique has not yet been replicated in commercially produced equipment, and it is not now widely used.

Electrochemical processes are not currently in regular use for fingermark enhancement in the United Kingdom. This is because some of the chemicals used in the processes are highly corrosive and there are health and safety issues associated with their use. However, processes such as gun blueing and palladium deposition have been shown to be more effective than cyanoacrylate fuming on brass cartridge cases either used on their own or as additional processes after a cyanoacrylate fuming treatment (Saunders and Cantu, 1995; Dominick and Laing, 2011; Girelli et al., 2015), and in many countries worldwide, they are more regularly used. More extensive studies into their relative effectiveness and optimum processing sequences are desirable before such techniques can be more widely exploited.

Recent comparative studies (Beresford et al., 2011) indicate that on stainless steel surfaces the electrodeposition of polymers may be at least as effective as alternatives such as cyanoacrylate fuming, powders and powder suspensions and further research may result in more widespread use of such processes in the future.

The rising trends in theft of copper-containing metal items for scrap value have raised a requirement for a rapid and cheap method of developing fingermarks on these articles. As a consequence there has been interest in adapting the electroless silver deposition process (Abbott et al., 2007; Gu et al., 2010) to the enhancement of fingermarks on copper and copper-based alloy surfaces, and comparative studies on this process are underway.

14.3   Etching

14.3.1   Outline history of the process

1976: Given included nitric acid as a fuming process for enhancing fingermarks on cartridge cases.

1978: Jones followed suggestions made by Belcher (1977) and investigated a range of etching and electrodeposition processes. Those utilising etching included nitric acid, which showed some preferential etching of nickel-based casings; copper sulphate, which also etched nickel; and hydrochloric, sulphuric and hydroiodic acids, which gave no useful results.

1998: Cantu et al. demonstrated that acidified hydrogen peroxide can be used to remove excess gun blue and also to visualise sebaceous prints on metal surfaces by selectively etching the background.

14.3.2   Theory

Etching processes operate by selective removal of material from the surface, with the difference in the removal rate between the regions of the fingermark ridge and the adjacent regions of the metal, providing sufficient contrast to visualise the fingermark. Marks may be revealed in two ways, outlined in the succeeding text.

When sebaceous marks are present, the deposits effectively act as a protective film, masking the metal underneath the ridges from the etching solution or vapours. As a consequence the surrounding metal is etched more than the metal underneath

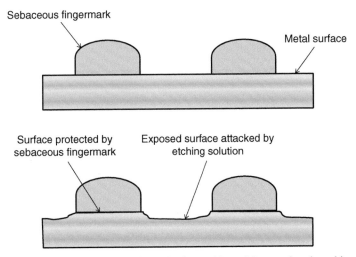

Figure 14.1 Schematic diagram showing selective etching of the metal and masking of regions under the ridges by a sebaceous mark.

the fingermark ridges (Figure 14.1) and may also differ in colour from the pristine metal. A similar effect can be obtained if the surface has initially been treated with a process building up an inert layer on the fingermark, such as cyanoacrylate fuming. In this case the polycyanoacrylate deposit acts as the mask instead of the sebaceous fingermark.

Where marks with high eccrine content are present on certain types of metal surface, corrosion may be initiated on the surface in the regions of the fingermark ridges. Once initiated, this corrosion may be accelerated by heating or by application of an etching solution, and the ridges become more deeply etched into the surface (Figure 14.2).

14.3.3 Etching processes

The most commonly used etching solution is acidified hydrogen peroxide, originally proposed for the removal of lead and excess gun blue from cartridge casings (Cantu et al., 1998). The formulation recommended is a single working solution made up as follows:

5% Acetic acid solution	14.1 mL
3% Hydrogen peroxide solution	20.0 mL

The process is most suited to application on brass surfaces. The item to be treated is immersed in the working solution until sufficient contrast is observed between mark and background and then immersed in a water bath to stop the reaction. Etched

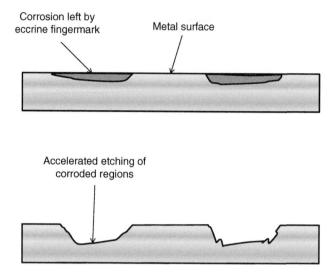

Figure 14.2   Schematic diagram showing selective etching of the corrosion initiated by the ridges of the eccrine mark.

regions are grey in colour. This reagent is thought to give a lower possibility of overdevelopment on brass surfaces compared with gun blueing.

The process may be used on latent marks, although it is also recommended as a secondary treatment for items that have previously been treated using cyanoacrylate fuming.

14.4   Corrosion visualisation

14.4.1   Outline history of the process

2001: Williams and McMurray first observed that the SKP technique, traditionally used for detecting the onset of corrosion in metals, can be applied in the direct detection of fingermarks on metal surfaces. The process is found to remain effective even after the mark has been wiped from the surface.

2008a: Bond proposed a combination of heating, electrostatic charging and powdering as an alternative means of visualising the corrosion left on the metal surface by the fingermark.

2010: Bleay et al. showed that disulphur dinitride sublimation can be used to enhance fingermarks on wiped metal surfaces, indicating that this process also targets residual corrosion.

2011: Wightman and O'Connor further investigated the potential use of heating to enhance marks on a range of metal surfaces, in some cases utilising colour changes in the surface oxidation layers to increase contrast.

14.4.2   Theory

The theory behind all corrosion visualisation processes is that the corrosion initiated on the surface by an eccrine fingermark produces a region that has different electrical characteristics from the adjacent, pristine regions (Figure 14.3).

It is proposed by Bond (2008a) that corrosion is locally initiated on the metal surface by the action of chloride ions in the eccrine fingermark residues. In general, the process operating is

$$M^{Z+} + Z.Cl^- + Z.H_2O \rightarrow M(OH)_Z + Z(H^+ + Cl^-)$$

Sebaceous fingermarks can also locally modify the electrical properties, effectively acting as a thin insulating layer over the conducting metal surface.

The corrosion visualisation processes all visualise marks in different ways. In the SKP method proposed by Williams et al. (2001), the subtle differences in the electrical properties of the surface are directly imaged using a probe that is scanned across the metal surface. The probe used is a fine vibrating gold electrode that is brought into close proximity to the metal surface, but not placed in contact with it. The theory associated with the SKP process is outlined in the succeeding text.

The vibrating tip of the gold probe and the metal surface act as the two plates of a parallel plate capacitor. Any material in the space between them, which includes air and any insulating layers on the surface, acts as the dielectric in the capacitor.

If a Volta potential difference (ΔV) exists between the probe tip and the metal surface, the vibration of the probe tip will cause a periodic change in the capacitance, and this in turn generates an alternating current, $i(t)$, in an external circuit. A DC bias voltage E is applied to cancel the alternating current $i(t)$, and the measured value of E can therefore be directly related to the value of ΔV. The circuit is illustrated in Figure 14.4.

It can therefore be seen that as the probe tip is scanned across the surface, any slight changes to the electrical properties of the material between the probe tip and metal surface, or in the metal surface itself, can result in changes to ΔV. By continuously recording and displaying the measured values as the probe is scanned, a Volta

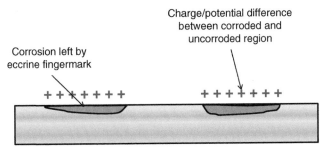

Figure 14.3   Schematic diagram showing differences in electrical properties between the region of the fingermark and the uncorroded surface.

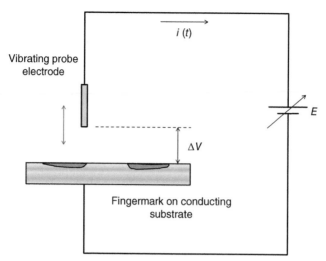

Figure 14.4   Schematic diagram showing principle of operation of scanning Kelvin probe.

potential map of the surface can be generated, and the presence of the fingermark revealed by differences in Volta potential of the ridges and adjacent background. Both eccrine and sebaceous fingerprints can be detected by this method because they can locally modify the surface properties as described previously (Figure 14.5a). By conducting a topographical scan prior to the scan to measure Volta potential, it is possible to obtain images of marks on surfaces with more complex shapes (Figure 14.5b).

In the technique proposed by Bond (2008a), the method used to visualise the residual corrosion is different. The metal surface is first heated to accelerate corrosion and oxidation of the surface. This step alone may produce sufficient contrast between the fingermark and the pristine metal for the mark to be seen without any further treatment (Wightman and O'Connor, 2011). An electrostatic charge of 2.5 kV is then applied to the surface, creating a difference in charging characteristics between the corroded and uncorroded regions (as for the ESDA process, Section 8.4). This charge pattern is then visualised by applying carbon-coated spherical beads (as used in the ESDA process) to the surface, the carbon toner particles preferentially adhering to the more highly charged regions of the mark. This technique is unlikely to be effective in visualising sebaceous marks because corrosion is not initiated by sebaceous residues.

14.4.3   Corrosion visualisation processes

The nature of corrosion visualisation processes means that specialised equipment is required for their application. Williams and McMurray (2007) constructed apparatus for the scanning of cylindrical items such as cartridge casings, mounting the

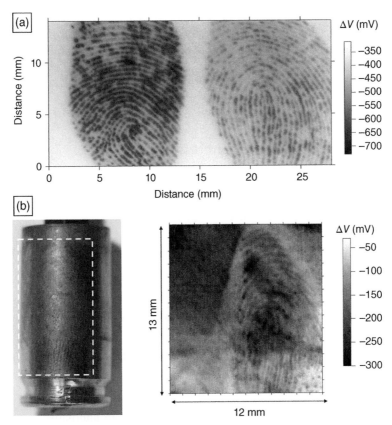

Figure 14.5 Scanning Kelvin probe images. (a) Greyscale interpolated Volta potential maps produced by substantially eccrine (left) and sebaceous (right) fingermarks on a planar iron surface. Scans were carried out at room temperature and ambient humidity using a 0.1 mm diameter profiled gold wire probe and scanning at a probe to sample height of 0.05 mm using a data point density of 20 pts/mm, and (b) fresh sebaceous fingermark deposited on 9 mm Luger calibre bullet, fired using a Smith & Wesson model 5903 handgun. Visual image of scanned surface along with SKP-derived Volta potential maps recorded 12 days after firing. Images reproduced courtesy of Swansea University.

cartridge casing on a spindle and rotating it underneath the vibrating gold probe. An initial scan was carried out to register sample topography prior to conducting Volta potential measurements so that measurements could be corrected for irregularities in surface profile. It has also been shown that it is possible to enhance the difference in Volta potential between the fingermark and the background by depositing thin metal layers over the surface (e.g. by vacuum metal deposition) prior to carrying out SKP (Dafydd et al., 2014). There are commercial suppliers of SKP equipment, but none have yet been adapted for fingermark visualisation.

Commercial equipment has also been produced using the principles published by Bond (2008a). This also utilises a spindle for the mounting of cartridge cases, which are electrostatically charged and then rotated underneath a stream of toner powder to visualise the mark.

14.5   Electrodeposition

14.5.1   Outline history of the process

1977: Belcher experimented with different methods of visualising fingermarks on heated metal surfaces, including gun blueing of steel surfaces and brown photographic toner solutions for enhancing marks on copper.

1978: Jones investigated a further range of deposition processes including 5% selenic acid, which gave the 'gun blueing' effect on brass with some results on steel and nickel, and a solution of antimony in hydrochloric acid, which plated antimony onto the metal surfaces.

1980: Belcher proposed potassium permanganate solution as an alternative method for enhancing marks on copper.

1995: Saunders and Cantu published results of tests using a modified physical developer, acidified silver nitrate and gun blueing on unfired cartridge casings and also compared cyanoacrylate fuming and gun blueing on a range of fired cases.

1995: Migron et al. proposed palladium deposition as an alternative process for enhancing marks on cartridge cases.

1996: Bentsen et al. tested further electrodeposition techniques on fired cartridge cases including solutions of copper, nickel, chromium and tin sulphate at different concentrations, comparing results with 4% selenious acid (the principal constituent of gun blueing solutions). Selenious acid was found to have the highest sensitivity.

2001: Smith and Kauffman reported the use of alternative selenious acid-based formulations such as aluminium black incorporating a range of other chemicals, making them more suited for enhancing marks on aluminium.

2001: Bersellini et al. proposed electropolymerisation of pyrroles as a means of visualising sebaceous marks on metal surfaces.

2010: Beresford and Hillman utilised electropolymerisation of aniline to visualise fingermarks and showed that the electrochromic properties of the polymer can be further used to change the contrast between the fingermark and the metal surface.

2013: Qin et al. reported the deposition of thin films of Prussian blue for visualising fingermarks on metal surfaces.

2015: James and Altamimi used cold patination fluid as a means of enhancing marks on unfired ammunition.

14.5.2 Theory

A wide variety of different electrodeposition processes have been proposed, resulting in the deposition of both metallic and polymeric films on the surface. All processes utilise the same fundamental principle in that a sebaceous fingermark (or mark developed using a prior treatment such as cyanoacrylate fuming) acts as a mask on the surface. The reaction that results in the deposition of the film on the surface is able to occur where exposed metal is present, but not in regions that are masked by the fingermark (Figure 14.6). Fingermarks are revealed by the differences in growth rate of the film on the ridges and on the background.

The specific reactions that result in film formation differ and some of those that are utilised are outlined as follows:

Silver nitrate: Silver nitrate can be used on brass or copper surfaces, where a reaction occurs between the silver in solution and the copper in exposed regions of the surface. This results in the deposition of silver (as a grey deposit) on the surface according to the reaction

$$2Ag^+ + Cu \rightleftharpoons 2Ag + Cu^{2+}$$

Gun blueing: The gun blueing process principally utilises the reaction that occurs between selenious acid and metals, shown as follows:

$$H_2SeO_3 + 4H^+ + 4e^- \rightleftharpoons Se + 3H_2O$$

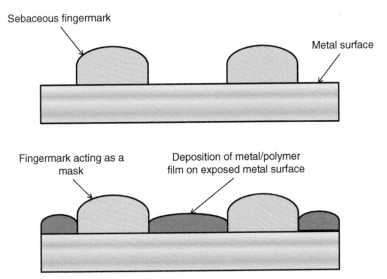

Figure 14.6   Schematic diagram showing fingermark enhancement by selective growth of surface films on a metal surface, with the fingermark acting as a mask.

Although this reaction can occur between selenious acid and a range of differ-ent metals, 'gun blueing' is most suited to the enhancement of marks on brass where parallel reactions can occur between copper and zinc as well as zinc and selenious acid. The outcome of these reactions is the formation of a black CuSe reaction product on the surface, which provides excellent contrast with the regions of metal masked by the fingermark:

$$Cu^{2+} + Zn \rightarrow Cu + Zn^{2+}$$

$$H_2SeO_3 + 4H^+ + 2Zn \rightarrow Se + 3H_2O + 2Zn^{2+}$$

$$Se + Cu \rightarrow CuSe$$

Palladium deposition: A range of palladium compounds have been investigated for use in the palladium deposition process. The principal reactions of those found most applicable to enhancing fingermarks on brass are shown in the suc-ceeding text. In both cases a coating of grey palladium metal is formed on the surface:

$$Zn / Cu + 2Na_2PdCl_4 \rightarrow Pd + ZnCl_2 + CuCl_2 + 4NaCl$$

$$2Zn / Cu + 2K_2PdCl_6 \rightarrow Pd + 2ZnCl_2 + 2CuCl_2 + 4KCl$$

Polyaniline: Polyaniline is a conducting polymer formed on metal surfaces from the electrochemical polymerisation of aniline from an aqueous solution according to the reaction shown in Figure 14.7.

The polymerisation reaction is irreversible. Polyaniline has important charac-teristics that are utilised in the process proposed by Beresford and Hillman (2010). It is an electrochromic polymer with three different redox states. By controlling the potential applied to the deposited polymer layer, it is possible to change its col-our through a range from clear/yellow to green to dark blue, the structural changes and their associated colours being shown in Figure 14.8. Once the polymer film has been formed, these differently coloured redox states can be continually and reversibly accessed.

An example of a mark enhanced using polyaniline deposition is illustrated in Figure 14.9.

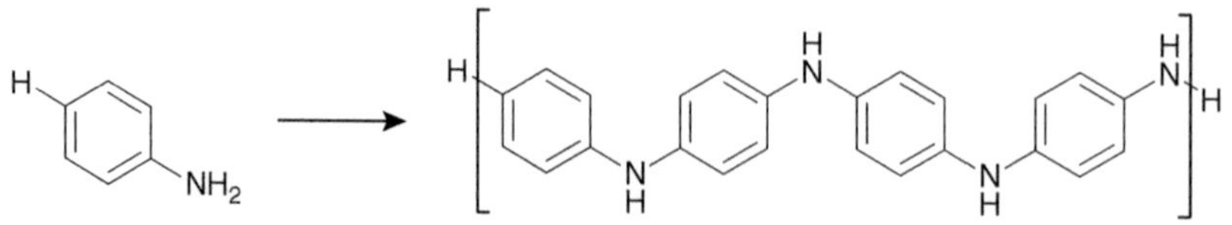

Figure 14.7   The polymerisation reaction of polyaniline.

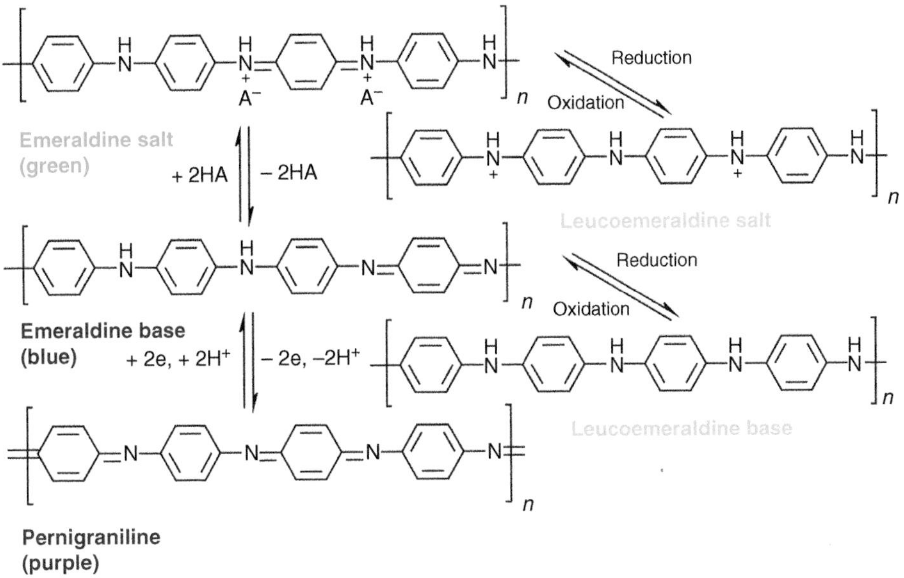

Emeraldine salt (green)

+ 2HA ‖ − 2HA

Leucoemeraldine salt

Reduction / Oxidation

Emeraldine base (blue)

+ 2e, + 2H⁺ ‖ − 2e, −2H⁺

$+ 2e, + 2H^+$ ‖ $- 2e, -2H^+$

Leucoemeraldine base

Reduction / Oxidation

Pernigraniline (purple)

Figure 14.8 The different oxidation states of polyaniline that can be utilised by electrochromic enhancement.

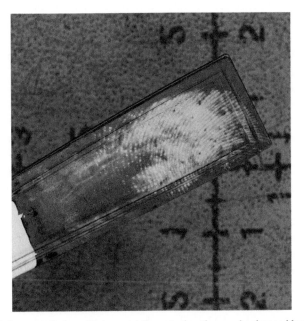

Figure 14.9 A fingermark deposited on stainless steel cutlery and enhanced by the electrodeposition of polyaniline. Image reproduced courtesy of the Home Office.

14.5.3   Electrodeposition processes

Gun blueing solutions can be made from chemicals; however because of the highly toxic nature of selenious acid, they are more often produced by dilution of commercial gun blueing solutions. A working solution used in recent comparative studies (Dominick and Laing, 2011) is given as follows:

Super blue liquid gun blue (Birchwood Casey)	2.3 mL
Distilled water	97.7 mL

Solutions for palladium deposition are made up as a single working solution as follows (Dominick and Laing, 2011):

Sodium chloride	2.93 g
Distilled water	50 mL
Palladium chloride	0.88 g

Both the aforementioned processes are applied by immersing the article to be treated into the working solution and directly observing development until optimum contrast is obtained between ridges and background, typically 30 s to 1 min. The article is then removed, rinsed in water to remove traces of the treatment solution and then dried.

Gun blueing results in the formation of a blue-black layer on the exposed metal surface, and palladium deposition results in a dark grey film. Examples of marks developed using gun blueing are illustrated in Figure 14.10.

Electrodeposition of polyaniline utilises a one-compartment three-electrode cell, which enables both the deposition of polyaniline and its subsequent electrochromic modification to be controlled electrochemically (Beresford et al., 2011).

The metal surface with fingermarks present on it is made the working electrode in the cell, with a platinum counter electrode and Ag/AgCl reference electrode. The electrolyte used in the cell is an aqueous acid solution with the aniline monomer, typically $1 M\ H_2SO_4$ or $0.2 M$ p-toluenesulphonic acid and $0.1 M$ aniline solution.

Polyaniline can be deposited potentiostatically using a voltage of 0.9 V or via cyclic voltammetry using a sweep rate of $20\ mV\ s^{-1}$ between 0.2 and 1.2 V.

Selective electrodeposition of poly-3,4-ethylenedioxythiophene (PEDOT) has been achieved in a similar way (Brown and Hillman, 2012).

The process proposed by Qin et al. (2013) for deposition of thin films of Prussian blue also utilised a one-compartment three-electrode cell using the metal item bearing fingermarks as the work electrode, platinum foil as the counter electrode and Ag/AgCl (saturated with $0.1 M$ KCl) as the reference electrode. The thin film of Prussian blue was electrodeposited from an aqueous $5\ mM$ solution of $K_3[Fe(CN)_6]$ and $5\ mM\ FeCl_3$ in $1\ mM$ HCl using cyclic voltammetry. During film deposition the electrode potential was cycled at a sweep rate of $50\ mV\ s^{-1}$ between 0.1 and 1.2 V.

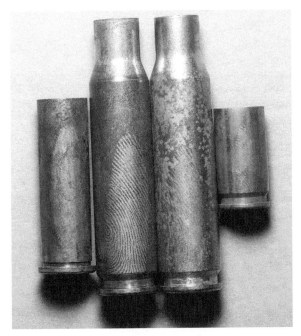

Figure 14.10 Fingermarks on brass and nickel cartridges developed using gun blueing.

References

Abbott A P, Nandhra S, Postlethwaite S, Smith E L, Ryder K S, 'Electroless deposition of metallic silver from a choline chloride-based ionic liquid: a study using acoustic impedance spectroscopy, SEM and atomic force microscopy', Phys Chem Chem Phys, vol 9(28), (2007), p 3735–3743.

Belcher G L, 'Methods of casting and latent print recovery', Fingerprint Identif Mag, vol 59(1), (1977), p 14–15.

Belcher G L, 'Developing latents on copper-coated casings', Fingerprint Whorld, vol 6(22), (1980), p 39.

Bentsen R K, Brown J K, Dinsmore A, Harvey K K, Kee T G, 'Post firing visualisation of fingerprints on spent cartridge cases', Sci Justice, vol 36, (1996), p 3–8.

Beresford A L, Hillman A R, 'Electrochromic enhancement of latent fingerprints on stainless steel surfaces', Anal Chem, vol 82, (2010), p 483–486.

Beresford A L, Brown R M, Hillman A R, 'Comparative study of electrochromic enhancement of latent fingerprints with existing development techniques', J Forensic Sci, vol 57, (2011), p 93–102.

Bersellini C, Garofano L, Giannetto M, Lusardi F, Mori G, 'Development of latent fingerprints on metallic surfaces using electropolymerization processes', J Forensic Sci, vol 46(4), (2001), p 871–877.

Bleay S M, Kelly P F, King R S P, 'Polymerisation of S_2N_2 to $(SN)_x$ as a tool for the rapid imaging of fingerprints removed from metal surfaces', J Mater Chem, vol 20, (2010), p 10100–10102.

Bond J W, 'Visualisation of latent fingerprint corrosion of metallic surfaces', J Forensic Sci, vol 53(4), (2008a), p 812–822.

Bond J W, 'The thermodynamics of latent fingerprint corrosion of metal elements and alloys', J Forensic Sci, vol 53(6), (2008b), p 1344–1352.

Bond J W, Heidel C, 'Visualisation of latent fingerprint corrosion on a discharged brass shell casing', J Forensic Sci, vol 54(4), (2009), p 892–894.

Brown R M, Hillman A R, 'Electrochromic enhancement of latent fingerprints by poly(3,4-ethylenedioxythiophene)', Phys Chem Chem Phys, vol 14, (2012), p 8653–8661.

Cantu A A, Leben D A, Ramotowski R, Kopera J, Simms J R, 'Use of acidified hydrogen peroxide to remove excess gun blue from gun blue-treated cartridge cases and to develop latent prints on untreated cartridge cases', J Forensic Sci, vol 43(2), (1998), p 294–298.

Dafydd H, Williams G, Bleay S, 'Latent fingerprint visualization using a scanning Kelvin probe in conjunction with vacuum metal deposition', J Forensic Sci, vol 59(1), (2014), p 211–218.

Dominick A J, Laing K, 'A comparison of six fingerprint enhancement techniques for the recovery of latent fingerprints from unfired cartridge cases', J Forensic Identif, vol 61(2), (2011), p 155–165.

Girelli C M A, Lobo B J M, Cunha A G, Freitas J C C, Emmerich F G, 'Comparison of practical techniques to develop latent fingermarks on fired and unfired cartridge cases', Forensic Sci Int, vol 250, (2015), p 17–26.

Given B W, 'Latent fingerprints on cartridges and expended cartridge casings', J Forensic Sci, vol 21(3), (1976), p 587–594.

Gu C D, Xu X J, Tu J P, 'Fabrication and wettability of nanoporous silver film on copper from choline chloride-based deep eutectic solvents', J Phys Chem C, vol 114, (2010), p 13614–13619.

James R M, Altamimi M J, 'The enhancement of friction ridge detail on brass ammunition casings using cold patination fluid', Forensic Sci Int, vol 257, (2015), p 385–392.

Migron Y, Mandler D, Frank A, Springer E, Almog J, 'Is a fingerprint left on a fired cartridge? The development of latent fingerprints on metallic surfaces by palladium deposition', Proceedings of the International Symposium on Fingerprint Detection and Identification, 26–30 June 1995, Ne'urim, Israel, p 217–226.

Migron Y, Mandler D, 'Development of latent fingerprints on unfired cartridges by palladium deposition: a surface study', J Forensic Sci, vol 42(6), (1997), p 986–992.

Qin G, Zhang M-Q, Zhang Y, Zhu Y, Liu S-L, Wu W-J, Zhang X-J, 'Visualization of latent fingerprints using Prussian blue thin films', Chin Chem Lett, vol 24, (2013), p 173–176.

Saunders G C, Cantu A A, 'Evaluation of several techniques for developing latent fingerprints on unfired and fired cartridge cases', Proceedings of the International Symposium on Fingerprint Detection and Identification, 26–30 June 1995, Ne'urim, Israel, p 155–160.

Smith K, Kauffman C, 'Enhancement of latent prints on metal surfaces', J Forensic Identif, vol 51(1), (2001), p 9–15.

Wiesener S, Springer E, Argaman U, 'A closer look at the effects of the shooting process on fingerprint development on fired cartridge cases', Proceedings of the International Symposium on Fingerprint Detection and Identification, 26–30 June 1995, Ne'urim, Israel, p 161–178.

Wightman G, O'Connor D, 'The thermal visualisation of latent fingermarks on metallic surfaces', Forensic Sci Int, vol 204(1–3), (2011), p 88–96.

Williams G, McMurray H N, Worsley D A, 'Latent fingerprint detection using a scanning Kelvin microprobe', J Forensic Sci, vol 46(5), (2001), p 1085–1092.

Williams G, McMurray N, 'Latent fingerprint visualisation using a scanning Kelvin probe', Forensic Sci Int, vol 167, (2007), p 102–109.

Further reading

Bond J W, 'Visualisation of latent fingerprint corrosion of brass', J Forensic Sci, vol 54(5), (2009), p 1034–1041.

Nizam F, Knaap W, Stewart J D, 'Development of fingerprints using electrolysis: a technical report into the development of fingerprints on fired brass cartridge cases', J Forensic Identif, vol 62(2), (2012), p 129–142.

Sapstead R M, Corden N, Hillman A R, 'Latent fingerprint enhancement via conducting electrochromic copolymer films of pyrrole and 3,4-ethylenedioxythiophene on stainless steel', Electrochim Acta, vol 162, (2015), p 119–128.

Wightman G, Emery F, Austin C, Andersson I, Harcus L, Arju G, Steven C, 'The interaction of fingermark deposits on metal surfaces and potential ways for visualisation', Forensic Sci Int, vol 249, (2015), p 241–254.

15

Miscellaneous processes: lifting and specialist imaging

Stephen M. Bleay

Home Office Centre for Applied Science and Technology, Sandridge, UK

Key points

- Lifting is a versatile process for separating marks from the surface they have been deposited on. It has traditionally been used on marks developed using other processes (e.g. powders) but can also be effective on latent marks.

- A range of specialist imaging processes are available that utilise high energy radiation or particles to eject molecules or emit characteristic radiation from the surface.

- Analysis of the radiation/molecules emitted from the surface can provide a wealth of additional contextual information to the investigator.

15.1   Introduction

In addition to the range of processes described in the previous chapters, there is another set of processes that do not fit easily into any of the other categories. Many of these are specialist analytical techniques with imaging modes that can be used to obtain additional contextual information from marks that have already been developed using other processes.

The exception to this is lifting, traditionally used as a process for removing fingermarks developed using powders from a surface to make their visualisation easier and also as a means of recovering footwear marks. Recent observations that the black gelatin lifting media used to recover footwear marks are also highly effective in

---

Fingerprint Development Techniques: Theory and Application, First Edition.
Stephen M. Bleay, Ruth S. Croxton and Marcel de Puit.
© 2018 John Wiley & Sons Ltd. Published 2018 by John Wiley & Sons Ltd.

Table 15.1   Summary of the principal features of some of the specialist processes proposed for imaging and analysis of fingermarks.

Process	Analysis environment	Excitation source	Beam size	Emitted species
Scanning electron microscopy	Vacuum	Electron beam	10 nm	Secondary electrons Backscattered electrons X-rays Visible light
X-ray fluorescence	Ambient	X-rays	10–100 µm	X-rays
Secondary ion mass spectrometry	Vacuum (Ambient – for MeV systems)	Ions	<1 µm	Charged molecular fragments, neutral species, atoms
Matrix-assisted laser desorption/ionisation mass spectrometry	Ambient	Laser	10–100 µm	Charged molecular fragments

recovery of latent fingermarks, which have made the lifting process noteworthy in its own right. There are several circumstances where lifting followed by the use of specialist lighting techniques to visualise the lifted mark may be preferable to, or even more effective than, traditional chemical or physical processes.

Most of the processes used as specialist imaging techniques involve bombardment of the surface with some form of energetic particle or high energy electromagnetic radiation. As a result of this bombardment, electromagnetic radiation or molecular species that are highly characteristic of the surface regions are emitted, and these can be analysed to give additional chemical information about the donor of the mark. Processes falling into this category include scanning electron microscopy (SEM), X-ray fluorescence (XRF), secondary ion mass spectrometry (SIMS) and matrix-assisted laser desorption/ionisation mass spectrometry (MALDI-MS). A summary of the principal features of these specialist imaging processes is given in Table 15.1.

In addition to the processes outlined earlier, other mass spectrometry-based techniques have been proposed for analysis of fingermarks, including direct analysis in real time mass spectrometry (DART-MS) (Rowell et al., 2012) and desorption electrospray ionisation (DESI)-MS (Morelato et al., 2013).

Apart from the mass spectrometry-based techniques, attenuated total reflection Fourier transform infrared spectroscopy (ATR-FTIR) can also be used to analyse the chemical species present in a fingermark by determining wavelengths at which characteristic absorptions occur. This would not generally be of operational interest because such analysis relies on the fingermark being deposited directly on the imaging sensor; however it has been demonstrated that marks lifted from surfaces using lifting materials can also be analysed in this way (Ricci et al., 2006, 2007a).

All of the specialist techniques described earlier are only of use for fingermark visualisation because they can be operated in an imaging mode, with the capability of mapping the chemical information obtained from the fingermark and the surface. The three-dimensional spatial distribution of chemicals within the fingermark and surface can provide valuable contextual information to an investigation, for example, whether a person has handled drugs or explosives or the order of deposition of a mark and printed text.

15.2 Current operational use

Gelatin lifting has also been used for lifting of latent footwear marks and powdered fingermarks for many years. However, its use for the lifting of latent fingermarks, the application described in this chapter, is a more recent development. The use of gelatin lifts for recovery of latent fingermarks is increasing, and specialised imaging equipment has been developed to make imaging of the lifted marks easier (Bleay et al., 2011). Lifting may be preferable to powdering or chemical treatment in several situations, including recovery of marks from high value items (e.g. electrical equipment such as laptops, valuable antiques, etc.) that may be damaged by application of powders or chemicals or recovery of marks from areas that are not easy to access and where any developed marks would be difficult to see (e.g. on the inside of door handles).

In some circumstances specialist imaging processes may be capable of providing additional information about a fingermark, and their use should not be discounted.

With the specialist imaging processes available, SEM is a useful research tool for investigating fingermark development techniques and has primarily been used for this purpose in recent years. In some cases it has been augmented by other techniques including transmission electron microscopy and atomic force microscopy for cases where very high magnifications are required to explore fundamental interactions of fingermarks.

In practical terms, SEM is little used for casework because its application often requires a small area to be cut from the exhibit and coated with a conductive material to prevent the sample charging. However, there are situations where it may provide additional information or ridge detail, and it remains an invaluable tool for understanding the interactions between the fingermarks and the surfaces they are deposited onto.

XRF (and X-ray transmission) may be useful for practical application, and the development of fingermark reagents designed for X-ray functionality is feasible. However the cost of analytical equipment is high and currently beyond the reach of most police forces.

SIMS will normally be destructive to the item, because it requires cutting an area small enough to fit inside the chamber of an SIMS instrument. The high vacuum required may also be detrimental to the fingermark (Bright et al., 2013). In some circumstances SIMS may be capable of providing additional information about a fingermark or revealing additional ridge detail, but equipment is still highly specialised and not widely available.

MALDI-MS (and the closely related SALDI method) is also a specialist technique requiring expensive analytical equipment, but is less destructive to the item. Analysis requires the application of a medium to the surface and fingermark to enhance the effect of the laser and boost ejection of molecules from the surface for subsequent mass spectrometry analysis. Novel powders have been used to both develop the fingermark and act as an enhancer (Rowell et al., 2009; Ferguson et al., 2011; Francese et al., 2013).

ATR-FTIR is also conducted using specialist laboratory equipment, but lifted marks can be placed on the equipment for analysis, making the process compatible with marks recovered from crime scenes (Ricci et al., 2006, 2007a).

The full range of applications for these processes is still being established, and their operational use is very limited. Suitable analytical equipment can be found in several academic institutions and it may be possible to build partnerships giving police access to such facilities when circumstances demand. A challenge for the more widespread use of such technologies will be to produce them in a form more accessible to fingermark enhancement laboratories or that can be transported to the crime scene.

15.3   Lifting

15.3.1   Outline history of the process

1913: Crispo proposed the use of a paper coated with a gelatin/glycerol mix for lifting of marks powdered with lead acetate and subsequently treated with hydrogen sulphide.

Mid-20th century: Rubber lifters began to be used for the lifting of footwear marks.

Early 1970s: Widespread introduction of aluminium powdering and lifting using clear adhesive tape in the United Kingdom. Gelatin lifts were later used as an alternative means of lifting powdered fingermarks.

2005: Introduction of specialist imaging equipment for rapid imaging of black gelatin lifts increased interest in the gelatin lifting process for recovery of latent fingermarks.

15.3.2   Theory

The description given in this section specifically refers to the use of black gelatin lifts for the recovery of latent fingermarks. Black gelatin lifts have a combination of properties that make them well suited for this purpose, as outlined in the succeeding text.

The gelatin lifter is a relatively low tack adhesive material that is placed onto the surface bearing the fingermark followed by application of pressure. The gelatin is

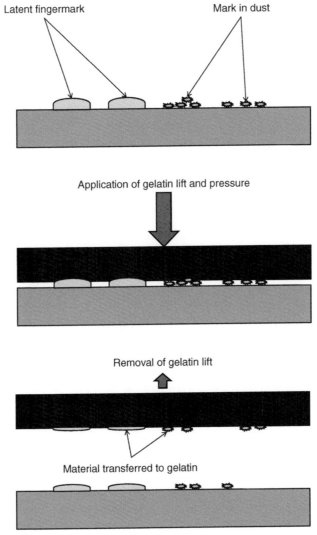

Figure 15.1 Schematic diagram showing how gelatin lifts can lift and reproduce surface features.

able to deform to the texture of the surface contours during application, and any air bubbles present are then smoothed out ensuring intimate contact across the entire surface. The slight adhesive nature of the surface means that on removal of the gelatin lift, a proportion of any grease and loose particulate matter present on the surface will be transferred to the surface of the gel (Figure 15.1). The gel may also retain some impression of the contours of the surface it has been applied to.

The surface features (grease, dust, etc.) retained on the lift represent regions that have different reflective properties from the high gloss, black background of the lift. By optimising the lighting conditions, the contrast between the surface features and

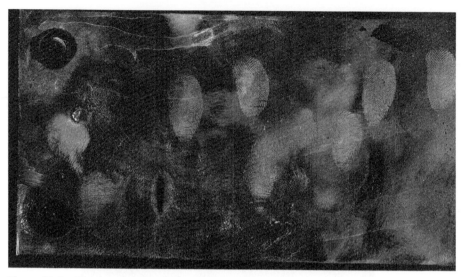

Figure 15.2   Fingermarks lifted from a metal push plate on a door using a black gelatin lift and imaged using specialist equipment. Reproduced courtesy of the Home Office.

the pristine black gelatin surface can be maximised. Specular lighting (Section 6.3.2.2) is generally most effective for this purpose. In the regions where nothing is present on the gel, the angle of the specular reflection from the surface means that light is reflected away from the imaging system and the background appears black. The particulates and grease on the surface scatter light and/or produce diffuse reflections, with the consequence that some light reaches the imaging system, and those regions appear lighter.

An example of a section of a gelatin lift taken from a push plate on a door and scanned using specialist imaging equipment producing controlled, specular lighting conditions is illustrated in Figure 15.2.

Gelatin lifts should also be examined under oblique lighting (Section 6.3.2.1) because any lifted marks in dust may not be prominent under the specular lighting conditions used to capture greasy deposits, but can scatter light strongly when oblique lighting is used.

15.3.3   The lifting process

The lifting process should be applied according to the gel manufacturer's instructions (BVDA, 2017), peeling the acetate from the gelatin lift and applying it to the surface being treated. The gel is then smoothed in place to remove air bubbles. It may be beneficial to leave the gel in place for several minutes or to warm it slightly, but the benefits of these approaches for lifting latent marks have not been conclusively demonstrated. The lift should then be peeled from the surface, removing the traces of the mark.

Once lifted, the gelatin lift should be stored without a cover material if practical and imaged as soon as possible. This is because the quality and clarity of any lifted latent marks will progressively degrade, and reapplication of a cover material exacerbates this and may introduce other artefacts (Bleay et al., 2011).

'Gelatin' lifts can be obtained from more than one manufacturer, but it is not possible to recommend a single type of lifter for all applications. In general higher tack lifts are most effective in lifting latent fingermarks, but in some cases may cause damage to the surface, for example, delamination. In these circumstances a lower tack lifter may be more appropriate, and the ultimate selection of lifter by the user must take these factors into account.

15.4   Scanning electron microscopy

15.4.1   Outline history of the process

1920s: First observations that beams of electrons could be focused by means of electrostatic or magnetic fields and that the short wavelength of electron beams offered significant improvements in both resolution and depth of field compared to light microscopy (Goodhew and Humphreys, 1988; McMullan, 2006).

1937: Von Ardenne produced the first electron microscope utilising a focused electron beam being scanned in a raster pattern to form an image (McMullan, 1988).

1965: Production of the first commercial scanning electron microscopes by the Cambridge Scientific Instrument Company, based on the research work of Oatley et al.

1971: Van Essen described the potential for using SEM including in combination with energy dispersive X-ray spectroscopy for forensic science applications, including studying hair and fibres and analysis of ink and paint composition.

1975: Garner et al. utilised SEM for the imaging of latent fingermarks on glass and metal surfaces.

1978–1979: Studies by Whelan (1978) and Reynoldson (1979) showed that SEM can also be utilised for imaging of marks developed using other processes, enabling ridges to be tracked across boundaries between dissimilar surface regions.

1980s: SEM enters operational use at the Metropolitan Police (Creer and Brennan, 1987).

15.4.2   Theory

In scanning electron microscope, an energetic (typically keV) beam of electrons is focused onto the surface. In common with optical processes in other regions of the electromagnetic spectrum, there are a number of interactions that can occur between

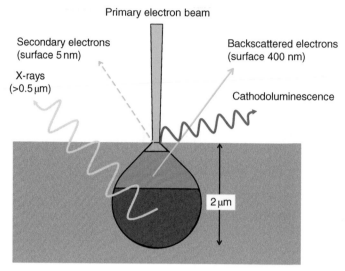

Figure 15.3 Principal interactions between electron beam and sample in scanning electron microscopy.

the electron beam and the surface. These interactions include transmission (if the sample is sufficiently thin) and diffraction by crystal lattices that may be present in the materials of the surface, both of which are of most relevance for transmission electron microscopy and are therefore not discussed further here.

The interactions of principal interest for SEM are illustrated schematically in Figure 15.3.

The normal mode of imaging is secondary electron imaging. Secondary electrons are produced as a consequence of inelastic collisions between electrons in the primary beam and atoms in the surface layers, and some have sufficient energy to escape the surface. In secondary electron imaging, a positive charge is applied to the detector, which attracts most of the negatively charged electrons emitted from the surface. As a result, the number of electrons received at the detector is relatively high, and the resultant image is not 'noisy'. The electron beam is scanned across the surface in a series of lines known as a raster, and the signal level recorded at each discrete point is represented by a pixel on a screen. Secondary electron imaging is particularly effective in resolving fingermarks where differences in topography or morphology exist between the ridges and the background.

Backscattered electron imaging is most useful where the elemental composition of the fingermark ridge and the background is different, particularly if one has a higher atomic number density than the other. Backscattered electrons occur where the incident electron from the primary beam undergoes a series of inelastic collisions with atoms in the sample and is scattered backwards out of the surface. Backscattered electrons are of high energy compared with secondary electrons. The number of backscattered electrons occurring is directly related to the atomic density of the surface being examined, regions of high atomic number being more likely to interact with the incident electrons and backscatter them.

Backscattered electron imaging is performed by biasing the detector with a slight negative charge, thus repelling the lower energy secondary electrons and only allowing the higher energy backscattered electrons to reach the detector. Because the number of electrons reaching the detector is reduced, backscattered electron images may be 'noisier' than secondary electron images. However, this imaging mode may be of use in resolving fingermarks developed using processes that result in high atomic number elements being preferentially deposited or absorbed by the ridges, such as vacuum metal deposition and both iodine fuming and iodine solution treatments.

The incident electrons can also promote emission of radiation of different wavelengths, in a process analogous to fluorescence in the visible region of the spectrum. Electrons in the atoms close to the surface can be promoted into excited states by the incident electrons, and as they decay back into their ground states, they do so with the emission of an X-ray of energy/wavelength that is characteristic of the element present. For certain materials, this emission of energy occurs at an energy/wavelength corresponding to the visible region of the spectrum. This is known as cathodoluminescence.

The X-rays that are emitted can be separated and analysed according to their characteristic wavelength or energy. In practice energy dispersive detectors are more compact than wavelength dispersive systems and are more commonly found on electron microscopes. X-ray spectroscopy can be carried out in a static mode, to determine the elemental composition of a particular location on the surface, or be used in mapping mode, scanning the beam across the surface and recording the types of X-rays emitted at each point. If a characteristic element is present in the fingermark, it may be possible to resolve the ridges from the background in this way.

15.4.3 The scanning electron microscopy process

SEM involves placing the region of the surface to be analysed into a vacuum chamber and evacuating the chamber and then scanning an energetic beam of electrons across the surface in a raster pattern. The imaging mode can be varied to record the secondary electrons, backscattered electrons, X-rays or visible radiation emitted as the electron beam is scanned.

The limited size of the sample chamber used in the scanning electron microscope means that the region of interest may need to be cut from the item. Unless the surface is conductive, it may be necessary to sputter a conductive coating onto the surface and to earth it in order to prevent charging effects on the surface disrupting the image. A thin layer of gold is most commonly used; however this can inhibit an X-ray spectroscopy of light elements, and if analysis of such elements is required, a coating of carbon can be used instead.

In most cases, the initial image is obtained in the secondary electron imaging mode, which may be sufficient to resolve ridges from the background by means of differences in their topography or morphology. It may also be useful to obtain spectra of the characteristic X-rays emitted from points on the fingermark ridge and the background to establish if any element is present in one region and not in the other. If such a difference is identified, X-ray mapping can then be used to obtain a clearer distinction between the two regions if required.

As indicated earlier, scanning electron microscopes are specialist pieces of equipment more likely to be found in research institutes than in police laboratories, and skilled operators are required to obtain optimum results.

15.5   X-ray fluorescence (and X-ray imaging)

15.5.1   Outline history of the process

1895: Röntgen conducted some of the first detailed studies of X-rays and demonstrated their use in a transmission mode to image the bones of the hand.

1928: Glocker and Schreiber first proposed the use of a primary X-ray beam to excite XRF from a surface.

1965: Graham and Gray considered the use of X-rays for revealing fingermarks on problematic surfaces such as patterned backgrounds and skin, using lead powder to develop the mark followed by X-ray electronography to image it.

2005: The use of XRF to reveal developed fingermarks on patterned backgrounds by mapping characteristic elements in the mark was reported (Home Office, 2005).

2006: Worley et al. reported that micro-XRF can also be used to reveal latent fingermarks by mapping characteristic elements that may be present in contaminants (e.g. sun cream).

15.5.2   Theory

The earliest application of X-rays to image fingermarks and to separate them from backgrounds was X-ray electronography (Graham, 1973). The reference given provides a detailed overview, and because this process is no longer in regular use, it will therefore not be described further.

The process more recently considered as a means of imaging and analysing both latent and developed fingermarks is XRF. In this process, the surface is irradiated with monochromatic X-rays, which promotes emission of X-rays characteristic to the elements present. This is directly analogous to fluorescence in the visible region of the spectrum and also equivalent to carrying out X-ray spectroscopy in the scanning electron microscope, except that in XRF X-rays instead of electrons are used to cause emission of the characteristic X-rays.

In XRF, a short wavelength beam of X-rays is used to irradiate the surface bearing the fingermark, promoting electrons in the surface atoms into excited states. As these electrons decay back to ground states, they emit longer wavelength X-rays that have energies characteristic of the elements present in the surface layers. As the X-ray beam is scanned across the surface, the distribution of a particular element can be mapped by recording the locations where X-rays of energy characteristic to that element are emitted. In cases where an element is known to be localised in the ridges of the fingermark, XRF can be used to reveal fingermark ridges against an otherwise distracting background.

15.5.3   The X-ray fluorescence process

The method of conducting XRF is very similar to that of SEM. The surface of interest is placed on a stage and areas of up to 100 mm × 100 mm scanned using a monochromatic beam of X-rays (e.g. generated at 20–60 kV from a rhodium target). Spot diameters of down to 10 μm diameter can be achieved with current instruments. The characteristic X-rays emitted from each point of the scan are recorded and can be displayed as maps showing the distribution of particular elements on the surface (Figure 15.4). Existing instruments are capable of detecting X-rays emitted from elements in the atomic number range from sodium to uranium.

The potential advantages of XRF over X-ray mapping within a scanning electron microscope are that larger areas can be examined and the surface being analysed does not have to be under vacuum and does not have to be coated with a conductive coating to prevent charging. As a consequence XRF is potentially less detrimental to the item. The principal disadvantage is that the costs of such equipment make it less accessible than SEM. Skilled operators will also be required to obtain optimum results.

Many instruments used for XRF also have an X-ray transmission mode that can sometimes also be used for fingermark imaging. In this mode the atomic density of an area determines the number of X-rays transmitted through the item and therefore the intensity of the signal reaching the detector. In regions where a high atomic number element is present, less X-rays are transmitted, and the area appears darker in the image. Processes that result in the fingermark ridges (or the background) being preferentially labelled with a high atomic number element may present the possibility of increasing contrast between the fingermark and the background by X-ray transmission. The use of this imaging mode and a comparison with conventional XRF imaging is shown for a mark treated with physical developer and further enhanced using iodide toning in Figure 15.5.

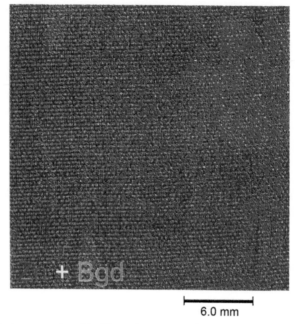

6.0 mm

Figure 15.4 An image produced by X-ray fluorescence from a mark developed on fabric using vacuum metal deposition, red signal = zinc from metal deposition, green signal = fabric background. Reproduced courtesy of HORIBA UK Ltd.

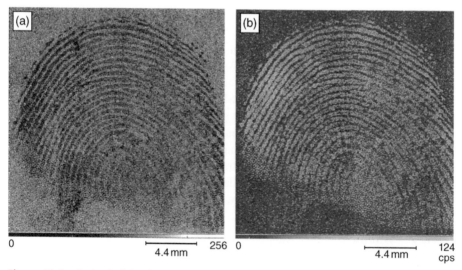

Figure 15.5 A physical developer mark on paper after iodide toning: (a) image of mark in X-ray transmission mode and (b) image formed from characteristic X-rays from iodine. Reproduced courtesy of HORIBA UK Ltd.

15.6   Secondary ion mass spectroscopy (SIMS)

15.6.1   Outline history of the process

1910: Thomson demonstrated that bombardment of a solid with ions produced emission of positive ions and neutral atoms from the surface.

1958: Honig developed the first practical SIMS instrument.

1969: Benninghoven developed and introduced the static SIMS method, using low primary ion currents to confine the analysis to the layers close to the surface.

1980s: The development of higher sensitivity detection systems allowed the use of lower energy primary beam currents and results in considerably less damage to the surface during analysis, making the process more feasible for surface analysis. The use of an imaging mode for mapping of molecular species across a surface was demonstrated (Brown and Vickerman, 1984).

1986: Brown used SIMS for imaging of latent fingermarks and mapping distributions of molecular fragments associated with fingermark constituents, including Na^+ and Cl^- ions, peaks indicative of the presence of both long- and short-chain aliphatic materials, silicones, alkoxy and phenoxy groups, and the main negative ion from myristic, palmitic and oleic acids.

2001: Koch et al. reported further studies into latent fingermark composition using SIMS.

2007: Szynkowska et al. started a series of studies using SIMS to analyse latent fingermarks (Szynkowska et al., 2007) and fingermarks containing contaminants of forensic relevance including drugs of abuse (Szynkowska et al., 2009) and gunshot residues (Szynkowska et al., 2010).

2012: The potential application of SIMS in determining the order of deposition of latent fingermarks and printing inks was demonstrated, both in imaging and depth profiling modes (Bright et al., 2012), and the possibility of extending this to developed marks was considered (Attard-Montalto et al., 2013).

2013: Bailey et al. showed that SIMS can be used to reveal fingermark ridge detail not visualised by other processes, utilising characteristic species still present in the fingermark ridges and not either targeted by previous processes or below their limits of detection.

15.6.2   Theory

The theory and method of application of the SIMS process to fingermark analysis and imaging have been described in Chapter 3 and will not be repeated here. An example of an image of a fingermark collected using SIMS is shown in Figure 15.6.

(a)

Field of view: 5000.0 × 5000.0 μm²

(b)

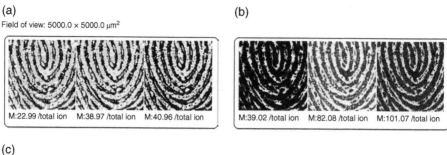

M:22.99 /total ion   M:38.97 /total ion   M:40.96 /total ion   M:39.02 /total ion   M:82.08 /total ion   M:101.07 /total ion

(c)

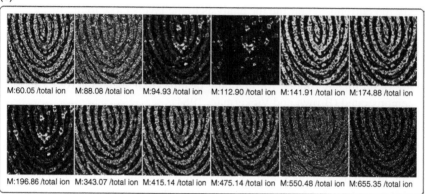

M:60.05 /total ion   M:88.08 /total ion   M:94.93 /total ion   M:112.90 /total ion   M:141.91 /total ion   M:174.88 /total ion

M:196.86 /total ion   M:343.07 /total ion   M:415.14 /total ion   M:475.14 /total ion   M:550.48 /total ion   M:655.35 /total ion

Figure 15.6   SIMS imaging of fingermarks. Positive ion images of an undoped fingermark deposited on a silicon wafer depicting (a) elemental ions (Na, K and either ^{41}K or CaH, respectively), (b) fragment ions originating from the substrate and (c) fragment ions originating from the fingermark. Image reproduced courtesy of the University of Surrey.

15.7   Matrix-assisted laser desorption/ionisation mass spectrometry (MALDI-MS)

15.7.1   Outline history of the process

1980s: First reported studies using practical MALDI systems (Karas et al., 1985; Beavis et al., 1989).

2004: Rowell develops and patents functionalised nanoparticles that can be used to both develop latent fingermarks (Theaker et al., 2008) and act as a matrix enhancer during subsequent MALDI-MS analysis (Rowell et al., 2009).

2009: Rowell et al. demonstrated that drugs of abuse and their metabolites can be detected within fingermarks developed using functionalised nanoparticles and analysed by MALDI-MS.

2009: Wolstenholme et al. demonstrated that MALDI-MS can be utilised in the compositional analysis of untreated, latent fingermarks.

2011: Ferguson et al. proposed a novel two-step method for MALDI analysis of latent fingermarks, utilising powdered MALDI matrix material as a means of developing latent marks.

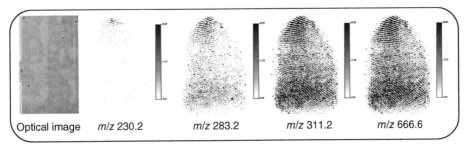

Optical image   *m/z* 230.2   *m/z* 283.2   *m/z* 311.2   *m/z* 666.6

Figure 15.7 The use of MALDI-MSI to reveal fingermark ridge detail. Optical image: a mark on the sticky side of a parcel tape processed with iron oxide powder suspension, exhibiting poor enhancement. Endogenous species imaged by MALDI reveal ridge detail, maps shown for 13-aminotridecanoic acid (*m/z* 230.2), oleic acid (*m/z* 283.2), eicosenoic acid (*m/z* 311.1), glycerophosphoserine (*m/z* 666.6). Reproduced courtesy of Sheffield Hallam University.

2012–2014: Broad-ranging exploration of the potential of MALDI-MS (and SAL-DI-MS) in obtaining additional contextual information from fingermarks, including separation of overlapping fingermarks (Bradshaw et al., 2012), detection of contaminants such as condom lubricants (Bradshaw et al., 2013a), drugs (Lim et al., 2013; Sundara and Rowell, 2014) and explosives (Rowell et al., 2012), as well as using MALDI-MS in sequence with conventional fingermark enhancement reagents (Bradshaw et al., 2013b).

15.7.2 Theory

The theory and method of application of the MALDI-MS process to fingermark analysis and imaging have been described in Chapter 3 and will not be repeated here. An example of an image of a fingermark collected using MALDI is shown in Figure 15.7.

15.8 Attenuated total reflection Fourier transform infrared spectroscopy (ATR-FTIR)

15.8.1 Outline history of the process

1967: Harrick described the principles of internal reflection spectroscopy in the infrared region of the spectrum.

2004: Williams et al. utilised IR microspectrometry to compare fingermarks of males, females, adults and children, investigating compositional differences between these groups and between eccrine and sebaceous deposits.

2005: Grant et al. used the same approach to locate and characterise particles of exogenous materials such as drug residues trapped in fingermark ridges.

2005: Tahtouh et al. utilised an FTIR focal plane array detector to scan a fingermark developed using cyanoacrylate fuming on a polymer banknote in a series of lines, stitching these together to form an overview final image. Characteristic absorptions associated with polycyanoacrylate and not found for the polymer substrate were used to separate the mark from the background.

2006: Chan and Kazarian demonstrated the use of a large sensor array linked to an ATR-FTIR instrument for rapid imaging and analysis of forensic traces. Ricci et al. refined this approach and showed that the process could be applied to traces lifted from surfaces on tapes and brought back to the laboratory for analysis.

2007: Ricci et al. (2007a) showed that rapid ATR-FTIR analysis could be applied to fingermark residues, both on marks deposited directly on the sensor and on latent marks lifted from a range of surfaces using gelatin lifts (2007b).

15.8.2   Theory

The theory and method of application of the ATR-FTIR process to fingermark analysis and imaging have been described in Chapter 3 and will not be repeated here. An example of an image of a fingermark collected using ATR-FTIR is shown in Figure 15.8.

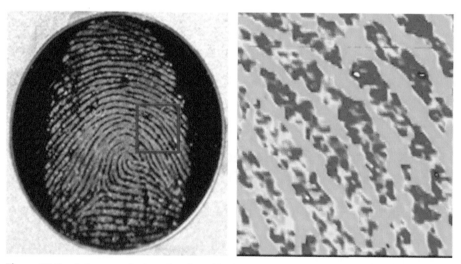

Figure 15.8   A fingermark viewed under white light and a small portion of the same fingermark imaged using ATR-FTIR. The 'heat map' represents the distribution and relative concentration of a lipid component of the fingermark. Image reproduced courtesy of Imperial College London.

References

Attard-Montalto N, Ojeda J J, Jones B J, 'Determining the order of deposition of natural latent fingerprints and laser printed ink using chemical mapping with secondary ion mass spectrometry', Sci Justice, vol 53(1), (2013), p 2–7.

Bailey M J, Ismail M, Bright N, Everson D, Costa C, De Puit M, Bleay S, Elad M L, Cohen Y, Geller B, Webb R P, Watts J F, 'Enhanced imaging of developed fingerprints using mass spectrometry imaging', Analyst, vol 138(21), (2013), p 6246–6250.

Beavis R C, Chait B T, Standing K G, 'Matrix-assisted laser-desorption mass spectrometry using 355 nm radiation', Rapid Commun Mass Spectrom, vol 3(12), (1989), p 436–439.

Benninghoven A, 'Analysis of sub-monolayers on silver by secondary ion emission', Phys Status Solidi, vol 34(2), (1969), p 169–171.

Bleay S M, Bandey H L, Black M, Sears V G, 'The gelatin lifting process: an evaluation of its effectiveness in the recovery of latent fingerprints', J Forensic Identif, vol 61(6), (2011), p 581–606.

Bradshaw R, Roa W, Wolstenholme R, Clench M R, Bleay S, Francese S, 'Separation of overlapping fingermarks by matrix assisted laser desorption ionisation mass spectrometry imaging', Forensic Sci Int, vol 222(1), (2012), p 318–326.

Bradshaw R, Wolstenholme R, Ferguson L S, Sammon C, Mader K, Claude E, Blackledge R D, Clench M R, Francese S, 'Spectroscopic imaging based approach for condom identification in condom contaminated fingermarks', Analyst, vol 138(9), (2013a), p 2546–2557.

Bradshaw R, Bleay S, Wolstenholme R, Clench M R, Francese S, 'Towards the integration of matrix assisted laser desorption ionisation mass spectrometry imaging into the current fingermark examination workflow', Forensic Sci Int, vol 232(1–3), (2013b), p 111–124.

Bright N J, Webb R, Hinder S J, Kirkby K J, Ward N I, Watts J F, Bleay S, Bailey M J, 'Determination of the deposition order of overlapping latent fingerprints and inks using secondary ion mass spectrometry (SIMS)', Am Chem Soc Anal Chem, vol 84(9), (2012), p 4083–4087.

Bright N J, Webb R P, Kirkby K J, Willson T R, Driscoll D J, Reddy S M, Ward N I, Bailey M J, Bleay S, 'Chemical changes exhibited by latent fingerprints after exposure to vacuum conditions', Forensic Sci Int, vol 230(1–3), (2013), p 81–86.

Brown A, 'Characterisation of fingerprints by static SIMS and SIMS imaging', Analysis Report, Surface Analysis Industrial Unit, UMIST, 22 March 1986.

Brown A, Vickerman J C, 'Static SIMS, FABMS and SIMS imaging in applied surface analysis', Analyst, vol 109, (1984), p 851–857.

BVDA International, 'BVDA Gel Lifter Manual', http://www.bvda.com/EN/prdctinf/en_gel_1.html (accessed 12 April 2017).

Crispo D, Bull Soc Chim Belg, vol 26, (1913), p 190–193.

Ferguson L, Bradshaw R, Wolstenholme R, Clench M R, Francese S, 'A novel two step matrix application for the enhancement and imaging of latent fingermarks', Anal Chem, vol 83(14), (2011), p 5585–5591.

Francese S, Bradshaw R, Flinders B, Mitchell C, Bleay S, Cicero L, Clench M R, 'Curcumin: a multipurpose matrix for MALDI mass spectrometry imaging applications', Anal Chem, vol 85(10), (2013a), p 5240–5248.

Garner G E, Fontan C R, Hobson D W, 'Visualisation of fingerprints in the scanning electron microscope', J Forensic Sci Soc, vol 15, (1975), p 281–288.

Glocker R, Schreiber H, 'Quantitative Röntgenspektralanalyse mit Kalterregung des Spektrums', Ann Phys, vol 390(8), (1928), p 1089–1102.

Goodhew P J, Humphreys F J, 'Electron Microscopy and Analysis', 2nd edition, Taylor & Francis, London, 1988, ISBN 0-85066-414-4.

Graham D, 'Use of X-Ray Techniques in Forensic Investigations', Churchill Livingstone, Edinburgh/London, 1973, ISBN 04430009414.

Graham D, Gray H C, 'X-rays reveal fngerprints', New Scientist, October 1965, p 35.

Grant A, Wilkinson T J, Holman D R, Martin M C, 'Identification of recently handled materials by analysis of latent human fingerprints using infrared spectromicroscopy', Appl Spectrosc, vol 59(9), (2005), p 1182–1187.

Harrick N J, 'Internal Reflection Spectroscopy', John Wiley & Sons, Inc., New York, 1967, p 342, ISBN 978-0-470-35250-2.

Home Office, 'Fingerprint Development and Imagining Newsletter', HOSDB Publication No. 47/05, October 2005.

Honig R E, 'Sputtering of surfaces by positive ion beams of low energy', J Appl Phys, vol 29, (1958), p 549–555.

Karas M, Bachmann D, Hillenkamp F, 'Influence of the wavelength in high-irradiance ultraviolet laser desorption mass spectrometry of organic molecules', Anal Chem, vol 57(14), (1985), p 2935–2939.

Koch C H, Augustine M R, Marcus H L, 'Forensic applications of ion-beam mixing and surface spectroscopy of latent fingerprints', Proc SPIE, vol 4468, (2001), p 65–77.

Lim A Y, Rowell F, Elumbaring-Salazar C G, Lokee J, Ma J, 'Detection of drugs in latent fingermarks by mass spectrometric methods', Anal Methods, vol 5, (2013), p 4378–4385.

McMullan D, 'Von Ardenne and the scanning electron microscope', Proc Roy Microsc Soc, vol 23, (1988), p 283–288.

McMullan D, 'Scanning electron microscopy 1928–1965', Scanning, vol 17(3), (2006), p 175–185.

Morelato M, Beavis A, Kirkbride P, Roux C, 'Forensic applications of desorption electrospray ionisation mass spectrometry (DESI-MS)', Forensic Sci Int, vol 226(1), (2013), p 10–21.

Oatley C W, Nixon W C, Pease R F W, 'Scanning electron microscopy', Adv Electron Electron Phys, vol 21, (1965), p 181–247.

Reynoldson T E, 'Imaging Fingerprints by Means of a Scanning Electron Microscope', HO PSDB Tech. Memo. No. 10/79, 1979.

Ricci C, Chan K L A, Kazarian S G, 'Combining the tape-lift method and Fourier transform infrared spectroscopic imaging for forensic applications', Appl Spectrosc, vol 60(9), (2006), p 1013–1021.

Ricci C, Bleay S, Kazarian S G, 'Spectroscopic imaging of latent fingermarks collected with the aid of a gelatin tape', Anal Chem, vol 79(15), (2007a), p 5771–5775.

Ricci C, Phiriyavityopas P, Curum N, Chan K L A, Jickells S, Kazarian S G, 'Chemical imaging of latent fingerprint residues', Appl Spectrosc, vol 61(5), (2007b), p 514–522.

Rowell F, Hudson K, Seviour J, 'Detection of drugs and their metabolites in dusted latent fingermarks by mass spectrometry', Analyst, vol 134(4), (2009), p 701–707.

Rowell F, Seviour J, Lim A Y, Elumbaring-Salazar C G, Loke J, Ma J, 'Detection of nitro-organic and peroxide explosives in latent fingermarks by DART- and SALDI-FOF-mass spectrometry', Forensic Sci Int, vol 221(1–3), (2012), p 84–91.

Sundara L, Rowell F, 'Detection of drugs in lifted cyanoacrylate-developed latent fingermarks using two laser desorption/ionisation mass spectrometric methods', Analyst, vol 139, (2014), p 633–642.

Szynkowska M I, Czerski K, Grams J, Paryjczak T, Parczewski A, 'Preliminary studies using imaging mass spectrometry TOF-SIMS in detection and analysis of fingerprints', Imaging Sci J, vol 55(3), (2007), p 180–187.

Szynkowska M I, Czerski K, Rogowski J, Paryjczak T, Parczewski A, 'ToF-SIMS application in the visualization and analysis of fingerprints after contact with amphetamine drugs', Forensic Sci Int, vol 184(1–3), (2009), p e24–e26.

Szynkowska M I, Czerski K, Rogowski J, Paryjczak T, Parczewski A, 'Detection of exogenous contaminants of fingerprints using ToF-SIMS', Surf Interface Anal, vol 42(5), (2010), p 393–397.

Tahtouh M, Kalman J R, Roux C, Lennard C, Reedy B J, 'The detection and enhancement of latent fingermarks using infrared chemical imaging', J Forensic Sci, vol 50(1), (2005), p 1–9.

Thomson J J, 'Rays of positive electricity', Philos Mag, vol 20, (1910), p 752–767.

Van Essen C G, 'The scanning electron microscope in forensic science', Phys Technol, vol 5, (1971), p 234–245.

Whelan P, 'The interpretation of secondary electron images of fingerprint films', HO PSDB Tech. Memo. No. 18/78, 1978.

Williams D K, Schwartz R L, Bartick E G, 'Analysis of latent fingerprint deposits by infrared microspectrometry', Appl Spectrosc, vol 58, (2004), p 313–316.

Wolstenholme R, Bradshaw R, Clench M R, Francese S, 'Study of latent fingermarks by matrix-assisted laser desorption/ionisation mass spectrometry imaging of endogenous lipids', Rapid Commun Mass Spectrom, vol 23, (2009), p 3031–3039.

Worley C G, Wiltshire S S, Miller T C, Havrilla G J, Majidi V, 'Detection of visible and latent fingerprints using micro-X-ray fluorescence elemental imaging', J Forensic Sci, vol 51(1), (2006), p 57–63.

Further reading

Bailey M J, Bright N J, Hinder S, Jones B N, Webb R P, Croxton R S, Francese S, Ferguson L S, Wolstenholme R, Jickells S, Jones B J, Ojeda J J, Kazarian S G, Bleay S, 'Chemical characterization of latent fingerprints by matrix-assisted laser desorption ionization, time-of-flight secondary ion mass spectrometry, mega electron volt secondary mass spectrometry, gas chromatography/mass spectrometry, X-ray photoelectron spectroscopy, and attenuated total reflection Fourier transform infrared spectroscopic imaging: an intercomparison', Anal Chem, vol 84(20), (2012), p 8514–8523.

Chan K L A, Kazarian S G, 'Detection of trace materials with Fourier transform infrared spectroscopy using a multi-channel detector', Analyst, vol 131, (2006), p 126–131.

Crane N J, Bartick E G, Perlman R S, Huffman S, 'Infrared spectroscopic imaging for non-invasive detection of latent fingerprints', J Forensic Sci, vol 52(1), (2007), p 48–53.

Creer K E, Brennan J S, 'The work of the Serious Crimes Unit', Proceedings of International Forensic Symposium on Latent Prints, FBI Academy, Quantico, VA, 7–10 July 1987, p 91–100.

De Koeijer J A, Berger C E H, Glas W, Madhuizen H T, 'Gelatine lifting, a novel technique for the examination of indented writing', J Forensic Sci, vol 51(4), (2006), p 908–914.

Ferguson L S, Creasey S, Wolstenholme R, Clench M R, Francese S, 'Efficiency of the dry-wet method for the MALDI-MSI analysis of latent fingermarks', J Mass Spectrom, vol 48, (2013), p 677–684.

Francese S, Bradshaw R, Ferguson L S, Wolstenholme R, Clench M R, Bleay S, 'Beyond the ridge pattern: multi-informative analysis of latent fingermarks by MALDI mass spectrometry', Analyst, vol 138(15), (2013b), p 4215.

Graham D, 'X-ray techniques in forensic science', Criminologist, vol 4, (1969a), p 171–181.

Graham D, 'Some technical aspects of the demonstration and visualisation of fingerprints on human skin', J Forensic Sci, vol 14(1), (1969b), p 1–12.

Graham D, Gray H C, 'The use of X-ray electronography and autoelectronography in forensic investigations', J Forensic Sci, vol 11(2), (1966), p 124–143.

Lail H A, 'Fingerprint recovery with electronography', The Police Chief, October 1975, p 34, 39–40.

Mooney D J, 'Fingerprints on human skin', Identif News, February 1977, p 5–8.

Shalhoub R, Quinones I, Ames C, Multaney B, Curtis S, Seeboruth H, Moore S, Daniel B, 'The recovery of latent fingerprints and DNA using a silicone-based casting material', Forensic Sci Int, vol 178(2), (2008), p 199–203.

Shor Y, Tsach T, Vinokurov A, Glattstein B, Landau E, Levin N, 'Lifting shoeprints using gelatin lifters and a hydraulic press', J Forensic Sci, vol 48(2), (2003), p 368–372.

Theaker B J, Hudson K E, Rowell F J, 'Doped hydrophobic silica nano- and micro-particles as novel agents for developing latent fingerprints', Forensic Sci Int, vol 174(1), (2008), p 26–34.

Theeuwen A B E, van Barneveld S, Drok J W, Keereweer I, Lesger B, Limborgh J C M, Naber W M, Schrok R, Velders T, 'Enhancement of muddy footwear impressions', Forensic Sci Int, vol 119(1), (2001), p 57–67.

Wiesner S, Tsach T, Belser C, Shor Y, 'A comparative research of two lifting methods: electrostatic lifter and gelatin lifter', J Forensic Sci, vol 56(Suppl 1), (2011), S58–S62.

Williams G, McMurray N, 'Latent fingerprint visualisation using a scanning Kelvin probe', Forensic Sci Int, vol 167, (2007), p 102–109.

Winstanley R, 'Recovery of latent fingerprints from difficult surfaces by an X-ray method', J Forensic Sci Soc, vol 17, (1977), p 121–125.

16

Evaluation and comparison of fingermark enhancement processes

Stephen M. Bleay

Home Office Centre for Applied Science and Technology, Sandridge, UK

Key points

- There is a requirement for standardised test methodologies that can distinguish between different processes in comparative trials.

- Such test methodologies should cover fundamental tests to establish process selectivity and sensitivity through to operational trials on live casework.

- Evaluation and monitoring should not cease after the operational implementation of a process, enabling any changes in effectiveness to be investigated in a timely manner.

16.1 Introduction

It is apparent from the wide range of fingermark enhancement processes that have been described in Chapters 6–15 that the selection of the most appropriate process for a particular scenario is not necessarily simple. The processes under consideration may enhance marks by very different mechanisms, and it is therefore important to have a standardised means of distinguishing between them in terms of their effectiveness. The increasing adoption of the ISO 17025 standard by fingermark enhancement

---

Fingerprint Development Techniques: Theory and Application, First Edition.
Stephen M. Bleay, Ruth S. Croxton and Marcel de Puit.
© 2018 John Wiley & Sons Ltd. Published 2018 by John Wiley & Sons Ltd.

laboratories around the world has provided another driver for the adoption of a standard method for evaluating fingermark enhancement processes (ISO, 2005). ISO 17025 places emphasis on the use of methods that have been validated and are fit for purpose. The validation of a fingermark enhancement process for operational use may include (amongst other tests) an assessment of its sensitivity and selectivity, establishing the range of surfaces that it is effective on and identifying where it can be used in a processing sequence.

The published literature on fingermark enhancement has varied significantly in the rigour of the approaches taken, with some publications basing conclusions on several 1000s of deposited marks and others using far fewer marks and deliberate 'grooming' by wiping the fingers on the nose and/or forehead. The fact that the outputs of both types of study can be given equal weight has been a cause of concern within the research community, and as a consequence there have been several papers that have aimed to propose standard approaches to comparisons of fingermark evaluation processes (Jones et al., 2001; Kent, 2010; Sears et al., 2012). This approach has been further supported by the publication of fingermark research guidelines by the International Fingermark Research Group (IFRG, 2014).

The processes that are in routine operational use have originated from many different sources, some from accidental observations of their action in developing marks and others from adaptations of processes used in other branches of science. As a consequence, the body of knowledge and evidence that exists for some of these processes in their application for fingermark enhancement is not necessarily complete. Attempts have been made to collate this knowledge for many existing processes (Bleay et al., 2012) to assist in demonstrating that they have been validated for operational use. However, as new processes emerge from academic research, there is a need to ensure that the evidence that is required for validation is captured at each stage of the research process and that these stages and the purposes of them are clearly understood.

One approach that has been widely adopted in many government departments, agencies and commercial organisations as a means of assessing the maturity of technologies in their progression from research and development towards operational implementation is the Technology Readiness Level (TRL). There is much synergy between the stages identified in the TRL system and the steps taken in evaluating and implementing a new fingermark enhancement process, and therefore the TRL has been proposed as a framework for taking novel processes from concept to operational use (Bandey, 2014; IFRG, 2014). The adapted scale that is proposed for fingermark research is shown in Table 16.1.

A more detailed description of the some of the methodologies proposed for research at TRLs 3 and above is provided in the following sections. A process at TRL1 or TRL2 is a concept that has not yet had any practical testing carried out on it, and therefore TRL3 represents the point at which laboratory assessment begins.

Table 16.1   Technology Readiness Levels as applied to fingermark research.

Technology Readiness Level	Fingermark context
1. Basic principles observed and reported	Published papers reporting synthesis of new chemicals or reporting principles of a novel optical technique
2. Technology concept and/or application formulated	Published papers or other references reporting reactions of chemicals that are relevant to the environment of a fingermark or physical interactions of optical techniques with surfaces
3. Analytical and experimental critical function and/ or characteristic proof of concept	Chemical spot tests using the process on individual fingermark constituents or on single marks to demonstrate feasibility or trials to establish that the optical technique is applicable to the constituents within a fingermark
4. Component and/or breadboard validation in laboratory environment	Chemical formulation and/or process optimisation using real fingermarks or trials to establish optimum optical environment for fingermark visualisation
5. Component and/or breadboard validation in relevant environment	Extensive laboratory trials using the process on samples covering a range of donors, substrates and ages of mark. Testing in this phase may be conducted for several reasons, and therefore experiments may vary according to end purpose
6. System/subsystem model or prototype demonstration in a relevant environment	Pseudo-operational trials using marks on realistically handled, operationally representative items and surfaces
7. System prototype demonstration in an operational environment	Operational trials on items and surfaces encountered in live casework
8. Actual system completed and qualified through test and demonstration	Publication of results obtained from tests covering TRL3–TRL7 and issue of processing instructions. Inclusion in processing manuals
9. Actual system proven through successful mission operations	Provision of supporting data for process in operational use obtained by monitoring performance over several years

16.2   Technology Readiness Level 3: Proof of concept

The objective of research at TRL3 is to provide confirmation of the scientific principles proposed in the literature for the novel process or to gather information about its scope. One important outcome of testing in this phase is to obtain information about the *selectivity* of the process.

For chemical processes, enhancement of fingermarks generally occurs by means of a reaction between chemicals in the reagent and chemical species in the fingermark. A method often used for investigating such processes is to use small quantities of fingermark constituents and to react them with the chemical under test to see if the predicted reactions occur (Cantu et al., 1993). Such testing may be conducted in the liquid phase using solutions of the constituents or on test spots deposited onto porous or non-porous substrates (e.g. Figures 7.21 and 9.33). In some cases the visible product is sufficient to confirm the expected reaction has occurred; in other cases this can be supported by additional structural analysis to establish the mechanism of the reaction and nature of the reaction products (Wilkinson, 2000) or by spectrofluorophotometry to assess the fluorescence characteristics of the products formed (Spindler et al., 2009).

Spot testing is a good means of providing evidence of the selectivity of a process, evaluating which naturally occurring constituents and/or contaminants processes are capable of interacting with (Garrett and Bleay, 2013; Gaskell et al., 2013). It can also be used to establish substances that may give false-positive reactions with the reagent under test (Cox, 1991).

The spot testing approach can also be used for physical and optical processes to confirm that the expected physical interactions are occurring, although such tests are likely to give considerably less discrimination between individual constituents (e.g. powders will adhere to all viscous lipids but not dry amino acid spots) than equivalent tests with chemical processes.

It is also important that tests at TRL3 do not just consider model fingermark constituents and extend to trials that show the results observed are replicated with actual fingermarks. Confirmatory testing should therefore be conducted with fingermarks deposited by a small selection of donors. Ideally, these fingermarks should be 'natural' fingermarks deposited by donors that have not washed their hands for at least 30 minutes and therefore contain a combination of natural sweat deposits and any contaminants picked up from any items handled during that period. It is also worth considering including marks that are deliberately loaded with eccrine and/or sebaceous sweat in addition to 'natural' marks, thus providing additional confirmation of which types of mark are most likely to be enhanced by the process. Eccrine marks can be obtained by washing the hands and then wearing powder-free rubber gloves until the hands become sweaty, and sebaceous marks obtained by washing the hands and then wiping the fingers across regions rich in sebaceous glands, such as the forehead and the sides of the nose. Some researchers have proposed the use of simulants as an alternative to deposition of natural fingermarks and as a means of providing greater consistency between marks. Although this may be beneficial in some circumstances, there are limitations (Zadnik et al., 2013), and therefore simulants should be used with caution.

In addition to assessing the fundamental reactions occurring between the enhancement process and the fingermark, research at TRL3 may also be necessary to establish the fundamental interactions that occur between the fingermark and the substrate it has been deposited onto, for example, to determine whether a particular substrate is likely to absorb a fingermark or chemically react with it. Studies of this type typically utilise microscopy techniques to reveal the interactions occurring at a micro- and nanostructural level (Almog et al., 2004; Bacon et al., 2013).

16.3 Technology Readiness Level 4: Process optimisation

Once confirmation has been obtained that the predicted interactions occur between fingermarks and the enhancement process under investigation, the next stage of the research is generally the optimisation of the processing parameters in order to maximise the number of fingermarks that can be detected. This stage of research therefore focuses on establishing the *sensitivity* of the process.

For chemical processes, the formulations used for proof of concept may contain several components, and their influences on the reaction outcome may not always be known. There may also be other parameters that affect the process such as temperature and humidity, and the effect of variations in such parameters may need investigation.

One method for conducting a rapid assessment of the effects of variations in formulation (such as changing dye concentration) and/or processing parameters is the 'quartered fingermark' (Garrett and Bleay, 2013). Samples are produced by a donor placing a single fingermark in the centre of a surface that is divided into four equal parts, with another set of fingermarks deposited across each of the four boundaries between quarters (Figure 16.1).

For such tests, it is important to make each fingermark compositionally similar by carefully rubbing fingertips together before deposition to spread the mixture of constituents evenly across all fingers. The surface is then divided into four, and each quarter is then processed using a different formulation or set of processing conditions, for example:

Quarter 1: Baseline formulation

Quarter 2: Baseline formulation, 75% dye concentration

Quarter 3: Baseline formulation, 50% dye concentration

Quarter 4: Baseline formulation, 25% dye concentration

or

Quarter 1: Baseline formulation, processed at normal temperature

Quarter 2: Baseline formulation, processed at 25°C above normal temperature

Quarter 3: Baseline formulation, processed at 50°C above normal temperature

Quarter 4: Baseline formulation, processed at 75°C above normal temperature

After processing the quarters are recombined and evaluated, looking for trends in the appearance of the enhanced marks with changes in the processing conditions. The assessment can either be conducted on a subjective basis or by using

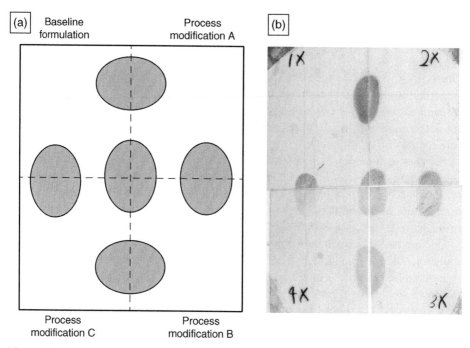

Figure 16.1 The 'quartered fingermark' concept used for investigating variations in processing parameters: (a) schematic diagram and (b) image of a comparison of different dye concentrations in a reagent under evaluation. Reproduced courtesy of the Home Office.

instruments such as reflection densitometers or fluorescence meters (Bicknell and Ramotowski, 2008) to obtain objective measurements from regions of the enhanced marks.

Ideally, experiments of this type should be repeated for marks deposited by a range of different donors to confirm that the trends observed are replicated across a sample of the population.

There may be situations where it is difficult to distinguish between different formulations of the same reagent using methods such as the quartered fingermark, or the process being evaluated may be required to enhance very low concentrations of a contaminant such as blood. In these circumstances, alternative tests using dilution series can be utilised to establish the relative sensitivity of the process (Figure 16.2).

In a 'dilution series', different concentrations of a solution of the model constituent (or contaminant) are deposited as a series of spots on an inert substrate. The spots are allowed to dry and then processed using the reagent. The lowest concentration value in the dilution series for which a visible and/or fluorescent reaction product is still discernible is recorded and compared to results from other reagents and/or variations on the same reagent (Sears et al., 2005). Research effort has

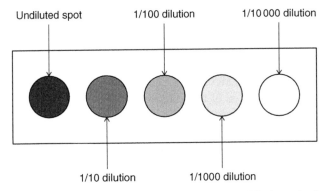

Figure 16.2 Schematic diagram of a dilution series concept used for investigating process sensitivity to particular constituents or contaminants.

been directed to the production of 'test strips' consisting of patterns printed using dilutions of mixtures of fingermark constituents (Kupferschmid et al., 2011). Although principally intended for use in confirming that processes are functioning properly in a laboratory environment, test strips can also be a useful means of comparing the effectiveness of different formulations.

The desired output of research at TRL4 is the generation of an optimised formulation and set of processing parameters for use in comparative trials with existing processes.

16.4 Technology Readiness Level 5: Laboratory trials

The research in the stages TRL3 and TRL4 is designed to establish the sensitivity and selectivity of the process in isolation. The studies conducted to demonstrate TRL5 should build on this knowledge base and extend testing to explore the *comparative* sensitivity and selectivity of the process.

Experiments in TRL5 generally use 'natural' fingermarks deposited under controlled conditions in a laboratory. Natural fingermarks are preferred because it is important to account for the variability in sweat composition between donors as part of the comparison. The exception to this general rule is where processes that are intended to target contaminants (e.g. blood or grease) are being investigated, in which case fingermarks produced by dipping the finger in the contaminant and depositing marks on a clean surface can be used.

There are several different types of experiments that can be used in laboratory trials, and which are actually selected will depend on what the trials are intended to establish. Some examples of the experiments that can be used and their general purpose are described in the following text.

16.4.1   Multiple donor trials

Multiple donor trials are a means of rapidly determining the ability of a process to develop fingermarks across a sample of a population. The test involves a large number of different donors placing a single fingermark on a test substrate, which is then aged for an appropriate period of time before being treated with the process under evaluation.

The number and quality of marks enhanced is recorded. Clearly, processes that are capable of enhancing marks of a good quality from the large numbers of donors are likely to be most beneficial in operational use, but these results should not be considered in isolation. It is also necessary to take into account tests that consider the sensitivity of the process, and processes that only develop small numbers of marks may be of use in sequential processing if these are marks from donors that are not enhanced by any other process. The use of processes in sequence is described in greater detail in Chapter 17.

Multiple donor studies can also be beneficial in establishing the typical response of individual donors to the process under test, enabling the researcher to identify pools of 'good', 'medium' and 'poor' donors for subsequent testing.

16.4.2   Depletion series

One limitation of multiple donor studies is that it only uses a single contact from each donor and therefore gives no information regarding sensitivity.

A means of obtaining information about sensitivity for deposited fingermarks is the 'depletion series', produced using the same finger to place a series of fingermarks on the test substrate. Each contact will result in the progressive transfer of material from the finger to the substrate, and therefore in theory fingermarks further down the depletion series contain a lower amount of the principal constituents. By obtaining depletion series from several different donors and then developing them, the sensitivity of the process can be established by observing how far down the depletion series marks continue to be developed. A test of this type can also provide information about inter-donor variability (Figure 16.3).

Although single panels with multiple depletion series can be used to compare the relative effectiveness of different processes, a meaningful comparison requires equivalent set of test substrates to be generated using the same set of donors, ideally one immediately after the other. This minimises the intra-donor variability between the depletion series deposited on each substrate. Variability can also be minimised by rubbing the fingers together before deposition to obtain an even distribution of constituents across all fingers. Tools have also been developed to ensure an even pressure and contact area between repeat contacts from the same finger (Fieldhouse, 2011), which may prove useful in studies of this type.

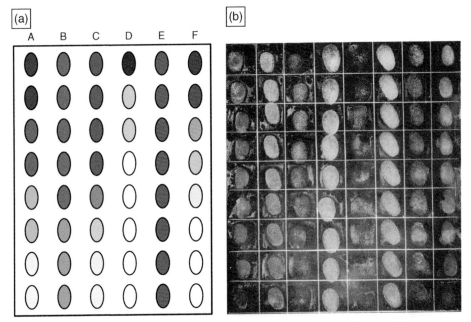

Figure 16.3 Depletion series deposited by several different donors, with variability between donors: (a) schematic diagram and (b) practical example showing fingermarks developed using cyanoacrylate fuming and fluorescent dye staining. Reproduced courtesy of the Home Office.

Despite all these methods of reducing variability between depletion series from different fingers of the same donor, it cannot be guaranteed that there is direct equivalence between test panels used to compare different processes. Where it is at all possible, the concept of a 'split depletion series' is recommended for direct comparisons between processes (Figure 16.4).

By using the same fingermark to conduct the comparison between processes, most issues associated with potential intra-donor variability can be overcome. There may be differences in pressure between one side of the deposited mark and the other during deposition; if it is suspected that this is influencing results, then the experiment should be repeated but reversing the sides of the depletion series treated with each process.

16.4.3 Evaluation of marks

For all comparative studies, it is essential to have a means of evaluating the marks developed by each process in order to determine their relative effectiveness. Several methods have been developed to assist in this comparison, using mainly subjective but increasingly objective measures of assessing marks.

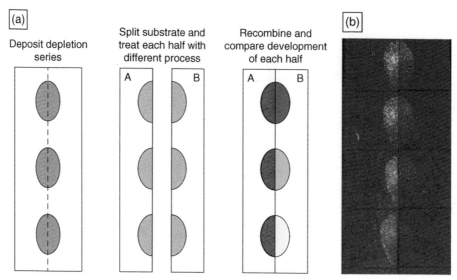

Figure 16.4 The concept of a split depletion series overcoming issues of intra-donor variability: (a) schematic diagram and (b) practical example comparing different formulations of 1,2-indandione. Reproduced courtesy of the Home Office.

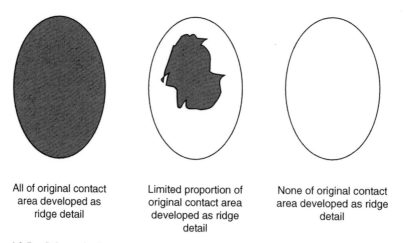

All of original contact area developed as ridge detail

Limited proportion of original contact area developed as ridge detail

None of original contact area developed as ridge detail

Figure 16.5 Schematic diagram showing the concept of using the proportion of area developed as visible ridge detail as a means of comparing marks.

For laboratory trials, such comparisons are made easier because of the fact that the mark is deposited under controlled conditions and the original contact area is largely known. As a consequence, one of the means used to evaluate marks is the proportion of the original contact area that is developed as visible ridge detail, as shown schematically in Figure 16.5.

This subjectively determined proportion of developed ridge detail can be converted to a numerical value that can be used in comparisons, an example of a

Table 16.2 Numerical grading scheme used for assessment of developed marks.

Score	Level of detail
0	No evidence of mark
1	Weak development; evidence of contact but no ridge detail visible
2	Limited development; up to one-third of original contact area developed with ridge detail but probably cannot be used for identification purposes
3	Strong development; between one-third and two-thirds of original contact area developed with ridge detail; identifiable fingermark
4	Very strong development; between two-thirds and all of original contact area developed with ridge detail; identifiable fingermark

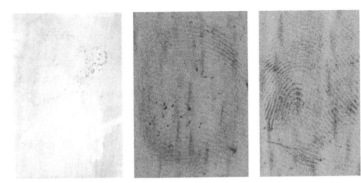

Figure 16.6 Examples of marks graded 1, 2, 3 and 4 using the grading scheme outlined above. Reproduced courtesy of the Home Office.

typical grading scheme being shown in Table 16.2 and illustrated using examples in Figure 16.6.

Scoring schemes of this type are subjective and rely on all the developed marks being graded by the same person (although studies have shown that reasonable consistency is usually obtained between assessors (Lewis, 2013)). The scheme earlier does not consider the numbers of minutiae that may be present, only the area of the mark that has been developed. There are several reasons for this: the majority of researchers conducting laboratory research are not skilled in fingerprint identification and not accustomed to counting points, point counting can be significantly more time consuming than assessing visible areas of ridge detail and small developed areas (e.g. near a delta or core) can contain large numbers of minutiae and thus skew results based on point counting alone.

More advanced schemes have been developed that assign secondary scores to clarity and continuity of ridge detail and the contrast between the ridges and the background. Such schemes may be required to properly discriminate between processes that give very similar levels of development, but, for example, one process gives ridges of higher contrast with the background.

Table 16.3 Comparative grading scheme used for assessment of developed marks.

Numerical value	Qualitative equivalent
−2	Significant decrease in enhancement when compared to mark developed using control process
−1	Slight decrease in enhancement when compared to mark developed using control process
0	No difference in enhancement when compared to mark developed using control process
+1	Slight increase in enhancement when compared to mark developed using control process
+2	Significant increase in enhancement when compared to mark developed using control process

An alternative means of discriminating between processes that is particularly appropriate where split marks are being used is the comparative method proposed by McLaren et al. (2010). In this method, a score is assigned based on the appearance of the half of the mark developed with the process under evaluation relative to the other developed using the control process (Table 16.3).

A scheme of this type provides a rapid means of identifying which process is more effective, but does not provide information about the quality of the marks that have been developed (a score of '0' could equally mean that both marks are developed very poorly or to a high quality). It should therefore be used in conjunction with a secondary assessment system if information about the quality of the marks is required.

Subjective assessment schemes are widely used in fingerprint research; however there has been increasing interest in finding more objective methods. Some of the approaches proposed have utilised quantified contrast differences between the developed ridges and the background (Humphreys et al., 2008; Vanderwee et al., 2011). Other research groups have considered tools that generate 'quality maps' based on an assessment of the clarity and contrast of the visible ridge detail and can output percentage scores or maps related to quality (Hicklin et al., 2011, 2013; Langenburg et al., 2012; Mattei et al., 2013). It is likely that such systems will find increasing application in research in the future.

16.4.4 Variables

In addition to the methodologies outlined previously, the influence of variables known to play a role in fingermark deposition (described in Chapter 2) and the ageing process post-deposition (described in Chapter 3) should be explored. Such variables include those associated with the fingermark, the substrate, the environment both are exposed to and the time elapsed since deposition. These are described in more detail hereafter.

16.4.4.1 The fingermark

In the majority of situations, processes are being evaluated on the basis that they are developing natural fingermarks. As a consequence, the influence of the natural variation in sweat composition between different individuals should be incorporated into experiments by using a range of donors. The donors can be selected in many ways, for example, a mixture of 'good', 'medium' and 'poor' donors selected from preliminary trials, a range of the typical population (e.g. a mixture of male, female, young, old, manual and office workers) or a targeted population (e.g. adult males 18–40 years old).

In cases where processes are being evaluated in terms of their ability to enhance contaminants, variation between individuals becomes irrelevant because the presence of the contaminant dominates fingermark composition. In such experiments a single donor can be used, producing fingermarks by dipping a finger into the contaminant and then placing marks on a clean surface. In cases of a specific contaminant such as blood, a single series of marks can be used, whereas if the process is intended to enhance a generic class of contaminant (e.g. 'fats'), then several sets of marks may be used, each produced from a different 'fatty' contaminant (e.g. Cadd et al., 2013).

16.4.4.2 The substrate

Very few processes are introduced with the purpose of developing fingermarks on a single, tightly defined type of substrate. It is generally desirable that a process develops marks on as broad a range of substrates as possible or at least a broad range within a generic class (e.g. 'plastics').

Laboratory trials should therefore aim to include an assessment of the variation in performance of the process across a range of operationally representative substrates. The substrates selected should consider the intended application of the process, for example, a process such as a powder intended for use on non-porous surfaces at crime scenes could consider glass, gloss painted wood, ceramic, laminates, metal and unplasticised PVC, all surfaces encountered in household interiors. A study on a process intended for use on paper items could include recycled printer paper, white and brown envelopes, newspaper, lined notebook paper, writing paper and banknotes. Although such substrates may appear nominally similar to each other, they can differ significantly in terms of chemical composition, fillers and additives used and porosity, all of which can lead to differences in the performance of the process. If there are any substrates for which the process is particularly good (or particularly poor), it is useful to identify this so that its scope of application can be selected accordingly.

For non-porous substrates in particular, the inclusion of nominally similar substrates with varying degrees of surface texture should be considered as a means of establishing the influence of surface texture on the effectiveness of the process. Again, the knowledge obtained from such testing can be used to establish the scope of application for the process.

16.4.4.3 The environment

During laboratory trials, tests are conducted under conditions that are reasonably controlled in terms of the temperature and relative humidity. Although such conditions may be replicated in indoor environments, many items and surfaces associated with crime scenes will experience environments that vary significantly from these 'standard' conditions (Figure 16.7).

Even without exposure to more extreme environments, there can be significant variations in climate from country to country and even within a single country. It can be difficult for this variability to be included in laboratory trials, and this aspect may only be properly explored in pseudo-operational and operational trials.

It is possible to explore more gross variations in environmental conditions on the effectiveness of processes, provided that exposure to such environments can be conducted in a controlled, reproducible way. Examples of environments that have been used in laboratory trials to examine the effect of extreme conditions on process effectiveness include:

- Water immersion (e.g. Nic Daeid et al., 2008)

- Heating to high temperatures (Dominick et al., 2009)

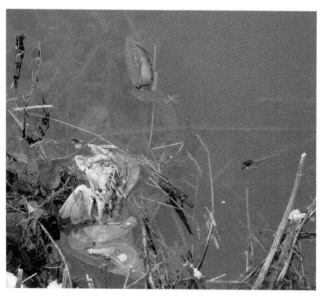

Figure 16.7 Plastic bags found in an environment where they have been subjected to water immersion.

- Exposure to ultraviolet radiation (Goode et al., 1979)
- Deposition of layers of greasy contaminants (Gaskell et al., 2013)
- Contact with drug contamination (Charlton et al., 2013)
- Exposure to gamma radiation (Ramotowski and Regen, 2005)
- Exposure to CBRN decontaminants (Zuidberg et al., 2014)

The range of environments that can be investigated is almost limitless, and there is no 'standardised' and widely accepted test of this type. In general, experiments incorporating assessments of the effect of the environment use customised methods, although equipment providing controlled environments (e.g. temperature controlled ovens, freezers, UV exposure cabinets) can be used to maintain control over exposure conditions.

16.4.4.4 Age of the mark

As has been previously described in Chapter 4, the composition and properties of fingermarks change after deposition, with some of these changes occurring within a few days and others occurring over a much longer period of time. As a consequence, laboratory trials should include fingermarks of different ages, for example:

- 1 day
- 1 week
- 1 month

These represent a reasonable range that is representative of the age of the marks encountered operationally: crime scenes may be attended within hours of the crime being committed, whereas some items may remain in exhibit stores for several weeks before treatment or before the crime is detected. After 1 month, any further changes in properties and composition occur at a much slower rate, and there is less benefit in including older marks in studies.

Obtaining information about the influence of the age of the mark on process effectiveness is beneficial, regardless of the outcome. Some processes are known to drop in effectiveness very rapidly as the fingermark ages. This does not mean that they are of no use in operational environments; if it is known that the crime has only recently been committed, such processes may be amongst the most effective available. Conversely, other processes may become more effective as the fingermark ages and are therefore more useful on items or surfaces that are only recovered or processed several days or weeks after the deposition of the mark.

16.4.4.5 *Distribution of constituents*

All of the experiments outlined previously assume a uniform distribution of finger-mark constituents across the ridges. This uniformity can be assisted by rubbing the hands and fingertips together before deposition of the marks, spreading constituents across all of the ridges.

Although this is suitable for experiments in this phase of testing, it should be recognised that in real scenarios there may be inhomogeneity in the distribution of constituents and/or contaminants across the fingertip. Such inhomogeneity may exist on the macro- or microscopic level (Figure 16.8).

In both of these scenarios, it is likely that the resultant fingermark will only be partly developed by a single process and application of another process will be required to reveal all of the ridge detail present. This is the principle behind sequential processing, which will be described in greater detail in Chapter 17. Marks of this type are difficult to generate reproducibly and are not generally used during this stage of testing. They may, however, be encountered during pseudo-operational and operational trials, as described hereafter.

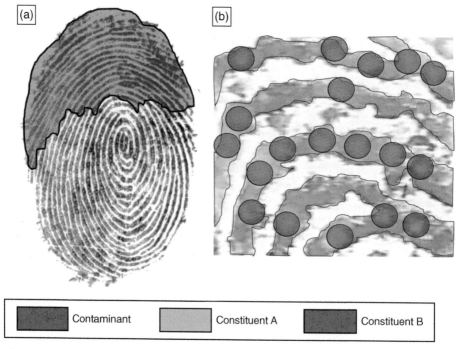

| Contaminant | Constituent A | Constituent B |

Figure 16.8 Examples of ways in which constituents/contaminants can be inhomogeneously distributed on a fingertip: (a) part of a finger covered in contaminant and (b) eccrine sweat constituents concentrated around pores with other constituents more evenly distributed along ridges.

16.5   Technology Readiness Level 6: Pseudo-operational trials

Once the performance of a fingermark enhancement process has been established across a range of substrates, donors and ages of mark in a laboratory environment, the next stage in its research should focus on more operationally representative scenarios.

There are several ways in which pseudo-operational material can be generated, including gathering of batches of material with unknown histories from waste bins, using sets of material known to have been handled in a similar manner (such as cheques or exam papers) (Figure 16.9), or from asking known donors to perform a given set of handing activities on a particular type of item. All of these methods give varying degrees of control over the deposition conditions and knowledge of the donors used but also share a common feature in that the marks deposited are likely to be partial and/or exhibit features such as movement or multiple touches.

Once the test material has been divided into batches that have either received equivalent, known amounts of handling or consist of nominally similar materials,

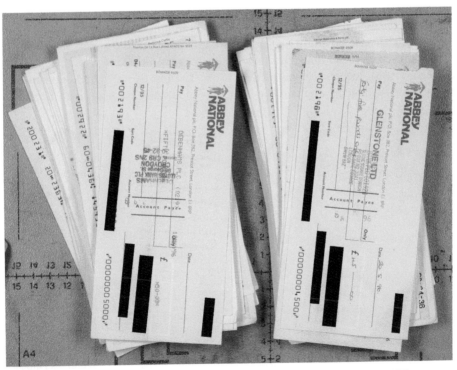

Figure 16.9   Equivalent bundles of cheques used for pseudo-operational trials on different processes.

each batch can be treated with a different process or formulation of the same process.

Because the initial contact area between the finger and the substrate is unknown and it is not generally possible to evenly split substrates around fingermarks whose location is uncertain, grading systems of the types proposed in Section 16.4 cannot be used. As a consequence, alternative ways of conducting comparative assessments on the marks developed are required.

One way of doing such assessments is to use a trained fingerprint examiner to assess the number of regions of developed ridge detail that are considered identifiable and to keep a cumulative total of these regions that are developed by each process.

Alternatively, measurements of the area of continuous, developed ridge detail can be used as a method of determining process effectiveness. This method does not require a trained fingerprint examiner and makes the assumption (based on previous consultation with examiners) that an area of $64\,\text{mm}^2$ generally contains a sufficient number of minutiae to be potentially identifiable. The area of developed ridge detail can be established by drawing around the developed region on a clear acetate sheet overlaid over the surface and then putting the clear acetate over graph paper (Figure 16.10).

Other potential means of assessing the ridge detail developed include the use of an Automated Fingerprint Identification System (AFIS) to auto-encode the regions of ridge detail and to include those that meet a minimum criterion for the number of minutiae. This will generally only be possible if the AFIS is a stand-alone system used for research rather than one connected to a live database.

Regardless of the assessment method used, the objective of pseudo-operational trials is to establish whether the process under assessment gives potential

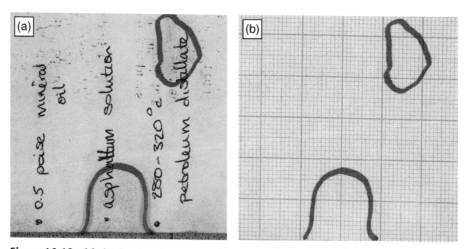

Figure 16.10   Marks developed on a paper document using ninhydrin in a pseudo-operational trial: (a) areas of continuous ridge detail drawn on clear acetate overlay and (b) acetate sheet placed over graph paper to enable area of ridge detail to be determined.

performance benefits over existing processes or whether it continues to develop significant numbers of marks on a previously difficult-to-treat substrate. The primary method of establishing these is by analysing the cumulative numbers of viable ridge detail developed over a wide range of items, which needs to be sufficiently large for trends to be seen. Examples of the types and quantities of materials used in pseudo-operational trials include batches of 75 fraudulently passed cheques (Hewlett and Sears, 1997; Hewlett et al., 1997) and collections of 100 plastic bags (Downham et al., 2012) to generate enough information for this phase.

16.6 Technology Readiness Level 7: Operational trials

The final experimental stage in the progression of a process from a paper concept to one that is in routine operational use is to verify that the results observed in the previous stages of assessment are reproduced in an operational environment.

Prior to initiating an operational trial, it may be necessary to obtain permissions from appropriate regulatory bodies. In the case of the United Kingdom, these include the Forensic Science Regulator and the Crown Prosecution Service. This is because of the risks that evidence may be lost when using experimental processes on live casework. The body of evidence obtained from previous experiments is important in demonstrating that the risks of losing evidence have been mitigated by conducting a thorough assessment of the process effectiveness prior to the operational trial.

Risks can be further mitigated by applying the process to items from real casework where the case is not going to be progressed before using items from live cases. The test methodology should be similar to that used in pseudo-operational trials, applying the test process(es) and the existing process to a broadly similar range of items and continuously monitoring the performance of each process in the trial. In operational trials, the assessment is conducted by a fingerprint examiner who evaluates the areas of ridge detail developed and records the number of identifiable marks enhanced by each process (Hewlett and Sears, 1999; Merrick et al., 2002). The trial should continue until a sufficiently large number of items have been treated and examined and also for a sufficiently long period for potential seasonal variations in the performance of the process to be identified (Wilkinson et al., 2003).

16.7 Technology Readiness Level 8: Standard operating procedures

If a process demonstrates clear benefits when included in an operational trial, it may be considered fit for operational use. To enable wider implementation of the process, instructions for its use should be prepared, and the results obtained in the previous phases of testing compiled to provide evidence that the process is fit for its intended purpose. This may include publication of these results in a peer-reviewed journal.

Laboratories wishing to implement the process may need to conduct a further limited amount of tests of its use in their specific laboratory environment and satisfy themselves that it performs as expected. They may also need to write local standard operating procedures around the equipment and facilities available and in accordance with any standards that the laboratory is working to, for example, ISO 17025.

16.8 Technology Readiness Level 9: Ongoing monitoring

Monitoring of the process should not cease once standard operating procedures have been drawn up and the process has entered operational use. The number of marks enhanced by the process should be continuously monitored, both to see whether the effectiveness of the process is changing over time and to build knowledge of its performance in operational use. By monitoring performance, any changes in effectiveness can be rapidly identified and the reasons for them explored. In some cases investigations into observed changes in performance have revealed batches of chemicals outside the requested specification, but in other cases more fundamental changes may be occurring over time, such as the progressive increase in recycled content in plastic bags that resulted in the fall in effectiveness of vacuum metal deposition on such items (Barras, 2009; Downham et al., 2012).

References

Almog J, Azoury M, Elmaliah Y, Berenstein L, Zaban A, '"Fingerprints" third dimension: the depth and shape of fingerprints penetration into paper – cross section examination by fluorescence microscopy', J Forensic Sci, vol 49(5), (2004), p 981–985.

Bacon S R, Ojeda J J, Downham R, Sears V G, Jones B J, 'The effects of polymer pigmentation on fingermark development techniques', J Forensic Sci, vol 58(6), (2013), p 1486–1494.

Bandey H L (ed.), 'Fingermark Visualisation Manual', Home Office, London, 2014.

Barras C, 'Recycled plastics giving criminals a break', New Scientist, 6 April 2009.

Bicknell D E, Ramotowski R S, 'Use of an optimized 1,2-indanedione process for the development of latent prints', J Forensic Sci, vol 53(5), (2008), p 1108–1116.

Bleay S M, Sears V G, Bandey H L, Gibson A P, Bowman V J, Downham R, Fitzgerald L, Ciuksza T, Ramadani J, Selway C, 'Fingerprint Source Book', Home Office, 6 June 2012, available online: https://www.gov.uk/government/publications/fingerprint-source-book (accessed 25 October 2017).

Cadd S J, Bleay S M, Sears V G, 'Evaluation of the solvent black 3 fingermark enhancement reagent: part 2, investigation of the optimum formulation and application parameters', Sci Justice, vol 53(2), (2013), p 131–143.

Cantu A A, Leben D A, Joullie M M, Heffner R J, Hark R R, 'A comparative examination of several amino acid reagents for visualising amino acid (glycine) on paper', J Forensic Identif, vol 43(1), (1993), p 44–67.

Charlton D T, Bleay S M, Sears V G, 'Evaluation of the multi metal deposition process for fingermark enhancement in simulated operational environments', Anal Methods, vol 5, (2013), p 5411–5417.

Cox M, 'A study of the sensitivity and specificity of four presumptive tests for blood', J Forensic Sci, vol 36(5), (1991), p 1503–1511.

Dominick A J, Nic Daeid N, Bleay S M, Sears V, 'The recoverability of fingerprints on paper exposed to elevated temperatures: part 1, comparison of enhancement techniques', J Forensic Identif, vol 59(3), (2009), p 325–355.

Downham R P, Mehmet S, Sears V G, 'A pseudo-operational investigation into the development of latent fingerprints on flexible plastic packaging films', J Forensic Identif, vol 62(6), (2012), p 661–682.

Fieldhouse S, 'Consistency and reproducibility in fingermark deposition', Forensic Sci Int, vol 207, (2011), p 96–100.

Garrett H J, Bleay S M, 'Evaluation of the solvent black 3 fingermark enhancement reagent: part 1, investigation of fundamental interactions and comparisons with other lipid-specific reagents', Sci Justice, vol 53(2), (2013), p 121–130.

Gaskell C, Bleay S M, Willson H, Park S, 'Enhancement of fingermarks on grease-contaminated, nonporous surfaces: a comparative assessment of processes for light and dark surfaces', J Forensic Identif, vol 63(3), (2013), p 286–319.

Goode G C, Morris J R, Wells J M, 'The application of radioactive bromine isotopes for the visualisation of latent fingerprints', J Radioanal Chem, vol 48, (1979), p 17–28.

Hewlett D F, Sears V G, 'Replacements for CFC113 in the ninhydrin process: part 1', J Forensic Identif, vol 47(3), (1997), p 287–299.

Hewlett D F, Sears V G, 'An operational trial of two non-ozone depleting ninhydrin formulations for latent fingerprint detection', J Forensic Identif, vol 49(4), (1999), p 388–396.

Hewlett D F, Sears V G, Suzuki S, 'Replacements for CFC113 in the ninhydrin process: part 2', J Forensic Identif, vol 47(3), (1997), 300–306.

Hicklin R A, Buscaglia J, Roberts M A, Meagher S B, Fellner W, Burge M J, Monaco M, Vera D, Pantzer L R, Yeung C C, Unnikumaran T N, 'Latent fingerprint quality: a survey of examiners', J Forensic Identif, vol 61(4), (2011), p 385–418.

Hicklin R A, Buscaglia J, Roberts M A, 'Assessing the clarity of friction ridge impressions', Forensic Sci Int, vol 226, (2013), p 106–117.

Humphreys J D, Porter G, Bell M, 'The quantification of fingerprint quality using a relative contrast index', Forensic Sci Int, vol 178(1), (2008), 46–53.

IFRG, 'Guidelines for the assessment of fingermark detection techniques', J Forensic Identif, vol 64(2), (2014), p 174–200.

ISO, 'ISO/IEC 17025:2005: General Requirements for the Competence of Testing and Calibration Laboratories', 2005, https://www.iso.org/standard/39883.html (accessed 25 October 2017).

Jones N E, Davies L M, Russell L M, Brennan J S, Bramble S K, 'A systematic approach to latent fingerprint sample preparation for comparative chemical studies', J Forensic Identif, vol 51(5), (2001), 504–551.

Kent T, 'Standardizing protocols for fingerprint reagent testing', J Forensic Identif, vol 60(3), (2010), p 371–379.

Kupferschmid E, Schwarz L, Champod C, 'Development of standardized test strips as a process control for the detection of latent fingermarks using physical developers', J Forensic Identif, vol 60(6), (2011), p 619–638.

Langenburg G, Champod C, Genessay T, 'Informing the judgements of fingerprint analysts using quality metric and statistical assessment tools', Forensic Sci Int, vol 219, (2012), p 183–198.

Lewis S, 'A large-scale donor trial to examine the performance of selected latent fingermark development techniques: preliminary considerations', presented at International Fingerprint Research Group Meeting, Ma'ala Hachamisha, 10 June 2013.

Mattei A, Cervelli F, Zampa F, Dardi F, 'Forensic traces quality analysis: a computer aided approach', presented at International Fingerprint Research Group Meeting, Ma'ala Hachamisha, 10 June 2013.

McLaren C, Lennard C, Stoilovic M, 'Methylamine pretreatment of dry latent fingermarks on polyethylene for enhanced detection by cyanoacrylate fuming', J Forensic Identif, vol 60(2), (2010), 199–222.

Merrick S, Gardner S, Sears V, Hewlett D, 'An operational trial of ozone-friendly DFO and 1,2-indandione formulations for latent fingerprint detection', J Forensic Identif, vol 52(5), (2002), p 595–605.

Nic Daeid N, Carter S, Laing K, 'Comparison of vacuum metal deposition and powder suspension for recovery of fingerprints on wetted nonporous surfaces', J Forensic Identif, vol 58(5), (2008), p 600–612.

Ramotowski R S, Regen E M, 'The effect of electron beam irradiation on forensic evidence: 1, latent print recovery on porous and non-porous surfaces', J Forensic Sci, vol 50(2), (2005), 298–306.

Sears V, Butcher C, Fitzgerald L, 'Enhancement of fingerprints in blood: part 3, reactive techniques, acid yellow 7 and process sequences', J Forensic Identif, vol 55(6), (2005), p 741–763.

Sears V G, Bleay S M, Bandey H L, Bowman V J, 'A methodology for finger mark research', Sci Justice, vol 52(3), (2012), p 145–160.

Spindler X, Stoilovic M, Lennard C, Lennard A, 'Spectral variations for reaction products formed between different amino acids and latent fingermark detection reagents on a range of cellulose-based substrates', J Forensic Identif, vol 59(3), (2009), p 308–324.

Vanderwee J, Porter G, Renshaw A, Bell M, 'The investigation of a relative contrast index model for fingerprint quantification', Forensic Sci Int, vol 204, (2011), p 74–79.

Wilkinson D, 'A study of the reaction mechanism of 1,8-diazafluoren-9-one with the amino acid, l-alanine', Forensic Sci Int, vol 109(2), (2000), p 87–102.

Wilkinson D, McKenzie E, Leech C, Mayowski D, Bertrand S, Walker T, 'The results from a Canadian National Field Trial comparing two formulations of 1,8-diazafluoren-9-one (DFO) with 1,2-indandione', Identif Canada, vol 26(2), (2003), p 8–18.

Zadnik S, Van Bronswijk W, Frick A A, Fritz P, Lewis S W, 'Fingermark simulants and their inherent problems: a comparison with latent fingermark deposits', J Forensic Identif, vol 63(5), (2013), p 593–608.

Zuidberg M C, van Woerkorn T, de Bruin K G, de Puit M, 'Effects of CBRN decontaminants in common use by first responders on the recovery of latent fingerprints – assessment of the loss of ridge detail on glass', J Forensic Sci, vol 59(1), (2014), p 61–69.

17

Sequential processing and impact on other forensic evidence

Stephen M. Bleay[1] and Marcel de Puit[2]
[1] Home Office Centre for Applied Science and Technology, Sandridge, UK
[2] Ministerie van Veiligheid en Justitie, Nederlands Forensisch Instituut, Digitale Technologie en Biometrie, The Hague, The Netherlands

---

Key points

- The broad range of fingermark enhancement processes available and the range of ways in which they enhance fingermarks make it possible to use multiple processes in sequence to maximise recovery.

- Fingermarks should be considered within the broader context of forensic evidence recovery, so the impact of fingermark recovery on other types of forensic evidence (and vice versa) should be assessed.

- Non-contact, non-destructive processes capable of locating multiple types of forensic evidence should always be considered at the beginning of forensic recovery sequences.

17.1 Sequential processing of fingermarks

One important differentiator between fingermark enhancement and the recovery of most other types of forensic evidence is the fact that it is possible to treat the same exhibit several times with different enhancement processes in order to maximise the amount of fingermark evidence recovered. This sequential approach to fingermark enhancement is made possible by the complexity of the chemical composition of fingermarks and the other physical properties that they possess.

Fingerprint Development Techniques: Theory and Application, First Edition.
Stephen M. Bleay, Ruth S. Croxton and Marcel de Puit.
© 2018 John Wiley & Sons Ltd. Published 2018 by John Wiley & Sons Ltd.

Sequential fingermark enhancement flow charts have been devised by several agencies for many different types of surface. An example of this type of processing chart is illustrated in Figure 17.1; in this case the chart for porous surfaces is produced by the Home Office Centre for Applied Science and Technology (Bandey, 2014).

The chart illustrates the order that the processes should be used in, the processes that are effective as single processes and may be appropriate for treating exhibits from volume crime and the effect of factors such as humidity, heat and surface texture on the effectiveness of each process in the sequence. Similar charts have been produced for a range of different surface types. The sequential processing charts all follow the same general approach of first proposing the use of non-contact, non-destructive processes and then progressing to processes that selectively deposit dry solid particles or material from the vapour phase and then liquid-based chemical and/or physical enhancement processes (with formulations based on organic solvents being generally less destructive than aqueous formulations and therefore used before them). By progressively selecting processes that target constituents that are still available to react after earlier treatments, it is possible to use multiple chemical/physical treatments and continue to develop additional marks after each one.

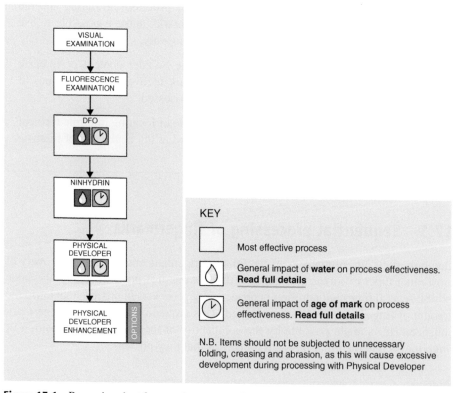

Figure 17.1 Processing chart for generic porous surfaces and associated key from the *Fingermark Visualisation Manual* (Bandey, 2014). Reproduced courtesy of the Home Office.

The way in which these processing charts are constructed is based on the results of experimental tests, the methodology of some of these being outlined in later sections. However, there is also a clear, logical rationale behind the selection of each process and the order in which to use them. This approach is evident when expanding upon the sequential processing chart for porous surfaces shown in Figure 17.1, and this can be seen in Table 17.1.

Theoretically, there are more enhancement processes that could be inserted into this sequence without significant detriment to the performance of those outlined previously. Table 17.2 shows the same sequence with some of these additional processes added.

Figure 17.2 provides a schematic representation of a processing sequence for porous surfaces, showing how each process in the sequence targets a different fingermark constituent.

Because additional processes could be incorporated into the sequence does not mean that they necessarily should be. The benefits in the number of additional marks that could be developed by the process must be weighed against the additional time and resources that are expended in applying it. This is where testing of candidate sequences becomes important as it can provide the supporting information to make informed decisions.

Not all processing charts give a continuous flow of processes that have little or no impact on subsequent treatments. An example of this situation can be seen in the equivalent processing chart for generic non-porous surfaces (Figure 17.3).

In this chart there are processes that are incompatible and cannot be used in sequence, and it may be necessary to make a decision as to which is likely to give the best results. The equivalent rationale behind the processing sequence suggested for non-porous surfaces is given in Table 17.3.

Table 17.1 A sequential processing route for porous surfaces.

Process	Rationale for selection
Visual examination	Non-contact, non-destructive. May reveal marks in visible contaminants such as dirt and ink
Fluorescence examination	Non-contact, non-destructive. May reveal naturally fluorescent marks or those deposited with fluorescent contaminants
DFO	Highly sensitive process reacting with amino acid constituents. Reaction with amino acids does not usually run to completion, leaving some available for reaction with subsequent processes. Non-amino acid constituents unaffected
Ninhydrin	Less sensitive than DFO, but capable of reacting with any residual amino acids and other some other constituents that may be present such as vitamins. Little impact on other constituents
Physical developer	Less sensitive than DFO and ninhydrin, but reacts with non-amino acid constituents (combinations of lipids and salts) remaining in the fingermark

Table 17.2 A modified sequential processing route for porous surfaces showing other processes (in italics) that could potentially be added.

Process	Rationale for selection
Visual examination	Non-contact, non-destructive. May reveal marks in contaminants such as dirt and ink
Fluorescence examination	Non-contact, non-destructive. May reveal naturally fluorescent marks or those deposited in fluorescent contaminants
UV reflection	*Non-contact, non-destructive (to fingermarks). May reveal marks in contaminants or rich in UV-absorbing amino acids*
ESDA	*No direct contact with surface, non-destructive. Marks developed by differences in electrostatic charge developed on fingermarks and background*
Iodine fuming	*Generally reversible process. Iodine vapour absorbed into lipids and water in fingermark, but resublimes over time. No permanent chemical reaction with fingermark constituents*
DFO	Highly sensitive process reacting with amino acid constituents. Reaction with amino acids does not usually run to completion, leaving some available for reaction with subsequent processes. Non-amino acid constituents unaffected
Ninhydrin	Less sensitive that DFO, but capable of reacting with any residual amino acids and other some other constituents that may be present such as vitamins. Little impact on other constituents
Physical developer	Less sensitive than DFO and ninhydrin, but reacts with non-amino acid constituents (combinations of lipids and salts) remaining in the fingermark
Oil Red O	*Less sensitive than DFO and ninhydrin. Stains lipids present in fingermarks; does not affect other water insoluble constituents*

In this sequence a decision point is reached where a choice needs to be made between the application of powder suspensions or cyanoacrylate fuming. Both processes are both highly effective enhancement processes and similar in terms of performance. However, they cannot be used in sequence because the application of one process adversely affects the other.

If powder suspensions are applied first, the aqueous components of the suspension and the water subsequently used to wash it from the surface will dissolve the salts and other soluble constituents that initiate the cyanoacrylate polymerisation reaction. If cyanoacrylate is used first, the thin layer of polycyanoacrylate deposited on the surface covers the residual fingermark deposit and prevents it from effectively interacting with the powder suspensions.

Neither process appears to totally inhibit the subsequent application of Basic Violet 3 to develop additional marks, but the decision regarding which process to use will depend on the individual circumstances of the case. The CAST chart is accompanied by notes that assist in the decision-making process, for example, the powder suspensions process is known to perform better on 1-week-old fingermarks

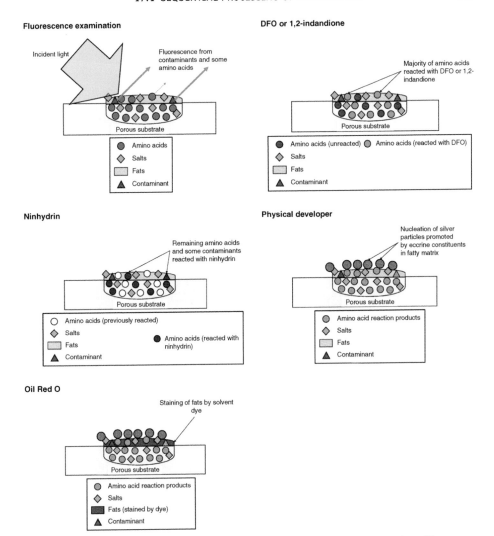

Figure 17.2   Schematic representation of a processing sequence for porous surfaces illustrating how fingermark constituents are successively targeted by different processes.

than it does on 1-day-old fingermarks, and this may suggest the use of cyanoacrylate fuming if exhibits have been recovered and are to be treated soon after the crime.

A schematic representation of the processing sequence utilising cyanoacrylate fuming is illustrated in Figure 17.4, again showing how each process targets different constituents in turn.

The enhancement of fingermarks on 'semi-porous' surfaces presents a complex scenario. On these surfaces there is the possibility that processes for both porous and non-porous surfaces could develop fingermarks and establishing the order in which these processes are applied will be critical.

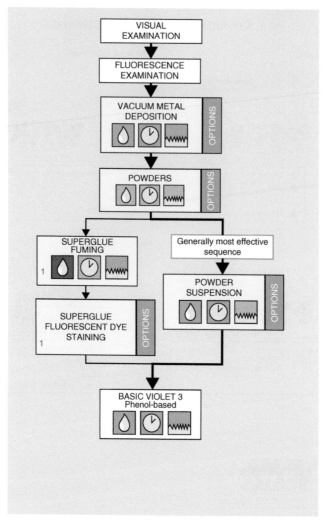

Figure 17.3 Processing chart for generic non-porous surfaces from the *Fingermark Visualisation Manual* (Bandey, 2014). Reproduced courtesy of the Home Office.

Table 17.3 A sequential processing route for non-porous surfaces.

Process	Rationale for selection
Visual examination	Non-contact, non-destructive. May reveal marks in contaminants such as dirt, ink or impressions in soft surfaces
Fluorescence examination	Non-contact, non-destructive. May reveal naturally fluorescent marks or those deposited in fluorescent contaminants
Powders	Utilise the adhesive properties of fingermark residues, selectively depositing dry powder on the fingermark but leaving chemical constituents unreacted
Cyanoacrylate fuming or	Initiated by water/salt constituents in fingermark residues
Powder suspensions	Precipitated by lipid/amino acid mixtures
Basic Violet 3	Stains fats and epithelial cells

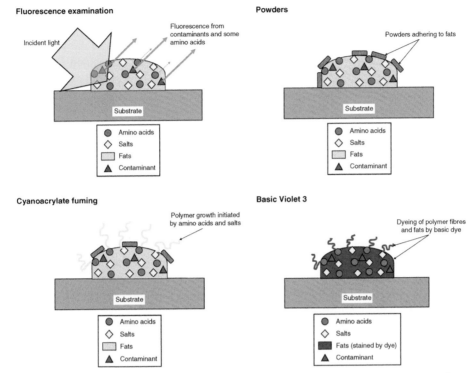

Figure 17.4   Schematic representation of a processing sequence for porous surfaces illustrating how fingermark constituents are successively targeted by different processes.

17.2   Test methodologies for developing processing sequences

In order to establish processing sequences, some means of testing the overall effectiveness of the sequence, the individual effectiveness of the processes within it and the impact of each process on subsequent processes is required. Some of the means by which this can be assessed are simple adaptations of the methods used to directly compare the effectiveness of individual processes in laboratory trials, and these are outlined in the succeeding text.

17.2.1   Sequential processing of multiple-donor panels

The 'multiple-donor' approach described in Chapter 16 can be adapted to the evaluation of sequential enhancement routines. In such an experiment a single fingermark is collected from many different donors, trying to obtain as representative a population of donors as possible. All of these fingermarks are deposited on a single substrate, which is then exposed to the desired environment for the selected period of time prior to the first enhancement process, and the number and quality of the fingermarks that are developed by that process is recorded.

The substrate is then exposed to the next enhancement process in the sequence under test, and the grading exercise is repeated. This process is repeated for all of the processes in the proposed sequence in turn. This should be repeated over a range of different surfaces and for marks of different ages, and if two candidate sequences are being compared, two surfaces of the same type should be prepared at the same time using the same donors. Figure 17.5 shows a set of fingermarks from different donors being put through a sequence of enhancement processes.

The overall effectiveness of the sequence is evaluated by assessing the number of the originally deposited fingermarks that are developed to a quality sufficient for identification. If a fingermark is developed by more than one of the processes in the sequence, it will only count as a single developed fingermark. The effectiveness of each individual process can be determined by recording the number of marks that are developed to an improved quality over the previous process, the number of additional marks it develops over the previous process and the number of unique marks it develops as part of the overall sequence. Such an analysis may enable the removal of a process from a sequence if it is demonstrated that it gives little benefit and develops no unique marks. Optimum sequences are those that develop the highest proportion of high quality fingermarks from the number originally deposited.

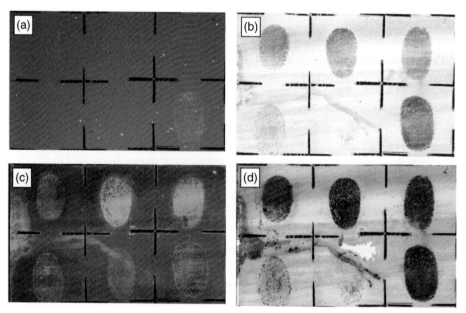

Figure 17.5   A series of photographs of a multiple-donor ceramic tile taken at different stages of a sequential processing study: (a) fluorescence examination using ultraviolet excitation, (b) black magnetic powder, (c) cyanoacrylate fuming/Basic Yellow 40 staining and (d) Basic Violet 3.

17.2.2   Sequential processing of split fingermarks

It is possible to investigate the potential impact of one enhancement process on the subsequent application of another by the 'split fingermark' method. This is particularly important where it is suspected that there is an incompatibility between two of the processes that are being proposed for use in the sequence or that the optimum order in which the two processes are to be used needs to be determined.

In this experiment, a depletion series of fingermarks are deposited down a centre line, on a surface that either is capable of being subsequently split (such as paper) or has been pre-split. The surface is divided and each half is exposed to a different treatment or sequence of treatments. In an example where processes A and B are being proposed for use in the sequence A–B, one half of the fingermark is treated using process B (the 'control' to establish how many fingermarks process B would develop) and the other treated by process A followed by process B (the test sequence). The two treated halves of the fingermark can then be recombined, and the effect of process A on process B determined. This is shown schematically and as results from an actual experiment in Figure 17.6.

By carrying out a series of these tests, it is possible to determine which processes are incompatible and which can be used in sequence without detrimental effects.

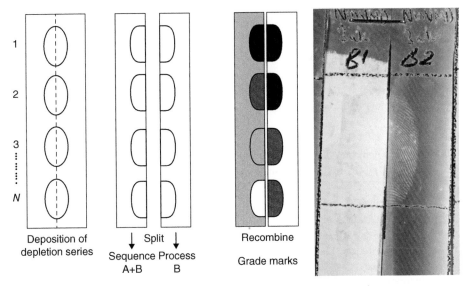

Figure 17.6   Schematic of a split depletion series used to establish processing sequences and an example showing where the prior application of ninhydrin has proved detrimental to subsequent treatment with vacuum metal deposition. Reproduced courtesy of the Home Office.

17.2.3   Sequential pseudo-operational trials

The pseudo-operational trial methodology described in Chapter 16 can also be extended to sequential processing, investigating the effectiveness of different sequences in their ability to recover the most marks overall and in establishing the effectiveness of individual processes in the sequence. Several examples of such studies have been reported for different substrates (Downham et al., 2012; McMullen and Beaudoin, 2013; Marriott et al., 2014). An example from a pseudo-operational trial demonstrating how the sequential use of processes can 'fill in' regions of previously undeveloped fingermark is shown in Figure 17.7.

An example of results generated from a pseudo-operational trial utilising sequential processing is given in Table 17.4.

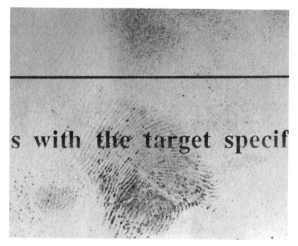

Figure 17.7   A fingermark from a pseudo-operational trial, initially treated with iodine solution (blue-black regions) and with further ridge detail revealed by ninhydrin (purple regions). Reproduced courtesy of the Home Office.

Table 17.4   The number of fingermarks developed on a mixture of 75 fraudulently passed cheques using the processes for porous surfaces in sequence in a pseudo-operational trial.

Process	Number of additional identifiable marks detected	Cumulative total
DFO (examined on day of treatment)	103	103
DFO (re-examined 14 days after treatment)	26	129
Ninhydrin (examined on day of treatment)	25	154
Ninhydrin (re-examined 14 days after treatment)	14	168
Physical developer	47	215

17.3   Integrated sequential forensic processing

17.3.1   Introduction

In the aforementioned sections, the only consideration in sequential treatments has been the potential impact of one fingermark enhancement process on another. In casework, fingermark recovery is rarely the only type of forensic evidence under consideration, and it is important to select the sequence of forensic recovery processes that will maximise evidential recovery whilst ensuring that the classes of evidence most critical to the case are preserved. It therefore becomes important to extend the understanding of sequential processing to the whole forensic process. In order to do this, it is necessary to utilise the understanding of what impact fingermark enhancement processes have on other methods of forensic evidence recovery, and vice versa.

Of critical importance in the devising of integrated forensic processing sequences are the range of non-contact, non-destructive processes that are available to the forensic scientist, several of which have the potential to simultaneously detect multiple evidence types. Visual examination using a range of white light sources and fluorescence examination using high intensity light sources of different wavelength outputs are of most practical use, and a summary of some of these useful wavelengths (expressed in terms of approximate colour) and their non-fingermark applications is given in Table 17.5.

Examination using short-wave ultraviolet (UV) radiation is not regarded as a truly non-destructive process although it is non-contact. This is because it is known that it has the potential to degrade DNA, potentially for exposure times of less than

Table 17.5   Some of the broader forensic applications of different types of light source.

Light source	Type of forensic evidence detected
White light	Footwear marks in dust (oblique lighting)
	Footwear marks (diffuse specular lighting)
	Fibres (oblique lighting)
	Indented writing (oblique lighting)
Long-wave ultraviolet	Footwear marks (absorbing or fluorescing contaminants)
	Document analysis (security features, alterations)
	Fibre detection
	Body fluid detection (semen, saliva, urine)
Blue	Body fluid detection (semen)
	Blood detection (background fluorescence)
Green	Fibre detection
Yellow	Fibre detection
	Erased ink marks (e.g. on skin)
Infrared	Blood detection (on dark surfaces)
	Document analysis (alterations, ink analysis, security features)

1 min depending on the power of the radiation source and its proximity to the DNA sample. If short-wave UV is being used for fingermark detection, its impact on potential DNA recovery will need to be taken into account.

Apart from the non-destructive processes outlined previously, which can generally be used on all types of evidence, the compatibility between fingermark enhancement and the other forensic recovery process needs to be considered for each forensic evidence type. A summary of the state of knowledge around other major types of forensic evidence is given in the following sections.

The use of any forensic recovery process and its impact on fingermark recovery can be assessed in terms of the triangle of interaction with the forensic recovery process being considered as the 'environment' that the fingermark and the surface are being exposed to.

17.3.2   DNA

Second only to fingermarks in terms of the number of identifications obtained, DNA is the one of the most important forms of identification evidence that can be recovered from crime scenes. The impact of fingermark recovery processes on the subsequent recovery of DNA has been investigated by several groups of researchers. The results of these studies are summarised in the succeeding text, but in general the application of a single fingermark enhancement process is rarely detrimental to subsequent DNA recovery. There is sometimes a misperception that fingermarks and DNA are exclusive evidence forms and that if one type of evidence is targeted, it will be detrimental to the other. In fact, fingermarks and DNA are complementary identification processes if used intelligently, and by using fingermark enhancement processes to show where articles have been handled, swabbing of contact areas for touch DNA can be more focused, thus saving time and resources and potentially increasing the success rates.

17.3.2.1   Effects of fingermark enhancement processes on DNA recovery

Because fingermarks and DNA are the two principal forms of forensic evidence that enable identification of individuals, it is not surprising that several studies have been conducted to establish the impact of recovering one type of evidence on subsequent recovery of the other. These have almost exclusively investigated the effect of fingermark enhancement processes on the recovery of DNA, and corresponding studies into the effect of DNA recovery on fingermark enhancement are currently lacking.

On the whole, the majority of studies that have been published agree that fingermark enhancement processes are not significantly detrimental to DNA recovery although there are some processes that are known to be more damaging than others. Of more importance is the need to avoid cross-contamination between DNA sources from different articles and different cases. As a consequence, DNA recovery may need to be conducted first in a clean environment, or precautions such as replacing reagents and cleaning surfaces between processing of each item taken to mitigate risks of cross-contamination.

Because DNA recovery was initially only possible from large biological stains, the first fingermark enhancement processes that began to be assessed in terms of their impact on DNA recovery were those that were in operational use for enhancement of fingermarks and/or footwear marks in blood. Some of the published studies are summarised in the succeeding text.

Stein et al. (1996) investigated DNA profiling of saliva and bloodstains on a range of different surfaces after treatment with superglue, ninhydrin and Basic Violet 3. No negative effect was observed on subsequent DNA typing. Anderson and Bramble (1997) evaluated the effect of light source examination on polymerase chain reaction (PCR)/short tandem repeat (STR) analysis of bloodstains. The light sources used included a several filtered high intensity light sources, an argon ion laser and both long- and short-wave UV sources. Most light sources had no appreciable effect on the results obtained from subsequent PCR analysis; however exposure of the bloodstains to short-wave UV light for more than 30 s precluded the acquisition of results from PCR analysis.

Roux et al. (1999) investigated the effect of commonly used fingermark enhancement processes on the subsequent DNA analysis of items potentially bearing both fingermarks and biological evidence. Bloodstains of varying ages were prepared on different operationally representative surfaces including white paper, glass, polyethylene bags, adhesive tape and stainless steel blades. It was considered that most fingermark enhancement processes did not have any adverse effects on DNA analysis, but some may have affected the quantity of DNA available by sticking the blood more strongly to the substrate. Multi-metal deposition was not recommended for use unless the blood had been fixed prior to application.

Studies specifically looking at blood enhancement reagents and their potential effect on STR DNA analysis were reported (Fregeau et al., 2000). Reagents investigated included Acid Black 1, Crowle's double stain, DFO, Hungarian Red, LeucoMalachite Green, luminol and ninhydrin, applied to fresh and aged fingermarks in blood deposited on both porous and non-porous surfaces. Enhancement of marks up to 54 days old was achieved with all reagents, with no adverse effects on the PCR amplification process. Continuous exposure of the blood to Crowle's double stain and Hungarian Red for 54 days slightly reduced the amplification efficiency of the larger STR loci, suggesting that long-term exposure to these chemicals may adversely affect DNA. The absence of a noticeable detrimental impact on DNA was confirmed by Grubwieser et al. (2003), with Coomassie blue, TMB and Leuco Crystal Violet being added to the range of blood reagents evaluated.

The possibility of recovering DNA from fingermarks in blood that had been treated with ninhydrin was demonstrated in an operational context in 2004 (Schulz et al., 2004). Finally, prior to the introduction of Acid Yellow 7 as an enhancement process for fingermarks in blood, a study was conducted to confirm that it had no detrimental impact on DNA recovery (Jordan, 2003).

Further studies investigated the effects of other fingermark enhancement processes including DFO (Zamir et al., 2000), 1,2-indandione (Azoury et al., 2002), VMD (Raymond et al., 2004), powders (Pesaresi et al., 2003) and powder suspensions (Jordan, 2003) on DNA recovery. None of these studies showed any one fingermark enhancement process to be significantly detrimental to DNA analysis.

As DNA analysis became more sensitive, studies began to consider the impact of fingermark enhancement processes on DNA recovery from latent marks using low template DNA analyses (Raymond et al., 2004; Leemans et al., 2006; Sewell et al., 2008; Bhoelai et al., 2011). For processes capable of targeting such small quantities of DNA, cross-contamination has become an increasing concern, and investigators are now considering whether fingermark enhancement processes can contribute to this.

A summary of some of the effects of commonly recommended fingermark enhancement processes on DNA recovery as determined in studies by the Home Office in conjunction with the Forensic Science Service in the early 2000s is given in Table 17.6.

As a consequence of the studies summarised in Table 17.6, some simple rules for maximising subsequent DNA recovery when carrying out fingermark enhancement treatments were generated. These are listed as follows:

Table 17.6 Potential impacts of fingermark recovery processes on DNA recovery.

Fingermark enhancement process	Potential effect on subsequent DNA recovery
Visual examination	None (possible cross-contamination if precautions not taken)
Fluorescence examination	None (possible cross-contamination if precautions not taken)
	Heating effect of high power light sources needs consideration
UV reflection	Degradation of DNA, potentially within seconds
Powdering	Cross-contamination issues with use of same brush and powder pot on multiple marks
	Brushing may remove some DNA from surface
	No inhibition recorded for standard powder types
DFO	None determined
Ninhydrin	None determined
Physical developer	Some detrimental effect of DNA recovery rates observed
Vacuum metal deposition	None determined
Superglue	None determined
Powder suspensions	None determined (when used to develop on adhesive tape)
Small particle reagent	None determined
Basic Violet 3	Some detrimental effects on DNA recovery rates observed
Solvent Black 3	None determined
Acid Black 1, Acid Yellow 7, Acid Violet 17	None determined

- All relevant anti-contamination precautions should be taken and best practice should be performed in the packaging and handling of the exhibit. Every possible precaution should be taken to reduce cross-contamination from sample to sample and from those handling the exhibit.

- DNA processing is best carried out as soon as possible after fingermark enhancement. This will optimise DNA recovery and help to limit the potential for cross-contamination.

- Low template DNA profiles are much more difficult to obtain from porous than non-porous surfaces. Full low template profiles from porous surfaces are not always achieved even on untreated articles.

- The use of a number of sequential fingermark treatments is likely to reduce DNA recovery and increase the potential for DNA cross-contamination. If both DNA and fingermark evidence are to be maximised, it may be prudent to select the single most effective fingermark enhancement process appropriate for the surface and immediately submit samples for DNA analysis.

- When aluminium powder is lifted, some DNA remains on the surface and some is lifted with the powder. Informative low template profiles have been obtained both from the surface after lifting and from the lift.

- Short-wave UV radiation is potentially destructive and should not be used if DNA recovery is required.

- The forensic provider should be informed which fingermark enhancement processes have been used so that the optimum method of DNA extraction may be selected accordingly.

As indicated previously, the increased sensitivity of DNA analysis techniques means that there is now a greater perceived risk of cross-contamination if articles are processed in a fingermark enhancement laboratory without clean room facilities. As a result, in many laboratories, DNA recovery tends to be carried out first in clean rooms and then the articles are sent for fingermark enhancement. Some laboratories conduct fingermark enhancement under clean room conditions, and equipment such as modified cyanoacrylate fuming chambers with sterilising UVC lamps are now available to enable cleaning between the processing of different samples.

In addition to the interaction between fingermark recovery and DNA, work has also begun to explore the impact of fingermark enhancement on the related area of body fluid detection. Simmons et al. (2014) considered the effect of different fingermark enhancement techniques on subsequent detection of semen, and a similar study has since been conducted by McAllister et al. (2016) for saliva. Both these studies have shown that some processes are more detrimental than others and this also needs to be taken into account when generating forensic recovery strategies.

Table 17.7 Potential impacts of DNA recovery processes on fingermark recovery.

DNA recovery process	Potential effect on subsequent fingermark enhancement
Wet swabbing	Removal of water-soluble fingermark constituents
	Physical damage to fingermark ridges
Dry swabbing	Physical damage to fingermark ridges
Flock swabbing	Physical damage to fingermark ridges
Taping	Removal of fingermark residues
Gelatin lifting	Removal of fingermark residues
Cutting of sample area	Total destruction of fingermark

17.3.2.2 Effects of fingermark enhancement processes on DNA recovery

It should be noted that almost all published studies to date have focused on the effect of fingermark enhancement processes on DNA recovery. What is often overlooked is the detrimental effect that DNA recovery may have on latent fingermarks. DNA recovery may involve quite aggressive processes such as rubbing of the surface with wet and dry swabs or applying and removing adhesive tape. Such processes may cause physical damage to fingermark residues, removing them completely or dissolving and redistributing some of the constituents. For these reasons speculative swabbing is not recommended for surfaces where fingermarks may be present. Some recent studies (Fieldhouse et al., 2016; Parsons et al., 2016) have begun to explore the impact of DNA recovery processes on fingermark enhancement and have identified that some processes (e.g. gelatin lifting) have less impact than others (e.g. nylon swabs and wet swabbing) that could be highly damaging. Some of the potential impacts are summarised in Table 17.7.

17.3.3 Digital forensics

A rapidly growing field of operational importance is that of digital forensics. The scope of this area is vast, but the principal area where potential conflicts exist between fingermark recovery and digital forensics is where there is the need to both extract digital information from storage media (e.g. computers, mobile phones, flash cards, USB sticks, CDs) and provide evidence regarding the people that have handled them. To extract the data from these items, it will be necessary to handle them, potentially damaging fingermarks. Conversely, there are several fingermark enhancement processes that may affect subsequent data recovery (Table 17.8).

By intelligent selection of the processes used and the order in which they are applied, it should be possible to obtain both types of evidence in the majority of cases, but as yet there are few published studies of this type or any detailed written guidance about which order processes should be applied and which processes should not be used. One published study by Jasuja et al. (2006) considered the impact of fingermark enhancement on subsequent data recovery from CDs and

Table 17.8   Potential impacts of fingermark recovery processes on digital evidence recovery.

Fingermark enhancement process	Potential effect on subsequent digital evidence recovery
Visual examination	None
Fluorescence examination	None
Powdering	May deposit metal powders on circuitry or within ports, resulting in shorting
Vacuum metal deposition	May deposit metal coatings on circuitry or within ports, resulting in shorting
	Beware of air trapped in batteries
Cyanoacrylate fuming	May bond moving parts together or deposit insulating material on contacts
Liquid phase processes	Should not be used – will potentially affect circuitry
Gelatin lifting	None on hardware. Possible delamination if used on CD label face

found that processes such as powdering, small particle reagent and iodine fuming where marks could be either easily washed from the surface or resublimed over time had no noticeable impact on subsequent reading of data. Cyanoacrylate fuming was observed to leave more permanent marks that could affect data recovery on some of the types of discs studied. With the rapid growth in the number and type of data storage devices now available, there is clearly the potential for further studies in this area so that more definitive guidance can be produced.

An example of the use of a lower impact process (gelatin lifting) to recover fingermarks from the screen of a tablet device prior to data extraction is given in Figure 17.8.

17.3.4   Footwear marks

There is a large degree of commonality between the processes that are used for developing footwear marks and those that are used to develop fingermarks (Bandey, 2008). It is not uncommon for footwear marks to be developed when treating exhibits for fingermarks, and fingermarks can also be developed when speculatively treating regions of flooring for footwear marks.

The principal difference between the two types of evidence is that whereas a fingermark usually consists of body secretions of which the approximate composition is generally known, footwear marks are often deposited in an unknown contaminant. Footwear enhancement processes therefore tend not to utilise chemical reactions unless there is evidence that suggests the presence of a particular contaminant such as blood.

The processes that are typically used for speculative searching of footwear marks, long-wave UV examination, oblique white light examination and electrostatic lifting apparatus (ESLA) are all non-destructive to fingermark deposits and may reveal

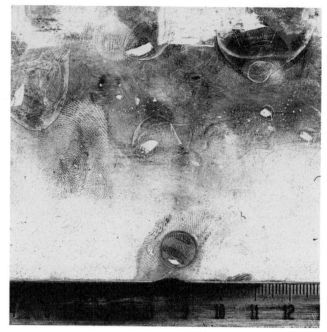

Figure 17.8   A gelatin lift taken from the screen of a tablet device, enabling fingermark recovery to take place before further handling for data extraction.

or develop fingermarks simultaneously with footwear marks. Subsequent processes that may be used in sequential footwear mark recovery, including gelatin lifting and powdering, are also capable of visualising fingermarks. For the most part, footwear and fingermark recovery is a simultaneous process rather than being a sequential one. There has been no reported study on the effects of chemical processes that are occasionally used for reacting with metal ions in soil (e.g. bromophenol blue and ammonium thiocyanate) on fingermark recovery. Tables 17.9 and 17.10 summarise what is known about the effects of fingermark enhancement processes on footwear marks and vice versa and the information regarding the effectiveness of fingermark processes in developing footwear marks originating from a study carried out by Law (2006) and summarised by Bandey (2008).

The primary exception to the general compatibility of the processes used for the different evidence types is where it is suspected that footwear marks in blood are present, and there is the possibility that fingermarks in blood may be present, too. Because footwear marks may be deposited over a large area, a reactive process giving a visible colour change or chemiluminescent reaction is often used to speculatively search for their presence. Reagents capable of being sprayed are used in this application, including Leuco Crystal Violet, Leuco Malachite Green and luminol. The acid dyes used for developing fingermarks in blood are best used to target small areas and are not useful for speculatively searching for footwear marks. The potential incompatibility arises if a process such as luminol is used to speculatively search

Table 17.9   Potential impacts of fingermark recovery processes on footwear mark recovery.

Fingermark enhancement process	Potential effect on subsequent footwear mark recovery
Visual examination	None – may detect footwear marks
Fluorescence examination	None – may detect footwear marks in some contaminants
Powdering	None – may develop footwear marks
DFO	Not known
Ninhydrin	Not known
Physical developer	Not known
Vacuum metal deposition	None – may develop footwear marks
Superglue	None – may develop footwear marks
Powder suspensions	None – may develop footwear marks
Small particle reagent	None – may develop footwear marks
Basic violet 3	Not known
Solvent black 3	None – may develop footwear marks in greasy contaminants
Iodine	None – may develop footwear marks in greasy contaminants

Table 17.10   Potential impacts of footwear mark recovery processes on fingermark recovery.

Footwear enhancement process	Potential effect on subsequent fingermark enhancement
Long-wave UV imaging	None – may detect absorbing and/or fluorescent fingermarks
Oblique lighting	None – may detect negative fingermark impressions in dust
ESLA	None – may lift fingermarks in dust
Gelatin lifting	May lift latent fingermarks with footwear marks
	Removal of material may reduce effectiveness of some processes
Powders	May simultaneously develop fingermarks
Powder suspensions	May simultaneously develop fingermarks
Bromophenol blue	Effect on fingermarks unknown
Ammonium thiocyanate	Effect on fingermarks unknown

for footwear and is applied over an area where fingermarks in blood are present. Luminol does not contain a fixing agent, and on non-porous surfaces repeat or over-vigorous applications, it may cause the ridge detail in the mark to run and become diffuse, as illustrated in Chapter 13.

17.3.5   Document examination

The general term 'document examination' covers a wide range of processes that may be applied to written or printed matter. These processes may be used to detect security features, to establish whether documents are altered or forged, to analyse handwriting, to establish the identity of the author or to reveal impressions left by writing on adjacent sheets of paper. When considering in which order document evidence should be processed, the information required from the exhibit should be assessed. By careful selection of the processes used, it may be possible to obtain all the required information from the document before any fingermark enhancement process is applied. Even if this is not possible, some reagents used for fingermark enhancement have been deliberately formulated to minimise their impact on subsequent document examination.

Some of the processes that may be employed in document examination are shown in Table 17.11, with information on any known effects on fingermark enhancement.

The process for which most ambiguity is seen is ESDA, which is capable of simultaneously detecting both indented writing and fingermarks. For this process the conditions used may require modification depending on whether detection of indented writing is of prime importance or subsequent fingermark recovery is a higher priority.

Studies have been carried out to establish the effect of the pre-humidification stage recommended to optimise detection of indented writing on subsequent fingermark recovery. Although Heath (1983) initially reported that pre-humidification may be beneficial to fingermark recovery, this was disputed by later researchers (Moore, 1988; Azoury et al., 2003), and pre-humidification is not recommended if fingermark recovery is required on the document. Pre-humidification is most detrimental to ninhydrin and 1,2-indandione, with DFO being less affected by the process although degradation still occurred for exposure time in excess of 60 min.

The fingermark enhancement processes that may be applied to porous exhibits and their potential effects on document examination are summarised in Table 17.12.

Early ninhydrin formulations based on acetone caused significant ink run and were incompatible with document examination. This was soon recognised, and by 1969 Crown had proposed a formulation using petroleum ether as the principal

Table 17.11   Potential impacts of document examination processes on fingermark recovery.

Document examination process	Potential effect on subsequent fingermark enhancement
White light examination (e.g. oblique, cross-polarised directional lighting)	None
Fluorescence examination	None – may detect latent fingermarks
IR examination (fluorescence and absorption)	None – may detect latent fingermarks
UV examination	Long-wave UV may detect latent fingermarks
	Short-wave UV may degrade some fingermark constituents (but may also detect latent fingermarks)
	Effect of mid-wave UV unknown
Handwriting analysis	None – provided exhibit handled with gloves
ESDA (detection of indented writing)	Pre-humidification of document may diffuse or remove marks
	Process may develop latent fingermarks
Gelatin lifting (detection of indented writing)	May damage surface of exhibit
	Process may lift fingermarks
Ink and paper analysis	Will be destructive to fingermarks

Table 17.12   Potential impacts of fingermark enhancement processes on document examination.

Fingermark enhancement process	Potential effect on subsequent document examination
Visual examination	None – may aid document examination
Fluorescence examination	None – may aid document examination
ESDA	None – conditions for fingermark enhancement may not be optimum for document examination
Powdering	May leave residue on surface that interferes with document examination
DFO	May cause some inks to run (dependent on formulation)
1,2-indandione	May cause some inks to run (dependent on formulation)
Ninhydrin	May cause some inks to run (dependent on formulation)
Physical developer	Will saturate paper with aqueous solutions and react away alkali fillers
	Deposition of silver particles on surface may interfere with document examination
Oil Red O	Will saturate paper with aqueous solutions
	Will stain background with pink colouration, may affect spectral analysis

solvent that significantly reduced ink running during treatment, and this philosophy was also adopted during research into the formulation based on CFC113 solvent (Morris and Goode, 1974). When this solvent was phased out, candidate formulations based on alternative solvents were tested to see what effect they would have on documents (Petruncio, 2000). The currently used ninhydrin formulation based on HFE7100 is both effective in developing fingermarks and in minimising the impact on subsequent document examination. An example showing the effect of a proposed 1,2-indandione formulation on a range of different inks is given in Figure 17.9.

It is not possible to totally remove any chance of inks running during fingermark enhancement, but most modern amino acid reagent formulations do take document examination into account and utilise solvents that have minimal impact.

17.3.6   Fibre analysis

In the case of fibre analysis, it is not the analysis process itself that may be detrimental to fingermarks, but it is the processes used to recover the fibres from the surface that may cause damage to the fingermark residues. The most commonly used process of fibre recovery is tape lifting (Robertson and Grieve, 1999), which may remove some fingermark residues from the surface and reduce the effectiveness of subsequent fingermark enhancement. Other recovery processes such as the use of vacuum are unlikely to be detrimental.

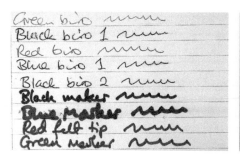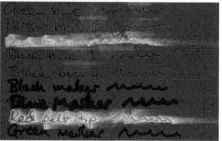

Figure 17.9 Writing in different inks on lined notepaper, treated with an experimental 1,2-indandione formulation and viewed under white light and fluorescence examination under green light. In this case, undesirable ink run has occurred.

Table 17.13 Potential impacts of fingermark enhancement processes on fibre analysis.

Fingermark enhancement process	Potential effect on subsequent fibre analysis
Visual examination	None – may detect fibres
Fluorescence examination	None – may detect fibres
Powdering	May remove fibres during brushing
Vacuum metal deposition	Vacuum system may draw off fibres
	Metal coating may obscure fibres
Superglue	Not known
Liquid phase processes	Fibres may be lost in solution
Gelatine lifting	None – may lift fibres for subsequent analysis

If fibre recovery needs to be considered in conjunction with fingermark enhancement, then visual examination and fluorescence examination should be considered first. Both these processes have the potential to reveal fingermarks and to locate fibres, which can enable them to be photographed *in situ* rather than on a tape lift. Other fingermark enhancement processes are potentially detrimental to fibre recovery, but this has not been extensively investigated. Some of the possible effects are summarised in Table 17.13.

17.3.7 Ballistic analysis

Ballistic analysis processes can be employed where it is necessary to link fired ammunition to a particular weapon and in the case of gunshot residue also to potentially link the firing event to a particular person. Fingermark evidence is capable of providing additional links to persons handling both guns and ammunition, and therefore by use of the forensic processes in the correct sequence, the amount of information recovered can be maximised. There are, however, potential conflicts between what is required from ballistic analysis and best practice for preserving fingermarks.

Processes used for ballistic analysis include weapon test firings, to establish the marks left by the gun on the bullet and cartridge casing during firing, and analysis of firing marks on discharged cartridge casings (Heard, 2013). The latter process has the potential to link casings from different crimes back to the same weapon. Both these analysis processes involve handling of the weapon and the cartridge casings with the potential of causing damage to any fingermarks that may exist on the surfaces unless precautions are taken to minimise this. Recovery of samples of gunshot residue is less problematic because this (in theory) can be carried out from the interior of the fired cartridge case without touching any surfaces that may potentially bear fingermarks.

It is similarly important to consider subsequent ballistic analysis if fingermark recovery is to be attempted first. Fingermark recovery rates on firearms and ammunition are generally low, and there are several reasons that may contribute to this such as weapons being deliberately wiped or covered in gun oil and fired cartridge casings being exposed to high temperature, abrasion and firing residues during the firing event. The most commonly used fingermark enhancement process that is applied to these items is cyanoacrylate fuming. The use of this process should be carefully considered if a weapon is to be test fired because the process has the potential to glue mechanisms within the weapon together. It may be possible to temporarily seal off parts of the weapon that could be affected by cyanoacrylate fuming during processing to mitigate this.

Fingermark enhancement processes used prior to firing mark analysis on cartridge casings should avoid heating or excessive deposition of any material that may reduce definition of the fine detail within the firing pin mark. There are no extensive reported studies of the effects of ballistic analysis on fingermarks and vice versa, but some of the anticipated effects of various fingermark enhancement processes are summarised in Table 17.14. It should be noted that some of the novel processes

Table 17.14 Potential impacts of fingermark enhancement processes on ballistic analysis.

Fingermark enhancement process	Potential effect on subsequent ballistic analysis processes
Visual examination	None
Fluorescence examination	None
Powdering	None on firearms
	Powder residue on ammunition may affect analysis of discharge residue
Vacuum metal deposition	None on firearms
	Metal layers deposited on ammunition, but should not preclude analysis of firing marks. May affect analysis of discharge residue
Superglue	None on ammunition
	May bond interior parts of firearms and affect test firings
Powder suspensions	Not known
Liquid phase processes	Firearms should not be immersed in liquids – may affect subsequent operation
Gelatin lifting	None

being developed for enhancement/visualisation of fingermarks on metals (scanning Kelvin probe, electrostatic powdering, disulphur dinitride) all utilise the residual change in the metal surface caused by the fingermark rather than relying on the presence of the fingermark residues themselves. This makes the 'fingermark' more resilient and may enable fundamental changes in fingermark recovery strategies for these types of exhibit.

References

Anderson J, Bramble S, 'The effects of fingerprint enhancement light sources on subsequent PCR-STR DNA analysis of fresh bloodstains', J Forensic Sci, vol 42(2), (1997), p 303–306.

Azoury M, Zamir A, Oz C, Wiesner S, 'The effect of 1,2-Indanedione, a latent fingerprint reagent on subsequent DNA profiling', J Forensic Sci, vol 47(3), (2002), p 586–588.

Azoury M, Gabbay R, Cohen D, Almog J, 'ESDA processing and latent fingerprint development: the humidity effect', J Forensic Sci, vol 48(3), (2003), p 564–570.

Bandey H L, 'Fingerprint and Footwear Forensics Newsletter: Special Edition – Footwear Mark Recovery', Publication No. 24/08, Home Office, May 2008.

Bandey H L (ed.), 'Fingermark Visualisation Manual', Home Office, London, 2014.

Bhoelai B, de Jong B J, de Puit M, Sijen T, 'Effect of common fingerprint detection techniques on subsequent STR profiling', Forensic Sci Int Genet Suppl Ser, vol 3, (2011), e429–e430.

Crown D A, 'The development of latent fingerprints with ninhydrin', J Crim Law Criminol Police Sci, vol 60(2), (1969), p 258–264.

Downham R P, Mehmet S, Sears V G, 'A pseudo-operational investigation into the development of latent fingerprints on flexible plastic packaging films', J Forensic Identif, vol. 62(6), (2012), p 661–682.

Fieldhouse S, Oravcova E, Walton-Williams L, 'The effect of DNA recovery on the subsequent quality of latent fingermarks', Forensic Sci Int, vol 267, (2016), p 78–88.

Fregeau C J, Germain O, Fourney R M, 'Fingerprint enhancement revisited and the effects of blood enhancement chemicals on subsequent Profiler Plus™ fluorescent short tandem repeat DNA analysis of fresh and aged bloody fingerprints', J Forensic Sci, vol 45(2), (2000), p 354–380.

Grubwieser P, Thaler A, Köchl S, Teissl R, Rabl W, Parson W, 'Systematic study on STR profiling on blood and saliva traces after visualization of fingerprint marks', J Forensic Sci, vol 48(4), (2003), p 733–741.

Heard B J, 'Forensic Ballistics in Court', Wiley-Blackwell, Hoboken, 2013, ISBN 1119962684.

Heath J S, 'The Effects of ESDA Examination and Photocopying on the Recovery of Latent Fingerprints on Documents', presented to the 3rd Scientific Meeting of the Australian Society of Forensic Document Examiners, Melbourne, Victoria, 25/26 June 1983.

Jasuja O P, Singh G D, Sodhi G S, 'Development of latent fingerprints on compact disc and its effect on subsequent data recovery', Forensic Sci Int, vol 156, (2006), p 237–241.

Jordan D, 'Report on the Effects of Acid Yellow 7 Fingerprint Enhancement on Subsequent DNA Profiling – A Collaborative Study by the FSS and the PSDB', British Crown Copyright, 2003.

Law W, 'Investigating the Possible Processes for Enhancement of Shoemarks', MSc thesis, University of Strathclyde, September 2006.

Leemans P, Vandeput A, Vanderheyden N, Cassiman J, Decorte R, 'Evaluation of methodology for the isolation and analysis of LCN-DNA before and after dactyloscopic enhancement of fingerprints', Int Congr Ser, vol 1288, (2006), p 583–585.

Marriott C, Lee R, Wilkes Z, Comber B, Spindler X, Roux C, Lennard C, 'Evaluation of finger-mark detection sequences on paper substrates', Forensic Sci Int, vol 236, (2014), p 30–37.

McAllister P, Graham E A, Deacon P, Farrugia K J, 'The effect of mark enhancement techniques on the subsequent detection of saliva', Sci Justice, vol 56(5), (2016), p 305–320.

McMullen L, Beaudoin A, 'Application of Oil Red O following DFO and ninhydrin sequential treatment: enhancing latent fingerprints on dry, porous surfaces', J Forensic Identif, vol 63(4), (2013), p 387–423.

Moore D S, 'The electrostatic detection apparatus (ESDA) and its effects on latent prints on paper', J Forensic Sci, vol 33(2), (1988), p 357–377.

Morris J R, Goode G C, 'NFN – an improved ninhydrin reagent for detection of latent finger-prints', Police Res Bull, vol 24 (1974), p 45–53.

Parsons R, Bates L, Walton-Williams L, Fieldhouse S, Gwinnett C, 'DNA from fingerprints: attempting dual recovery', CSEye, vol 6, (2016), p 8–17.

Pesaresi M, Buscemi L, Alessandrini F, Cecati M, Tagliabracci A, 'Qualitative and quantitative analysis of DNA recovered from fingerprints', Int Congr Ser, vol 1239, (2003), p 947–951.

Petruncio A V, 'A comparative study for the evaluation of two solvents for use in ninhydrin processing of latent print evidence', J Forensic Identif, vol 50(5), (2000), p 462–469.

Raymond J, Roux C, Du Pasquier E, Sutton J, Lennard C, 'The effect of common fingerprint detection techniques on the DNA typing of fingerprints deposited on different surfaces', J Forensic Identif, vol 54(1), (2004), p 22–44.

Robertson J R, Grieve M (eds), 'Forensic Examination of Fibres, Second Edition (International Forensic Science and Investigation)', CRC Press, Boca Raton, FL, 1999, ISBN 0748408169.

Roux C, Gill K, Sutton J, Lennard C, 'A further study to investigate the effect of fingerprint enhancement techniques on the DNA analysis of bloodstains', J Forensic Identif, vol 49(4), (1999), p 357–376

Schulz M, Wehner H, Reichert W, Graw M, 'Ninhydrin-dyed latent fingerprints as a DNA source in a murder case', J Clin Forensic Med, vol 11, (2004), p 202–204.

Sewell J, Quinones I, Ames C, Multaney B, Curtis S, Seeboruth H, Moore S, Daniel B, 'Recovery of DNA and fingerprints from touched documents', Forensic Sci Int Genet, vol 2, (2008), p 281–285.

Simmons R K, Deacon, P, Phillips, D, Farrugia K J, 'The effect of mark enhancement techniques on the subsequent detection of semen/spermatozoa', Forensic Sci Int, vol 244, (2014), p 231–246.

Stein C, Kyeck S H, Henssge C, 'DNA typing of fingerprint reagent treated biological stains', J Forensic Sci, vol 41(6), (1996), p 1012–1017.

Zamir A, Oz C, Geller B, 'Threat mail and forensic science: DNA profiling from items of evidence after treatment with DFO', J Forensic Sci, vol 45(2) (2000), p 445–446.

18

Interpreting the results of fingermark enhancement

Stephen M. Bleay

Home Office Centre for Applied Science and Technology, Sandridge, UK

Key points

- There are many reasons fingermarks may not be found after treatment.

- It is essential that fingerprint identification specialists are provided with images of any enhanced marks that are fit for the purposes of comparison.

- The image of the mark alone may not provide all of the information that is required by identification specialists and some additional contextual information may be needed.

- There are several scenarios where there is the potential to misinterpret the image of the fingermark unless appropriate additional information is provided.

18.1   Introduction

Even after use of all the possible enhancement processes in an appropriate sequence, there is no guarantee that any fingermarks will be enhanced. It is important to communicate this fact to those conducting the investigation and to provide possible explanations. In cases where it is declared that no fingermarks have been found, possible reasons that marks may not have been found and submitted for comparison include the following:

- The item or surface has not actually been handled.

- Little, if any, residue has been deposited on the surface. This situation may arise if the hands have recently been washed, the ambient temperature and humidity

---

Fingerprint Development Techniques: Theory and Application, First Edition.
Stephen M. Bleay, Ruth S. Croxton and Marcel de Puit.
© 2018 John Wiley & Sons Ltd. Published 2018 by John Wiley & Sons Ltd.

are low and sweating is not preferred, or the person handling the surface does not naturally leave much fingermark residue (some constituents of children's fingermarks often being more transient, and older people and females generally depositing less material than young males) (Noble, 1995; Williams et al., 2011; Lewis, 2013).

- The person handling the surface is wearing clean, non-porous gloves or another barrier material over their hands.

- The fingermark has been washed or rubbed from the surface after deposition. This may occur by deliberate means (e.g. an attempt to evade detection) or by accident (e.g. rubbing of the surface against the packaging material during transportation).

- Fingermarks are present, but they are in a contaminant that is not normally present in fingermarks and not targeted by any of the visualisation processes that have been used.

- Fingermarks are present and have been enhanced, but none of them are considered suitable for fingerprint comparison. This may be because they are partial, have discontinuous ridges or are blurred or smudged due to movement.

In cases where potentially identifiable marks have been enhanced, it becomes necessary to produce images of them that can be used in the comparison process. It should not be overlooked that the primary purpose of enhancing fingermarks and capturing images of them is to provide the identification specialist with all of the relevant information they need to conduct an initial assessment of the mark and to confirm an identification or exclusion (i.e. all of the appropriate stages of the ACE-V process (Vanderkolk, 2011) used for fingerprint comparison).

In order for the identification specialist to conduct the task to the best of their ability, the image supplied needs to be fit for the purposes of comparison and identification. It is also important to recognise that in many organisations, the person enhancing fingermarks and producing images of them is not the same person that conducts the fingerprint comparison. The person making decisions on what ridge detail will be marked up and photographed for submission to an identification specialist therefore needs an appreciation of what level of detail is regarded as sufficient for comparison. Without this understanding, it is possible for many marks that are suitable for comparison to be discarded or for too many low quality marks to be submitted resulting in resources being expended on work of no value (Earwaker et al., 2015).

In order to assist the assessment phase of ACE-V and minimise the risks of subsequent misinterpretation, it may be necessary to provide some additional contextual information in addition to the image of the mark on the transfer from the fingermark enhancement laboratory to the fingerprint identification bureau. However, the type of information provided needs to be carefully considered.

Research led by Dror (e.g. Charlton et al., 2010) has raised concerns about the provision of certain types of contextual information to the identification specialist, for example, the (potentially emotive) nature of the case that the fingermark originates from, because of the possibility that this may sway opinion regarding identification one way or another. This type of information is not critical to the ACE-V process used by the identification specialist and therefore need not be supplied to them. However, unlike many other classes of forensic evidence, the fingerprint identification specialist rarely examines the original fingermark *in situ*, and what is used during comparison may be a second-, third- or even fourth-generation representation of the mark. It may therefore be important to ensure that the identification specialist is given information that provides a comprehensive understanding of several factors associated with the mark, including

- Where the mark is located on the surface/item
- What type of substrate the mark has been developed on
- What type of constituent the mark is formed in
- What process has been used to enhance the mark
- What environment the mark and substrate have been exposed to
- What image processing may have been applied to the image prior to receipt by the expert

There is a risk that images of marks may be misinterpreted if some or all of this information is not provided, and this is discussed in the following sections.

18.2 Location of the mark

It has already been discussed in Chapter 1 that the location of the mark(s) on the item or surface may be important in establishing the way in which an item has been handled, which can provide support to (or contradiction of) a particular account of events.

The image of the fingermark on its own may not supply sufficient information to enable the location of the mark(s) to be established in a broader context. An image of the mark in isolation may provide little indication of its orientation, particularly, if the substrate it has been deposited on is relatively featureless. Equally, the position of the mark in relation to features such as door handles and so on may not be revealed by the image because it is not possible to include them in the frame and capture the mark at the required resolution. For most processes, the mark remains present on the substrate after enhancement, and this additional contextual information may be provided by means of overview shots of the scene or item (Figure 18.1) (Maceo, 2011).

Where marks have been developed using powders and subsequently lifted from the surface, different approaches may be required. Lifting is conducted for several reasons, with one advantage being that it removes the mark from potentially interfering backgrounds and makes imaging easier. However, because the mark has been removed from the surface, it is critical to maintain an accurate audit

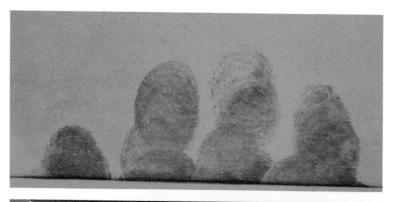

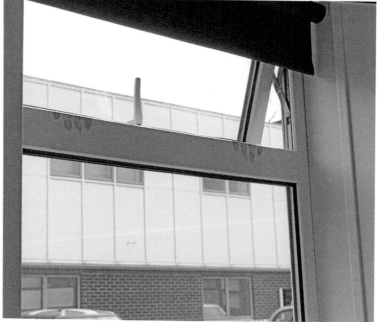

Figure 18.1 Close-up image of powdered marks and contextual overview shot showing the marks at a point of entry.

trail of which item/surface the lift has been taken from and the location of the mark on it. Although some indication of the texture of the surface may be carried over onto the lift, many surfaces are smooth, and the lift alone will not give information about the location of the marks. One means of providing this additional information is to include descriptions of the location that the mark has been recovered from on the lift itself (Figure 18.2).

The description of the location of the mark should be added immediately after the lift has been taken to minimise the possibility of subsequent mislabelling. The provenance of the lift has sometimes been an area of dispute, with differences of opinion arising about the surface the lift is claimed to have been taken from, including the cases involving McNamara (Cole, 2005) and van der Vyver (Altbeker, 2010).

18.3   Type of substrate

The identification specialist should also be made aware of the nature of the substrate the mark has been enhanced on. There are certain types of substrate that can contribute to the formation of marks that can be misinterpreted. Issues with interpretation may arise for a variety of reasons, with some examples given in the following text.

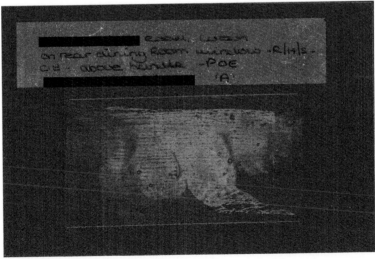

Figure 18.2   An example of information about the recovery location of the mark recorded on a lift of an aluminium powdered mark. Reproduced courtesy of the Home Office.

18.3.1   Thin, porous surfaces

When fingermarks are deposited on certain types of thin, porous substrate, it is possible for constituents of the mark to continue migrating through the substrate until they reach the reverse side (Figure 18.3).

The migration process may be accelerated by elevated temperature and pressure (Suzuki, 2013). This type of migration has been noted on tissue paper and also for some thin plastic bags. Although plastic bags may appear to be a non-porous surface, some are heavily recycled and contain significant amounts of porous additives such as chalk that can provide a pathway for migration of finger-mark constituents.

This issue with migration of fingermarks through the substrate is that it introduces ambiguity about the orientation of the mark. If the original surface that the mark is deposited on is unknown and the image of the developed mark is taken from what is actually the reverse surface, the identification specialist may search for the mark in the reverse of its correct orientation. By providing information about the substrate, this ambiguity can be taken into account by searching the mark in both orientations.

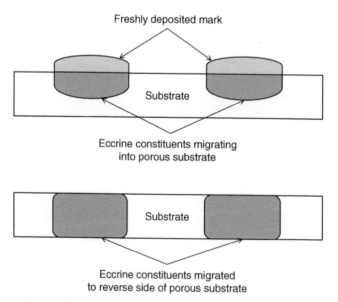

Figure 18.3   Schematic diagram showing penetration of fingermark constituents through the reverse side of a thin, porous substrate.

18.3.2 Adhesive or tacky surfaces

A separate but related issue can occur where marks are deposited on adhesive surfaces that are subsequently stuck down onto non-porous surfaces or on non-porous surfaces that are subsequently covered by an adhesive or tacky layer. In such cases it is possible for transfer to occur between the two surfaces, leaving sufficient material capable of being enhanced to potentially identifiable marks on both surfaces (Figure 18.4).

The transfer of materials may be influenced by several factors including the nature of the constituents, the age of the mark, the temperature, the pressure and the time that the surfaces are in contact.

The effect of this transfer is to again raise ambiguity about which surface the mark was originally deposited onto and therefore about the correct orientation of the mark. Identification specialists should be advised if the image of the fingermark that they are presented with has been developed on an adhesive surface or on an area that has previously been covered by an adhesive surface, thus enabling both orientations of the mark to be considered.

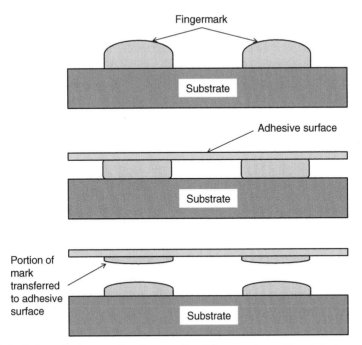

Figure 18.4 Schematic diagram showing transfer of fingermark constituents between an adhesive surface and a non-porous substrate.

Transfer may also occur where two surfaces that are tacky in nature (or are self-adhesive) come into contact with each other. An example of such a surface where marks have been transferred and subsequently developed in the reverse orientation is cling film (Figure 18.5) (Charlton et al., 2013).

18.3.3   Transparent, thin substrates

Another example of a substrate that may cause ambiguity in the interpretation of fingermarks is transparent, thin materials. On such materials, marks can be developed on both sides of the substrate (Figure 18.6).

Where marks are developed on both sides of the substrate, it may not be immediately obvious which side the mark is actually on, especially if the substrate is thin. It may be necessary to use alternative methods such as oblique lighting to determine this, and therefore if the correct side of the substrate (and orientation of mark) has been established, then it should be communicated to the identification specialist. If this ambiguity still exists, then the identification specialist should be advised that the mark is on a transparent substrate and could be in either of the two possible orientations.

18.3.4   Textured surfaces

Although most surfaces have an obvious texture associated with them, there are cases where a surface that may appear smooth to an initial examination may actually contain fine features that can either influence the process used to develop the mark or affect the appearance of the developed mark itself.

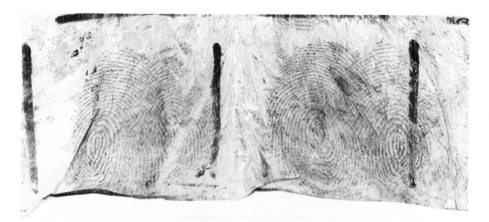

Figure 18.5 Marks developed using multi-metal deposition on cling film, showing evidence of transfer between tacky surfaces that have been in contact (marks originally deposited between gridlines).

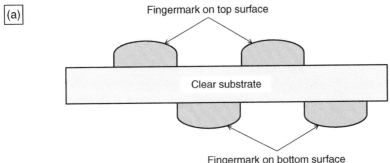

Fingermark on top surface

Clear substrate

Fingermark on bottom surface

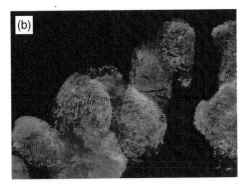
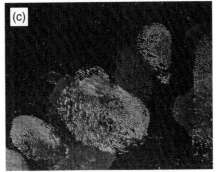

Figure 18.6 Development of fingermarks on both sides of a transparent, thin substrate: (a) schematic diagram illustrating a scenario, (b) fluorescence examination, revealing marks on both sides of a transparent substrate (acetate sheet) with no clear indication of correct orientation and (c) examination using oblique light, revealing only fingermarks on top surface in their correct orientation.

A practical example of this is gloss painted wood, which may contain fine particles of grit or fibre that become trapped in the paint layer during application. These may only be seen using methods such as oblique lighting, but have the potential to trap powder particles during powdering and appear as features on the surface. If such features occur with the ridge flow of a fingermark or close to its periphery, then there is the potential that they may be misinterpreted as features associated with the mark rather than the substrate (Figure 18.7).

On a coarser level, surfaces that may appear smooth may actually contain localised depressions where the finger does not make contact with the surface. This can result in the formation of marks of unusual appearance (e.g. irregular peripheral shapes). Mark Y7 in The Fingerprint Inquiry, Scotland, is an example of a mark where the role of the substrate in its formation was disputed, the irregular shape being variously attributed to multiple touches or to an irregular surface texture (Campbell, 2011).

The two-dimensional images provided to identification specialists are not able to convey information about whether the surface contains three-dimensional features,

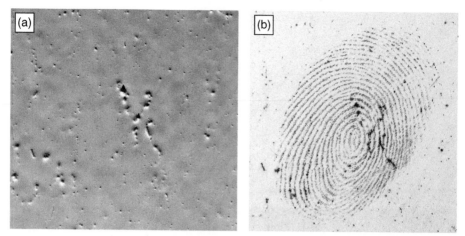

Figure 18.7 Texture affecting take-up of powder on surface, potentially giving false features within mark, (a) an apparently smooth surface lit using oblique lighting to reveal surface features and (b) mark deposited over the same area and subsequently developed using black granular powder.

and those developing marks and/or imaging them should record such information if they believe it would affect the subsequent comparison and the presence of such features is not evident in the image of the mark.

18.4 Constituents of the mark

In most situations, the constituents of the mark will have little impact on the way in which the image is interpreted and indeed in most cases will not be known. The main exception to this is where marks have been deposited in blood. Blood have several properties that make it behave very differently to natural constituents and many other potential contaminants. Although initially of relatively low viscosity, blood can coagulate and dry rapidly once out of the body, which can result in marks of significantly different appearance depending on the time the blood has been on the finger prior to deposition, the amount of blood on the finger and the pressure used during deposition (Langenburg, 2008).

There are also several scenarios that can be associated with the deposition of marks where blood is present, illustrated schematically in Figure 18.8.

Although several studies have investigated whether it is possible to determine which of these scenarios has actually occurred (Creighton, 1997; Huss et al., 2000; Praska and Langenburg, 2013), there is still no reliable way of doing this.

In addition, marks deposited in blood should always be examined with caution because there are several possible scenarios (e.g. high deposition pressure, thin layers of blood having dried out on the ridges but thicker layers in the furrows remaining wet) that can contribute to the resultant mark having less blood being

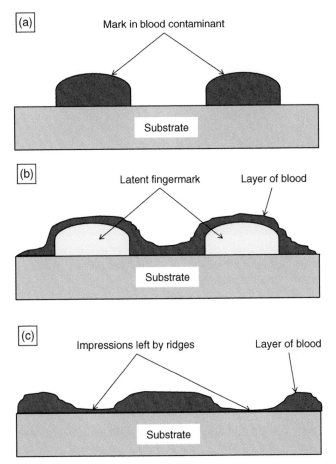

Figure 18.8 Possible scenarios where fingermarks may be associated with blood:
(a) fingermarks with blood contaminant on a clean surface, (b) latent fingermarks subsequently
covered by a layer of blood and (c) impressions left in a pre-existing layer of blood.

deposited on the ridges compared with the furrows. It is often difficult to determine
which feature is being viewed, an example of ambiguity between ridges and furrows being shown in Figure 18.9.

If the features that constitute the ridges are misinterpreted as furrows and vice
versa, potential identifications may be missed. This very issue has been a point of
dispute in the case of R v Smith[1] (2011), where different identification specialists
provided varying opinions on whether features in a mark left on a door handle were
ridges or furrows.

The provision of colour images of marks in addition to the greyscale image
traditionally used for comparison may be one means of providing additional

---

[1] '(a) ridges and furrows – what lines were the ridges and what lines were the furrows on the
print or prints left on the door handle'.

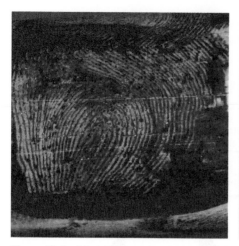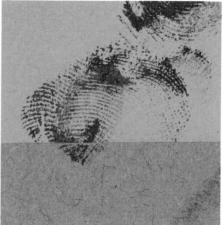

Figure 18.9   Mark in blood developed using Acid Violet 17 showing ambiguity between ridges and furrows and Acid Black 1 showing development of ridges as 'positive' and 'negative' regions within the same cluster of ridge detail.

information to the identification specialist. There may also be benefit in consulting a specialist in blood pattern analysis for an additional opinion on how the mark has been formed.

18.5   Enhancement process

Identification specialists should also be provided with information about the process that has been used to develop the mark. Although most processes used to enhance marks give a consistent outcome (e.g. marks developed using ninhydrin will nearly always give marks with purple-coloured ridges), there are some processes that may produce ridges that can vary in appearance, sometimes being lighter or sometimes being darker than the background. In some cases this may be observed for different marks on the same substrate or even on different regions within the same mark.

The most widely reported example of this behaviour is for marks that have been developed using vacuum metal deposition. Research has shown that the mode of development can vary from 'normal' (with little metal deposition on ridges and high deposition on the background) to 'reverse' (with higher levels of deposition occurring on the ridges than on the background). Several factors can influence which form of development is observed, including the type of polymer substrate (Jones et al., 2001a, 2001b), the age of the mark and whether any contaminants are present in the fingermark. Some examples of each type of mark are shown in Figures 7.12 and 7.14 and further illustrated in Figure 18.10.

Identification specialists need to be aware of the fact that both types of development may be observed with a single process, so that the mark can be searched taking into account that the ridges in the image may appear lighter than or darker than the furrows.

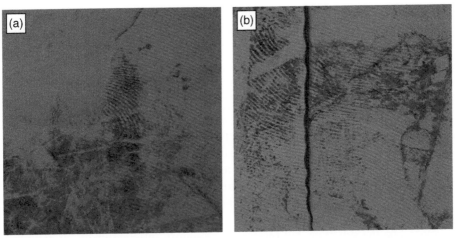

Figure 18.10 Examples of both (a) 'normal' and (b) 'reverse' developments of ridge detail on different areas of the same plastic bag by vacuum metal deposition.

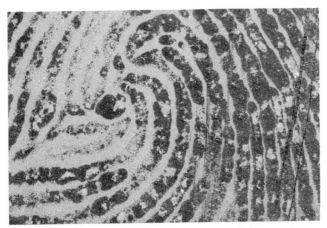

Figure 18.11 Example of a 'reverse' developed mark produced using cyanoacrylate fuming followed by fluorescent dye staining on a contaminated surface where material has been removed by the finger. The ridges in this image are darker than the background. Reproduced courtesy of the Home Office.

'Reverse' development may also be observed with other enhancement processes, although this may be less affected by the enhancement process used and more by the condition of the surface. An example of this is where the surface is coated with a thin layer of contaminant, which is removed by contact with the finger. If the contaminant itself is enhanced by the process, then a 'reverse developed' mark can occur, as shown for cyanoacrylate fuming in Figure 18.11.

Again, potential issues associated with misinterpreting this type of mark could be minimised by providing the identification specialist with colour images. Such images would give a better understanding of the enhancement process used, thus raising awareness that marks have been enhanced using a process that could give reverse development.

18.6   The environment

Another important factor that may affect the interpretation of fingermark is the environment that the marks and the substrate have been exposed to. This can be particularly important where substrate materials with limited thermal stability (such as thermoplastic polymers) are exposed to elevated temperatures. Such temperatures can be high enough to cause shrinkage/distortion of substrates, yet not high enough to destroy the fingermark. In such situations fingermarks can be developed on the substrate, but these may be significantly shrunken, or distorted in one or more axes, from the dimensions of the mark that was originally deposited. An example of the type of distortion that can potentially occur is shown in Figure 18.12.

It should be noted that although such heat distortion is most likely to arise from exposure to environments at the crime scene, it can also occur if care is not taken

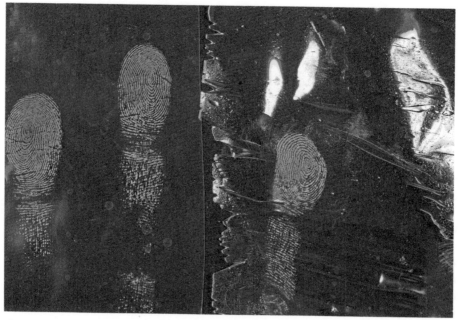

Figure 18.12   Sequence of fingermarks on a polymer substrate: left-hand side kept at ambient temperature and right-hand side heated in an oven at 100°C for 20 min before processing with cyanoacrylate fuming.

during normal chemical processing (e.g. some plastic windows on envelopes may melt and/or distort at the prolonged elevated temperatures used in the DFO and 1,2-indandione processes) or if certain surfaces are exposed to laser illumination for long periods of time.

If the identification specialist is not made aware that distortion and/or dimensional changes could have occurred to the mark, then subsequent comparison and matching will be made considerably more difficult. The effect of heat distortion on automated matching of marks has been studied and found to be detrimental (Dominick et al., 2011). Although search algorithms are designed to account for a reasonable amount of distortion associated with flexibility of the skin, natural movement and so on, they may not be able to account for the more extreme amounts of distortion and shrinkage that can arise on exposure to high temperatures, and therefore the identification specialist needs to be able to manually adjust for this.

18.7   Image processing

Once an image of the fingermark has been captured, it may be processed in several ways before it is presented to an identification specialist for comparison. Almost all images now captured are digital, and the type of processing that may be applied to the image includes conversion from colour to greyscale, adjusting greyscale levels, contrast and brightness and sharpening (Blitzer and Jacobia, 2002; Comber et al. in Ramotowski, 2013).

It is essential for evidential purposes that an audit trail be maintained that records the nature and order of any changes that have been made to the 'as captured' image of the mark (which should be preserved as a 'master copy') to produce the final image that is presented in court (Home Office, 2007). It is also important that the identification specialist is also made aware of the prior image processing history of any mark that is presented to them.

One area where there is the potential for misinterpretation if this information is not properly communicated is in the imaging of fluorescent marks. Most marks revealed by fluorescence examination have ridges that are fluorescent and thus appear brighter than the background. The colour of the fluorescence associated with marks enhanced using known processes is characteristic, and it should therefore be evident from a colour image which are ridges and which are furrows. When colour images of these marks are converted to greyscale, the fluorescing ridges thus appear white against a dark grey/black background. However, because identification specialists are more familiar with conducting comparisons against sets of 'inked' fingerprints where the ridges are black and the background white, it is common (but not universal) practice for images of fluorescent marks to be greyscale inverted (i.e. produced as a 'negative') so that the ridges in the image of the mark also appear black.

The identification specialist needs to be informed whether or not the image they are presented with has been greyscale inverted so that they can confirm that they are comparing the ridges in the mark with the ridges in the set of reference fingerprints. Examples of marks that either have been or may have been misinterpreted because of ambiguity about whether they had been greyscale inverted emerged during the Scottish Fingerprint Inquiry (Campbell, 2011). During the inquiry it was stated that mark QD2 had at one point been misinterpreted by a set of Danish experts because they failed to appreciate it was an image of a fluorescent mark developed using DFO that had not been greyscale inverted and examined it on the assumption that it was a visible mark developed using ninhydrin. Subsequent to the publication of the inquiry report, additional concerns were expressed that mark QI2 may have been misinterpreted by several identification specialists because they did not realise that it was a fluorescent mark developed by cyanoacrylate fuming and dye staining that had not been greyscale inverted (Kent, 2012) and the ridges were therefore the light regions.

These examples highlight the need for good communication between the enhancement laboratory (or crime scene practitioner), imaging unit and the fingerprint bureau, and the need to keep accurate audit trails of what processing has been applied. In common with several other examples given previously, the potential for this type of misinterpretation could be reduced by providing additional colour images of the mark. Because the colours associated with marks developed using standard processes are characteristic and well known, colour images remove much of the ambiguity about which process has been used to develop the mark. If a colour image of the mark has for whatever reason been colour inverted to produce a 'negative', it is generally obvious on a colour image because the colours of the ridges will not resemble any of the regularly used processes.

Another issue that may arise during the image processing stage is the overuse of image processing tools. The order in which image processing functions are applied to an image can have a significant influence on the final image, and the application of tools in the wrong order may in extreme circumstances introduce artefacts into the image that maybe misinterpreted as features in the mark. The identification specialist should be made aware of which processing tools have been used, particularly where many tools have been utilised to produce the final image and/or advanced tools such as fast Fourier transforms for subtraction of background patterns have been applied. A fuller description of the importance of appropriate application of image processing tools is given by Comber et al. in Ramotowski (2013).

18.8   Image capture

The previous sections have discussed the ways in which images of marks may be misinterpreted if insufficient information is provided with the image. It should not be overlooked that the image of the mark must also be fit for purpose and those producing the image should take the following factors into consideration during capture of the image. These factors are discussed in greater detail in specialist texts on forensic imaging (Marsh, 2014).

18.8.1 Resolution

Capturing the mark at a sufficiently high resolution is critical in enabling the identification specialist to utilise all of the detail present in the mark. Identification specialists conduct comparisons in a holistic way, utilising information associated with first-, second- and third-level details in forming their conclusions. Although first-level detail will readily be captured by all but the lowest resolution images, reproduction of second-level detail requires the image to be captured at a resolution of at least 500 pixels per inch (and >800 ppi if the image is captured in colour and converted to greyscale). If third-level detail is present and the identification specialist wishes to utilise it in comparison, then images of at least 1000 ppi should be captured. Examples of a mark captured at different resolutions are illustrated in Figure 18.13.

18.8.2 Focus and depth of field

It goes without saying that images should be captured in focus, because out-of-focus images cannot be corrected by subsequent sharpening functions and will inhibit the ability to conduct comparisons. For marks on flat surfaces, it should be easily possible to ensure all of the mark is in focus. However, on curved surfaces the depth of field becomes a consideration because by selecting capture conditions with limited depth of field, it is possible to capture images with part of the mark in focus and the remainder, out of focus. To avoid this, images should be captured using

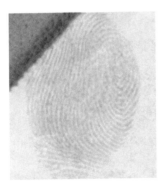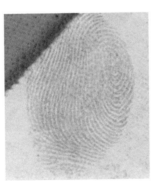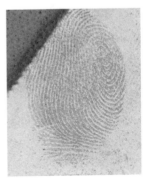

Figure 18.13 Images of a fingermark captured at 250, 500 and 2000 ppi, showing the differences in the levels of detail that can be discerned. Reproduced courtesy of the Home Office.

small apertures to give a greater depth of field. This will increase the exposure time and reinforces the need to maintain stability of the imaging system during capture by use of a copy stand or tripod.

18.8.3 Scales

It is also important that the image contains a scale, preferably an 'L'-shaped scale displaying measurements in two perpendicular axes. Not only does this provide a means of accurately displaying the dimensions of the mark, it also provides a reference that can be used if it is necessary to resample the image to a particular resolution (e.g. for input to a fingerprint database with set requirements for image size).

A perpendicular scale also provides an indication to the identification specialist if there are any issues associated with the image being captured at an unusual angle. Although in ideal circumstances every mark will be captured with the imaging system perpendicular to the mark, there are situations due to sample geometry, reflections from the surface or limited access where this is not possible, and the image is captured at an angle away from perpendicular. The fact that the scale is no longer a perfect 'L' shape in the resultant image indicates that the features of the mark may be slightly distorted, and this may need to be compensated for during comparison. Several software programs are now available that can correct for this distortion by using the scale as a reference and restoring it to an 'L' shape in the corrected image.

Colour scales can also be used in cases where it is necessary to correct images for any colour casts. They are generally less relevant for routine imaging of fingermarks because the image is usually converted into greyscale. However, colour scales can be very useful to imaging specialists utilising advanced imaging processing functions where very subtle colour differences can be used to separate marks from the background.

18.8.4 Optics

Many types of device can be used to capture images of fingermarks that are suitable for the purposes of comparison. The optics used for image capture will have a small but potentially significant influence on the image produced. It is generally recommended that macro (rather than zoom) lenses are used to capture images of fingermarks because these produce images that exhibit minimal distortion across the entire field of view. Other types of optics may produce a 'pin cushion' distortion in the image of the mark (the extreme case being observed for a 'fisheye' lens), with features towards the extremities of the image being most distorted. For the vast majority of images, this distortion is imperceptible and has negligible effect on subsequent comparison, but it is possible to apply corrections if such distortion is suspected to be affecting the image of the mark.

In summary, the identification specialist should act as an 'intelligent customer' for the outputs received from the crime scene investigator, the fingermark enhancement laboratory and/or the imaging unit. They should receive an appropriate level of supporting information about the mark, including any circumstances that may affect the way in which it is subsequently compared. They should also have a knowledge on potential influencing factors and be able to request clarification where they suspect information may be lacking. In many cases the enhancement, imaging and identification functions of fingerprints are regarded as separate disciplines, but ideally they should be regarded as stages in an end to end process with the boundaries between them blurred by greater interaction and communication. By increasing understanding of the full process by all concerned, the risks of misinterpretation of fingermarks can be minimised.

References

Altbeker A, 'Fruit of a Poisoned Tree', Jonathan Ball, South Africa, 2010, ISBN 9781868423330.

Blitzer H L, Jacobia J, 'Forensic Digital Imaging and Photography', Academic Press, San Diego, 2002.

Campbell A, 'Part 4 The Opinion Evidence – Chapter 27 XF and Various "Q" Marks Attributed To Mr Asbury', The Fingerprint Inquiry Scotland Report, 2011. https://www.webarchive.org.uk/wayback/archive/20150428160012/http:/www.thefingerprintinquiryscotland.org.uk/inquiry/21.html (accessed 29 October 2017).

Charlton D, Fraser-Mackenzie P, Dror I E, 'Emotional experiences and motivating factors associated with fingerprint analysis', J Forensic Sci, vol 55(2), (2010), p 385–393.

Charlton D T, Bleay S M, Sears V G, 'Evaluation of the multimetal deposition process for fingermark enhancement in simulated operational environments', Anal Methods, vol 5, (2013), p 5411–5417.

Cole S A, 'More than zero: accounting for error in latent fingerprint identification', J Crim Law Criminol, vol 95(3), (2005), p 985–1078.

Creighton J T, 'Visualisation of latent impressions after incidental or direct contact with human blood', J Forensic Identif, vol 47(5), (1997), p 534–541.

Dominick A J, NicDaeid N, Gibson A P, Bleay S M, 'Search results of heat-distorted fingerprints using sagem metamorpho AFIS', J Forensic Identif, vol 61(4), (2011), p 341–352.

Earwaker H C, Morgan R, Harris A, Hall L, 'Fingermark submission decision-making within a UK fingerprint laboratory: do experts get the marks that they need?', Sci Justice, vol 55(4), (2015), p 239–247.

Home Office, 'Digital Imaging Procedure v2.1', HOSDB Publication 58/07, 2007.

Huss K, Clark J, Chisum W J, 'Which was first – fingerprints or blood?', J Forensic Identif, vol 50(4), (2000), p 344–350.

Jones N, Stoilovic M, Lennard C, Roux C, 'Vacuum metal deposition: factors affecting normal and reverse development of latent fingerprints on polyethylene substrates', Forensic Sci Int, vol 115, (2001a), p 73–88.

Jones N, Mansour D, Stoilovic M, Lennard C, Roux C, 'The influence of polymer type, print donor and age on the quality of fingerprints developed on plastic substrates using vacuum metal deposition', Forensic Sci Int, vol 124, (2001b), p 167–177.

Kent T, 'Apparent misinterpretation of fingermark QI 2 (Ross) in evidence given to the Scottish Fingerprint Inquiry', Fingerprint Whorld, vol 38(148), (2012), p 112–116.

Langenburg G, 'Deposition of bloody friction ridge impressions', J Forensic Identif, vol 58(3), (2008), p 355–389.

Lewis S, 'A Large-Scale Donor Trial to Examine the Performance of Selected Latent Fingermark Development Techniques: Preliminary Considerations', presented at International Fingerprint Research Group Meeting, Jerusalem, Israel, 9–14 June 2013.

Maceo A V, 'Chapter 10 – Documentation of Friction Ridge Impressions: From the Scene to the Conclusion', in The Fingerprint Sourcebook, NIJ, Washington, DC, 2011.

Marsh N, 'Forensic Photography: A Practitioner's Guide', Wiley-Blackwell, London, 2014, ISBN 978-1119975823.

Noble D, 'Vanished into thin air: the search for children's fingerprints', Anal Chem, vol 67, (1995), p 435A–438A.

Praska N, Langenburg G, 'Reactions of latent prints exposed to blood', Forensic Sci Int, vol 224, (2013), p 51–58.

Ramotowski R (Ed.), 'Lee and Gaensslen's Advances in Fingerprint Technology', 3rd Edition, CRC Press, Boca Raton, 2013.

Smith R. v (Rev 1) [2011] EWCA Crim 1296 (24 May 2011).

Suzuki S, 'Studies on the Transmission of Latent Fingerprints to Reversed Surface of Plastic Sheet', presented at 10th International Fingerprint Research Group Meeting, Jerusalem, Israel, 9–14 June 2013.

Vanderkolk J R, 'Chapter 9 – Examination Process', in The Fingerprint Sourcebook, NIJ, Washington, DC, 2011.

Williams D K, Brown C J, Bruker J, 'Characterization of children's latent fingerprint residues by infrared microspectroscopy: forensic implications', Forensic Sci Int, vol 206(1–3), (2011), p 161–165.

Index

Fingerprint Development Techniques: Theory and Application, First Edition.
Stephen M. Bleay, Ruth S. Croxton and Marcel de Puit.
© 2018 John Wiley & Sons Ltd. Published 2018 by John Wiley & Sons Ltd.

Printed and bound by CPI Group (UK) Ltd, Croydon, CR0 4YY